The Impact of Culture and Faith in Dementia Care

The Impact of Culture and Faith in Dementia Care:

Psycho-Social-Spiritual Healing

Edited by

Michael Silbermann and Ann Berger

Cambridge Scholars Publishing

The Impact of Culture and Faith in Dementia Care:
Psycho-Social-Spiritual Healing

Edited by Michael Silbermann and Ann Berger

This book first published 2023

Cambridge Scholars Publishing

Lady Stephenson Library, Newcastle upon Tyne, NE6 2PA, UK

British Library Cataloguing in Publication Data
A catalogue record for this book is available from the British Library

ISBN (10): 1-5275-4001-4
ISBN (13): 978-1-5275-4001-9

To my beloved wife, Gisela, who has been struggling for years courageously and tenaciously with this cruel disease: Dementia, and my two daughters Anat and Ronit who served as the family's pillar throughout.

Special thanks go to Ronit, whose patience, understanding and encouragement made this publication possible.

- Michael Silbermann

Technion - Israel Institute of Technology, Haifa, Israel

To my spouse and children: Carl, Stephan and Rebecca. Whose love and support have made my work possible.

- Ann Berger

Pain and Palliative Care. Bethesda, Maryland, USA

TABLE OF CONTENTS

II. Palliative Care for the Patient with Dementia

III. Religion, Spirituality and Cultural Aspects in Dementia Care

FOREWORD

We are living longer and healthier. We hear that "seventy is the new fifty" and read about exceptional centenarians who run marathons or begin a new chapter of their life. The numbers broadcasted by demographers and epidemiologists confirm the feeling that we are aging better and longer than before.

These changes followed substantial improvements in living conditions, successful preventive strategies, and better care of chronic diseases. Not surprisingly, the extraordinary accomplishment of longer life is celebrated by the media, as the success of humans overcoming the entropic forces of nature. And yet, people are realizing in their everyday lives that longer life come with baggage. Over the last century, what we have gained of total life expectancy have been shared almost equally before the healthy life and the life that we live burdened by chronic disease and disability. Though, every man and woman affected by severe morbidity will tell you that the years of disability feel longer than those of healthy life.

At the population level, there is a substantial expansion of the percentage of people in the population who live with some disability. At the personal level, every single one of us has somebody ill and/or disabled in their family, and while we are often asked to help, we feel inadequate and unprepared to address this challenge. The reality is that we live with the completely unfounded certainly that both us and our close relatives will live for long time and never get ill or disabled. How to deal with the physical or cognitive disability that affect everybody at the end of life is not part of our culture, worse than pornography, a topic to be avoided and to keep away from our mind, and certainly not to be part of the formal and informal education of our children. The illusion that our parents or our friends will live many beautiful years and then.... suddenly disappear in a flash, is borne from fear that, if confronted by reality, will not know how to handle the situation. At the extreme, developing dementia is the feared nightmare for both patients and member of a surrounding family.

In most cases the response to dementia is denial. Children refuse to recognize that those "strange behaviors" are part of the pathology, which often results in long conflicts. Shifting the attention from an interpersonal to a medical problem is another avoidance strategy. Attempting expensive and complex diagnostic procedures and treatment regiments that we know well are unlikely to improve function and independence are a frequent response. Yet, it is not true that there is nothing that we can do. Years ago, when I was a geriatrician working "from the trench", I learned that talking to patients who are becoming aware that their mental capacity is getting shaky or to families and informal caregivers who are caring for a person with dementia can be extremely effective. The trick is to understand what dementia is, what does to the brain and how it changes the relationship with others and reshuffle the rank of priority for individuals and those around him. Understanding is key, and the more dimensions are brought into the picture, and the better the network of people involved can find some sort of equilibrium. In my experience, understanding is a powerful tool, much more effective than any drug that we have identified so far. This is why the arguments conveyed by this book are so important, because they improve our understanding of the dyadic relationship between the person with dementia and the surrounding personal and architectural environment. The call to spirituality can be amazingly powerful, especially if rooted in experiences of previous life.

This book reminds me of Moyra Jones, an extraordinary therapist that I met many years ago when I was visiting the health care system for the elderly in British Columbia. Moyra had an insightful understanding of people suffering from dementia and emphasized the need of looking after the whole person; body, mind, and soul. She rejected any treatment program aimed at modifying behavior and instead encouraged caregivers and institutions to make the journey through Alzheimer's Disease as untraumatic as possible. Her program, called *Gentlecare* focused on attitudes, grooming to communication, find way to adapt the environment to the person instead of the person to the environment. It looks for ways to cherish the person whose mind is turning in some unexpected direction. This is not an easy journey but may be quite rewarding in the quality of care provided but also in the gaining of understanding on the person we care for and, perhaps more profoundly, our own mind. Perhaps even more important, the right approach cannot be universal, because the journey though cognitive decline is infused by the many cultural elements and tradition that a person have been breathing over a lifetime. Thus, the careful evaluation of how Religion, Spirituality and Culture should shape and inform the management and care of patients suffering from dementia is one of the key to success. From this perspective, the chapters referring how different religions may affect the complex, reciprocal relationship between caregivers and people who are cognitively impaired are innovative and represents a singularity of this book, that hopefully will stimulate more research in this field.

Someone would think that the solution is to find a drug treatment that prevent or cure the different clinical forms of dementia. Of course, as a scientist and as a Geriatrician, I would not disagree. However, until then, studying the clues provided by this book are pearls to researchers, caregivers and health providers.

Luigi Ferrucci, MD, PhD
Intramural Research Program of the National Institute on Aging
National Institutes of Health, Baltimore, MD- USA

PREFACE

PSYCHO-SOCIAL-SPIRITUAL HEALING: THE IMPACT OF CULTURE AND FAITH IN DEMENTIA CARE

MICHAEL SILBERMANN AND ANN BERGER

Most of the relevant books contain very little about the process of aging, which precedes the outset of dementia, and how it affects those around them. With time patients with dementia grows depressed and enfeebled, while friends and colleagues avoid them. Only when we encounter such a case within the family, we the professionals realize how unready we are to help them. But admitting this and helping the patient cope with it seems beyond us. We, therefore, are able to offer only very limited comfort or guidance.

Nowadays, people live longer all over the world, and the management of aging and its consequences is currently handled by health care professionals who, for the most part, are not prepared for it due to the lack of health care providers trained in geriatrics and palliative care and trained to treat people with dementia. When the medical profession faces a situation that can be cured or managed, it has the means to do it. But if it cannot? The fact that to date we have no adequate solution to the difficult issues associated with dementia is troubling and causes extraordinary suffering to both the patient and his caregivers.

By and large, modern medicine has succeeded in postponing the fatal moment of many diseases farther into the future. Patients with certain cancers, for example, can continue their active life quite long after their diagnosis. Their cancer becomes a chronic disease whereby their symptoms come under control. Yet their disease, while slowed, continues progressing. However, in a matter of months or a few years, the body becomes overwhelmed. That is unfortunately the case with neuro-life threatening diseases such as dementias. This book provides the reader with a deeper understanding of the symptom burden, difficulties in caregiving, palliative care and the psycho-social-spiritual assessment and treatment of dementia patients by medical, paramedical and volunteer personnel. In doing so, the hope is this book will strengthen palliative care services by improving upon the existing ones and stimulating further research in this field.

The book offers an overview of how to deal with the various psychological-social and spiritual based therapy options for patients with dementia at different stages of their disease. It addresses the unique role of different cultures throughout the world and how this impacts psycho-social –spiritual healing. As an up-to-date text on psycho-social-spiritual and cultural care for patients with dementia, this book is an invaluable resource for professionals in most parts of the globe. All chapters in this book are written by experts in their fields and include the most current clinical and scientific information available. The book takes a multidisciplinary and global approach, providing insightful models of care and integrates clinical, psycho-social-spiritual and cultural data for practical management to enhance the efficacy of treatment while relieving suffering.

I

Medical Dimensions and Symptoms in Dementia

1

NON-PHARMACOLOGICAL ASPECTS OF PALLIATION IN ADVANCED-STAGE DEMENTIA PATIENTS

AANCHAL SATIJA, PHD[1]

Abstract

Dementia is a clinical syndrome caused by a heterogeneous group of disorders and characterized by a gradual, progressive impairment of cognition. People living with dementia experience a multitude of distressing symptoms during the course of their illness that affect their quality of life, such as eating problems, neuropsychiatric symptoms, pain, dyspnea, and cachexia. This chapter discusses the non-pharmacological therapies that may be provided to them for palliation of symptoms. Overall, these interventions have a potential for relieving patients' symptoms, but high-quality research is required to generate conclusive evidence. Meticulous assessment of symptomatic needs and an individualized approach to the delivery of non-pharmacological therapies can provide holistic healing for patients.

Keywords: Advanced dementia; Behavior; Cognition; Non-pharmacological; Palliative care

Introduction

Dementia affects more than 55 million people globally and is the seventh-leading cause of death in the world, with approximately 10 million new cases reported every year. Of these, more than 60% are in low- and middle-income countries (World Health Organization 2022). Dementia is usually a late-life disease that affects women more frequently than men. Because of

---

[1] Consultant, Indian Council of Medical Research, New Delhi- 110029

the increase in the elderly population, its prevalence is estimated to double every five years and is projected to increase to nearly 153 million cases in 2050 (GBD 2019 Dementia Forecasting Collaborators 2022). Dementia is a clinical syndrome characterized by a gradual and progressive impairment of cognition across various cognitive domains such as memory, reasoning and judgement, visuospatial ability, language functions, and personality or behavioral change. The cognitive impairment is manifested as a significant decline from the previous level of functioning. It is not a usual consequence of aging process and cannot be explained by other psychiatric illnesses (McKhann et al. 2011).

Of the various forms of dementia, Alzheimer's disease is the most common, followed by other forms such as vascular dementia, frontotemporal dementia, and dementia with Lewy bodies (World Health Organization 2022). Dementia progression may be categorized according to the severity of the disease. The need for assistance with activities of daily living increases as dementia progresses. Features of advanced dementia include extreme memory deficits and inability to ambulate independently, to perform activities of daily living, maintain urinary and fecal continence, and communicate with others. Individuals with advanced dementia experience severe disability and eventually become completely dependent for their daily activities in the final year of life (Mitchell 2015).

Palliative care needs in advanced dementia

Common symptomatic needs of patients with advanced dementia are eating problems (such as oral or pharyngeal dysphagia), cachexia, urinary or respiratory infections, pain, dyspnea, and neuropsychiatric symptoms (such as psychosis, agitation, or depression). This is accompanied by other significant concerns such as advanced care planning, institutionalization, place of death, and caregiver support (Mitchell 2015; Navia and Constantine 2022). Recognizing the life-limiting nature of advanced dementia, it may be considered a terminal illness. The goals of care should be, therefore, mainly palliative rather than curative, i.e., providing comfort and improving quality of life, which can be achieved via both pharmacological and non-pharmacological interventions (Eisenmann et al. 2020). The purpose of this chapter is to provide an evidence-based overview of the use of non-pharmacological interventions (NPIs) for the symptomatic management of patients suffering from advanced dementia.

Non-pharmacological interventions for dementia

It is important to understand that the goal of NPIs is not to cure dementia but to improve or maintain cognitive function, quality of life, and overall well-being of the individual (Lodha 2019). Interestingly, NPIs or non-drug treatments clearly specify what treatments are not included but do not distinctly define what interventions are included under this heading. The umbrella term "NPI" includes numerous treatment approaches, such as behavioral or psychosocial therapies, complementary or alternative medicines, nutritional interventions, physical exercise training, etc. Apparently, it is difficult to provide a mutually exclusive classification of the plethora of interventions that are covered under NPIs (Sikkes et al. 2021).

Broadly, the NPIs for managing dementia can be classified into four categories: (1) cognitive/emotion-oriented interventions such as validation therapy, reminiscence therapy, and simulated presence therapy; (2) sensory stimulation interventions such as aromatherapy, acupuncture, music therapy, light therapy, massage or touch therapy, sensory garden intervention, transcutaneous electrical nerve stimulation, and Snoezelen multisensory stimulation; (3) behavior management techniques; and (4) other interventions such as animal-assisted interventions, movement-based interventions, and energy therapies and spiritual interventions.

Cognitive/emotion-oriented interventions

Validation therapy

Developed by Naomi Feil, validation therapy is based on the typical principle of validation, i.e., to accept and confirm one's feelings or experiences (Neal and Barton Wright 2003). The therapist empathizes with the emotions and meaning of the behavior and speech of people with dementia (Lodha 2019). This is usually attained via use of simple words spoken in an empathic and clear voice, rewording indistinct words, and responding to actions through the effective use of non-verbal and verbal communication techniques (Abraha et al. 2017). An earlier systematic review to evaluate the efficacy of validation therapy did not provide sufficient evidence for use in people with dementia (Neal and Barton Wright 2003); however, recently it has proven beneficial in reducing stress and behavioral disturbances (Berg-Weger and Stewart 2017).

Reminiscence therapy

Reminiscence therapy is based on the fact that recent memories (e.g., a meal taken a little while ago) are impaired to a greater extent than remote ones (e.g., the wedding of a close family member). Using prosthetic memory aids such as photographs, videos, audios, or other familiar items of personal importance, the patients are motivated to talk about events and experiences from their past life (Cammisuli et al. 2016). Such conversations with the patients help them feel more socially connected, overcome loneliness, and develop an empathetic bond with the caregiver. Recent meta-analyses revealed that reminiscence therapy may be effective in reducing neuropsychiatric symptoms and depression and improves cognition and quality of life in people with dementia (Thomas and Sezgin 2021; Saragih et al. 2022).

Simulated presence therapy

Audio-video recordings consisting of cherished memories or conversations from earlier life are played to the dementia patient. It aims to stimulate old memories and make the patient's environment more familiar, thereby reducing behavioral symptoms (Abraha et al. 2017; Lodha 2019). However, well-designed studies assessing the effect of simulated presence therapy for managing behavioral symptoms are lacking, and quality of evidence is poor (Abraha et al. 2020).

Sensory stimulation interventions

People with cognitive impairment are less likely to probe their surroundings for sensory inputs; hence, appropriate sensory stimulation is not achieved. The latter, in turn, may lead to behavioral and psychological disturbances (Chung et al. 2002). Sensory stimulation interventions use various approaches to stimulate either single or multiple senses to treat a range of symptoms such as agitation, anxiety, pain, stress, mood, sleep, cognition, and quality of life in the advanced stage of dementia (Strøm, Ytrehus, and Grov 2016; Prins et al. 2020).

Aromatherapy

Aromatherapy is an olfactory sensory stimulation intervention that involves the use of aromatic plant oils such as lavender, rosemary, or lemon via topical application on skin, inhalation, or ingestion (Smith and D'Amico

2020). Individual studies have demonstrated its potential for reducing agitation and challenging behavior; however, a Cochrane review did not offer conclusive evidence for the same (Ball et al. 2020).

Acupuncture

Acupuncture is an age-old Chinese intervention based on the principle of harmonizing *yin* and *yang* energies. Hair-thin needles are inserted at acupoints and then stimulated manually or through various means such as electricity, heat, or laser (Satija and Bhatnagar 2017). Studies have demonstrated its beneficial effect on cognitive performance, activities of daily living, sleep quality, nocturnal behavioral disturbances, and quality of life in dementia patients (Prins et al. 2020; Ma et al. 2021). However, compliance and tolerance of dementia patients for acupuncture may be diminished.

Music therapy

Music affects our thoughts and emotions, and hence can impact body functions in multiple ways. The use of music as an NPI is relatively new (Satija and Bhatnagar 2017). Music interventions, e.g., listening to songs or musical instruments, singing, or music with movement, activate the limbic system and subcortical circuits, thereby eliciting feelings of pleasure (Strøm, Ytrehus, and Grov 2016; Moreno-Morales et al. 2020). It has been observed that dementia patients retain their ability to respond to music even when they are not able to communicate verbally (Moreno-Morales et al. 2020). A recent systematic review and meta-analysis by Moreno-Morales et al. demonstrated that music therapy has a positive impact on cognitive function, long-term depression, and quality of life for six months after the intervention. However, continuous and progressive therapy is recommended for sustained therapeutic benefit (Moreno-Morales et al. 2020).

Light therapy

Often, general sensory output is reduced in people with dementia, and they are less exposed to environmental bright light. Additionally, dementia progression causes degenerative changes in the suprachiasmatic nucleus of the hypothalamus, which generates the circadian rhythm responsible for regulating rest-activity and sleep-wake cycles. Light therapy comprises providing additional controlled light through different modes such as light boxes, ceiling lights, a light visor worn on the head, or dawn-dusk simulation. The additional light may stimulate neurons in the suprachiasmatic nucleus and reverse disturbances of the endogenous circadian rhythm (Forbes et al. 2014). Light therapy has been demonstrated to have a positive effect on the management of challenging behavior and on the reduction of affective symptoms and sleep disturbances (Cibeira et al. 2020; Kolberg et al. 2021; Tan et al. 2022).

Massage or touch therapy

Massage or touch therapy is a tactile sensory stimulation intervention that involves application of pressure to different body parts such as the hands, feet, or back by a trained therapist using rubbing, rolling, stroking, pressing, kneading, or other movements (Satija and Bhatnagar 2017; Margenfeld, Klocke, and Joos 2019). It stimulates the pressure receptors, thereby increasing vagal activity and decreasing cortisol levels. It promotes blood circulation and relaxation of muscles, and reduces stress and pain, and hence is widely accepted in the general population for a variety of medical conditions (Satija and Bhatnagar 2017; Field 2016; Kapoor and Orr 2017). Margenfeld et al. demonstrated evidence for the use of massage therapy in improving behavioral and psychological symptoms in individuals with dementia. The use of aroma oil during massage therapy showed better outcomes. Massage may also be used to relieve pain in people with dementia (Margenfeld, Klocke, and Joos 2019).

Sensory garden intervention or horticulture therapy

In general, both passive and active involvement with nature has a pleasant effect on human beings. Gardening is a multisensory intervention that is increasingly appreciated as a means to improve health outcomes. Gardens designed for gardening interventions come in several forms: there are "sensory gardens", which stimulate the senses through touch, smell, sight, and hearing (Gonzalez and Kirkevold 2014); "healing or therapeutic gardens", where therapeutic benefits are anticipated, such as reduction in stress and restoration of physical and mental well-being (Momtaz 2017); and "wander gardens", which provide a safe environment for patients with high elopement risk (Detweiler et al. 2008). The term "horticultural therapy" is often used interchangeably with "therapeutic horticulture" and is based on the use of plants or plant-related activities for improving the overall well-being of participants through their passive or active involvement (Gonzalez and Kirkevold 2014). The use of gardens and gardening interventions may improve affect, behavior, sleep, well-being, incidents of falls, and use of psychotropic drugs. So far, limited research has been performed in this field, yet the results seem promising (Gonzalez and Kirkevold 2014; Murroni et al. 2021).

Transcutaneous electrical nerve stimulation

Transcutaneous electrical nerve stimulation (TENS) intervention consists of application of electric current generated by the TENS machine via electrodes attached to intact skin surface (Johnson et al. 2022). It is primarily used for pain management and seldom for neuro-psychiatric ailments such as depression, headache, and alcohol or drug abuse. Early researchers believed that TENS could retard neural degeneration and stimulate regeneration by modifying the activity of cholinergic, noradrenergic, or serotonergic neurotransmitters. It was suggested that TENS may improve physical and psychosocial functioning, verbal fluency, short- or long-term memory, and the circadian rhythm of patients (Cameron, Lonergan, and Lee 2003). TENS can decrease pain arising due to pressure and improve gait ability, balance, and muscle strength, thereby demonstrating functional enhancement in patients with dementia (Hahm, Suh, and Cho 2019). While TENS may provide short-lived beneficial effects, more research is required to reach definite conclusions for its usage in dementia patients (Cameron, Lonergan, and Lee 2003; Hahm, Suh, and Cho 2019).

Snoezelen multisensory stimulation

The term "Snoezelen" is a combination of two Dutch words *"snoezel"* and *"doezelen"*, i.e., to sniff and to doze respectively. The Snoezelen approach is a multisensory stimulation intervention that provides a balance between restful and sensorial activity (Lotan and Gold 2009). The intervention is provided in a custom-designed space known as a "Snoezelen room" by a trained facilitator. It allows controlled stimulation of auditory, visual, olfactory, and tactile senses of the participant by modalities such as calming music, light effects, aromatic oils, textured balls, fiber-optic cables, and colored water columns (Maseda et al. 2018). Studies conducted to demonstrate its effect on behavior, mood, interaction, and perceptual abilities of dementia patients have not provided conclusive evidence. Though short-term benefits can be observed, more studies need to be conducted to establish long-term therapeutic effectiveness (Smith and D'Amico 2020).

Behavior management techniques

Difficult behaviors of dementia patients are associated with caregiver strain, and the behavior of stressed caregivers may further elicit more challenging behaviors of dementia patients. Therefore, interventions targeted at managing behavior can focus on either the patient, or at times, caregiver attitudes (National Collaborating Centre for Mental Health (UK) 2007). These include a host of interventions such as cognitive-behavioral therapy, communication training, functional analysis of specific behaviors, habit training, token economies, and personalized behavioral reinforcement approaches (O'Neil et al. 2011). Though earlier systematic reviews found limited evidence for the use of behavior management techniques (O'Neil et al. 2011; Moniz Cook et al. 2012), recent reviews of systematic reviews depicted their effectiveness and suggested using functional-analysis based interventions as the first line of NPIs for managing behavioral symptoms in dementia patients (Abraha et al. 2017; Dyer et al. 2018).

Other interventions

Animal-assisted interventions

Animal-assisted interventions involve human-animal teams for the therapeutic benefit of humans. They include both informal human-animal interaction and well-designed interventions. The International Association of Human-Animal Interaction Organisations (IAHAIO) has defined animal-assisted therapy as "goal oriented, planned and structured therapeutic intervention directed and/or delivered by health, education or human service professionals, including e.g., psychologists and social workers" with a focus "on enhancing physical, cognitive, behavioral and/or socio-emotional functioning of the particular human recipient either in the group or individual setting" (IAHAIO 2018). These interventions help the recipient develop a bond and companionship, thereby feeling socially integrated, which decreases feelings of boredom, loneliness, or isolation (Lai et al. 2019). While dogs are the most common intervention animal studied, any animal can serve as the intervention such as cats, horses, or fish (Yakimicki et al. 2019). The picture below demonstrates a cow-assisted activity, where a 90-year-old woman living with dementia is feeding the cows at the *"gowshala"* or cowshed (Fig. 1).

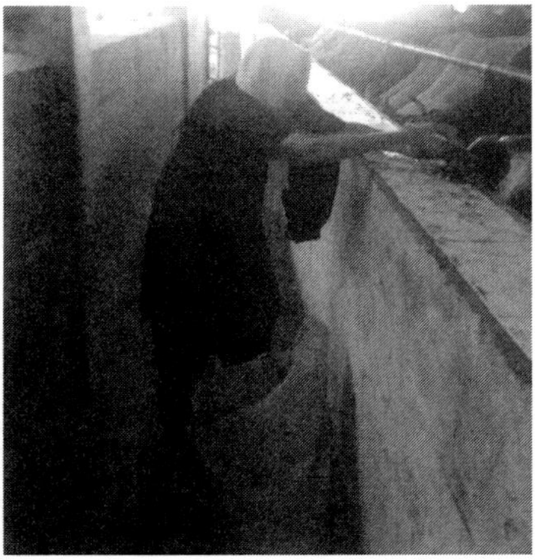

Fig 1: A 90-year-old woman living with dementia is feeding the cows at a *gowshala* during the last days of her life

Interactive and therapeutic pet-robot interventions are being used as an alternative to animal-assisted interventions (Park et al. 2020). The literature provides significant evidence for the effectiveness of animal-assisted interventions in reducing behavioral and psychological symptoms—especially depression—in dementia patients. Significant improvements were not observed for cognitive function, agitation, quality of life, and activities of daily living (Park et al. 2020; Chen et al. 2022). However, strict supervision is necessary to guard against possible infection risk and animal aggression (Lai et al. 2019).

Movement-based interventions

People with severe dementia are weak and frail, for the most part, yet display agitated and wandering behaviors. They can be trained and motivated to "move" to obtain improvement in daily functioning. Movement-based interventions include any interventions that involve bodily movements. These may be simple, interactive physical activities such as passing a ball or clapping hands, or structured and assisted activities such as walking, dance, aerobic exercises, yoga, or tai chi (Holliman, Orgassa, and Forney 2001; Barreto et al. 2015; Ojagbemi and Akin-Ojagbemi 2019). The preventive and therapeutic benefits of physical activities and exercise are well established for both healthy and diseased populations. Exercise considerably affects vascular and neuronal health by maintaining cerebral perfusion, promoting neurogenesis, and regulating neuroplasticity (Forbes et al. 2015). Many studies have investigated the effects of exercise or physical activity on outcomes such as activities of daily living, cognitive function, neuropsychiatric symptoms, and quality of life in dementia patients. Significant improvements have been observed in the ability to perform activities of daily living, cognition, and depression (Forbes et al. 2015; Barreto et al. 2015; Jia et al. 2019).

Energy therapies and spiritual interventions

Various cultures across the globe believe that the human body is made of subtle energy, also known as ch'i, qi, prana, or spirit. Energy or biofield field therapy involves the use of specific techniques by a skilled practitioner to modulate this subtle energy in order to promote intrapersonal and interpersonal healing for the self and other individuals. Such therapies impart physical, emotional, mental, and spiritual balance by cleansing the energy centers of the body, thereby providing holistic healing. They includes practices such as reiki, qigong, healing or therapeutic touch, johrei, and pranic healing (Satija and Bhatnagar 2017; Jain et al. 2015). The limited understanding of the mechanism through which these therapies operate restricts their use in clinical practice (Jain et al. 2015; Henneghan and Schnyer 2015). A review by Henneghan et al. demonstrated potential benefits of energy therapies in providing symptomatic relief and improving quality of life during end-of-life care (Henneghan and Schnyer 2015). It included three studies on people with dementia: two randomized control trials of the use of therapeutic touch (Woods, Beck, and Sinha 2009; Hawranik, Johnston, and Deatrich 2008) and a report on case studies (Meland 2009) of the use of reiki in dementia patients. The studies found lower levels of restlessness, distress, and anxiety in the study group.

Both cognitively intact and cognitively impaired individuals have spiritual needs, which if unmet during serious illness such as advanced dementia can lead to negative outcomes. The spiritual needs of dementia patients are not adequately understood. Only after understanding their spiritual needs, specific spiritual care interventions can be designed for this population (Camacho-Montaño et al. 2021; Palmer et al. 2022).

Only a few studies have been conducted on the use of energy therapies and spiritual interventions for dementia patients. Advanced dementia patients are unable to express their unmet needs and are completely dependent on the caregiver. In such a scenario, energy healing provided by other therapists may have favorable outcomes. However, research in this field is still nascent and the issue needs to be understood, explored, designed, and planned.

The Way Ahead

This chapter has provided an overview of the commonly used NPIs for symptomatic management in dementia patients. Along with the management of behavioral symptoms, NPIs have also been used for managing pain in dementia patients, though the evidence is not conclusive (Liao et al. 2021; Bao and Landers 2022). Multimodal NPIs may have a better effect on the symptomatic profile of patients, and hence are strongly recommended (Sharew 2022). NPIs definitely have a promising potential in reducing symptom burden in dementia patients. They usually have no major adverse effects and are well tolerated by the patients, and therefore healthcare professionals are encouraged to recommend NPIs in their routine practice. However, "one size does not fit all". Consequently, there is a need for a personalized approach, which in itself is challenging while conducting large-scale studies (National Collaborating Centre for Mental Health (UK) 2007). The DICE approach—Describe the behavior, Investigate the underlying causes, Create intervention, and then Evaluate the intervention—may be used by healthcare professionals to systematically identify and manage the distressing symptoms (Kales et al. 2017).

A plethora of literature, including case reports, primary studies, systematic reviews, reviews of systematic reviews, and meta-analyses, is available to evaluate the effectiveness of NPIs in dementia patients. Because of the heterogeneity of the studies in terms of methodology, intervention, and target population (i.e., patient, caregiver, or the patient-caregiver dyad), it is difficult to determine first-line NPIs for people living with advanced dementia. There is a dire need for a global consensus document that would provide guidance for the classification and implementation of NPIs and for conducting methodologically sound research to generate conclusive evidence for the use of NPIs in people with dementia. Additionally, the prevalence of dementia might increase in the post-pandemic era because of the long-term impact of the SARS-CoV-2 infection on cognitive function (Pyne and Brickman 2021; Liu et al. 2022). Therefore, healthcare workers, policymakers, and dementia care experts across the globe must come together to strategically plan the systematic implementation of NPIs.

In conclusion, the promising potential of NPIs must be acknowledged and utilized. A careful assessment of the unmet palliative care needs of dementia patients will help clinicians identify relevant interventions to reduce suffering and improve quality of life during the advanced stage of this illness.

References

Abraha, Iosief, Joseph M. Rimland, Isabel Lozano-Montoya, Giuseppina Dell'Aquila, Manuel Vélez-Díaz-Pallarés, Fabiana M. Trotta, Alfonso J. Cruz-Jentoft, and Antonio Cherubini. 2020. "Simulated Presence Therapy for Dementia." *The Cochrane Database of Systematic Reviews* 4 (4): CD011882. https://doi.org/10.1002/14651858.CD011882.pub3.

Abraha, Iosief, Joseph M. Rimland, Fabiana Mirella Trotta, Giuseppina Dell'Aquila, Alfonso Cruz-Jentoft, Mirko Petrovic, Adalsteinn Gudmundsson, et al. 2017. "Systematic Review of Systematic Reviews of Non-Pharmacological Interventions to Treat Behavioural Disturbances in Older Patients with Dementia. The SENATOR-OnTop Series." *BMJ Open* 7 (3): e012759. https://doi.org/10.1136/bmjopen-2016-012759.

Ball, Emily L, Bethan Owen-Booth, Amy Gray, Susan D Shenkin, Jonathan Hewitt, and Jenny McCleery. 2020. "Aromatherapy for Dementia." *The Cochrane Database of Systematic Reviews* 2020 (8): CD003150. https://doi.org/10.1002/14651858.CD003150.pub3.

Bao, Zhuming, and Margaret Landers. 2022. "Non-Pharmacological Interventions for Pain Management in Patients with Dementia: A Mixed-Methods Systematic Review." *Journal of Clinical Nursing* 31 (7–8): 1030–40. https://doi.org/10.1111/jocn.15963.

Barreto, Philipe de Souto, Laurent Demougeot, Fabien Pillard, Maryse Lapeyre-Mestre, and Yves Rolland. 2015. "Exercise Training for Managing Behavioral and Psychological Symptoms in People with Dementia: A Systematic Review and Meta-Analysis." *Ageing Research Reviews* 24 (Pt B): 274–85. https://doi.org/10.1016/j.arr.2015.09.001.

Berg-Weger, Marla, and Daniel B. Stewart. 2017. "Non-Pharmacologic Interventions for Persons with Dementia." *Missouri Medicine* 114 (2): 116–19.

Camacho-Montaño, Lucía Rocío, Jorge Pérez-Corrales, Marta Pérez-de-Heredia-Torres, Ana María Martin-Pérez, Javier Güeita-Rodríguez, Juan Francisco Velarde-García, and Domingo Palacios-Ceña. 2021. "Spiritual Care in Advanced Dementia from the Perspective of Health Providers: A Qualitative Systematic Review." *Occupational Therapy International* 2021: 9998480. https://doi.org/10.1155/2021/9998480.

Cameron, M., E. Lonergan, and H. Lee. 2003. "Transcutaneous Electrical Nerve Stimulation (TENS) for Dementia." *The Cochrane Database of Systematic Reviews* 2003 (3): CD004032. https://doi.org/10.1002/14651858.CD004032.

Cammisuli, D. M., S. Danti, F. Bosinelli, and G. Cipriani. 2016. "Non-Pharmacological Interventions for People with Alzheimer's Disease: A Critical Review of the Scientific Literature from the Last Ten Years." *European Geriatric Medicine* 7 (1): 57–64. https://doi.org/10.1016/j.eurger.2016.01.002.

Chen, Hongyu, Yuanyuan Wang, Minyi Zhang, Ning Wang, Yao Li, and Yan Liu. 2022. "Effects of Animal-Assisted Therapy on Patients with Dementia: A Systematic Review and Meta-Analysis of Randomized Controlled Trials." *Psychiatry Research* 314: 114619. https://doi.org/10.1016/j.psychres.2022.114619.

Chung, J. C., C. K. Lai, P. M. Chung, and H. P. French. 2002. "Snoezelen for Dementia." *The Cochrane Database of Systematic Reviews* 2002 (4): CD003152. https://doi.org/10.1002/14651858.CD003152.

Cibeira, Nuria, Ana Maseda, Laura Lorenzo-López, José L. Rodríguez-Villamil, Rocío López-López, and José C. Millán-Calenti. 2020. "Application of Light Therapy in Older Adults with Cognitive Impairment: A Systematic Review." *Geriatric Nursing (New York, N.Y.)* 41 (6): 970–83. https://doi.org/10.1016/j.gerinurse.2020.07.005.

Detweiler, Mark B., Pamela F. Murphy, Laura C. Myers, and Kye Y. Kim. 2008. "Does a Wander Garden Influence Inappropriate Behaviors in Dementia Residents?" *American Journal of Alzheimer's Disease and Other Dementias* 23 (1): 31–45. https://doi.org/10.1177/1533317507309799.

Dyer, Suzanne M., Stephanie L. Harrison, Kate Laver, Craig Whitehead, and Maria Crotty. 2018. "An Overview of Systematic Reviews of Pharmacological and Non-Pharmacological Interventions for the Treatment of Behavioral and Psychological Symptoms of Dementia." *International Psychogeriatrics* 30 (3): 295–309. https://doi.org/10.1017/S1041610217002344.

Eisenmann, Yvonne, Heidrun Golla, Holger Schmidt, Raymond Voltz, and Klaus Maria Perrar. 2020. "Palliative Care in Advanced Dementia." *Frontiers in Psychiatry* 11: 699. https://doi.org/10.3389/fpsyt.2020.00699.

Field, Tiffany. 2016. "Massage Therapy Research Review." *Complementary Therapies in Clinical Practice* 24 (August): 19–31. https://doi.org/10.1016/j.ctcp.2016.04.005.

Forbes, Dorothy, Catherine M. Blake, Emily J. Thiessen, Shelley Peacock, and Pamela Hawranik. 2014. "Light Therapy for Improving Cognition, Activities of Daily Living, Sleep, Challenging Behaviour, and Psychiatric Disturbances in Dementia." *The Cochrane Database of Systematic Reviews*, no. 2 (February): CD003946. https://doi.org/10.1002/14651858.CD003946.pub4.

Forbes, Dorothy, Scott C. Forbes, Catherine M. Blake, Emily J. Thiessen, and Sean Forbes. 2015. "Exercise Programs for People with Dementia." *The Cochrane Database of Systematic Reviews* 2015 (4): CD006489. https://doi.org/10.1002/14651858.CD006489.pub4.

GBD 2019 Dementia Forecasting Collaborators. 2022. "Estimation of the Global Prevalence of Dementia in 2019 and Forecasted Prevalence in 2050: An Analysis for the Global Burden of Disease Study 2019." *The Lancet. Public Health* 7 (2): e105–25. https://doi.org/10.1016/S2468-2667(21)00249-8.

Gonzalez, Marianne T., and Marit Kirkevold. 2014. "Benefits of Sensory Garden and Horticultural Activities in Dementia Care: A Modified Scoping Review." *Journal of Clinical Nursing* 23 (19–20): 2698–2715. https://doi.org/10.1111/jocn.12388.

Hahm, Suk-Chan, Hye Rim Suh, and Hwi-young Cho. 2019. "The Effect of Transcutaneous Electrical Nerve Stimulation on Pain, Muscle Strength, Balance, and Gait in Individuals with Dementia: A Double Blind, Pilot Randomized Controlled Trial." *European Journal of Integrative Medicine* 29 (August): 100932. https://doi.org/10.1016/j.eujim.2019.100932.

Hawranik, Pamela, Pat Johnston, and Judith Deatrich. 2008. "Therapeutic Touch and Agitation in Individuals with Alzheimer's Disease." *Western Journal of Nursing Research* 30 (4): 417–34. https://doi.org/10.1177/0193945907305126.

Henneghan, Ashley M., and Rosa N. Schnyer. 2015. "Biofield Therapies for Symptom Management in Palliative and End-of-Life Care." *The American Journal of Hospice & Palliative Care* 32 (1): 90–100. https://doi.org/10.1177/1049909113509400.

Holliman, Diane C., Ute C. Orgassa, and Jennie Pillion Forney. 2001. "Developing an Interactive Physical Activity Group in a Geriatric Psychiatry Facility." *Activities, Adaptation & Aging* 26 (1): 57–69. https://doi.org/10.1300/J016v26n01_04.

IAHAIO. 2018. "The IAHAIO Definitions for Animal Assisted Intervention and Guidelines for Wellness of Animals Involved in AAI." https://doi.org/10.1016/B978-0-12-815395-6.15001-1.

Jain, Shamini, Richard Hammerschlag, Paul Mills, Lorenzo Cohen, Richard Krieger, Cassandra Vieten, and Susan Lutgendorf. 2015. “Clinical Studies of Biofield Therapies: Summary, Methodological Challenges, and Recommendations.” *Global Advances in Health and Medicine* 4 (Suppl): 58–66. https://doi.org/10.7453/gahmj.2015.034.suppl.

Jia, Rui-Xia, Jing-Hong Liang, Yong Xu, and Ying-Quan Wang. 2019. “Effects of Physical Activity and Exercise on the Cognitive Function of Patients with Alzheimer Disease: A Meta-Analysis.” *BMC Geriatrics* 19 (1): 181. https://doi.org/10.1186/s12877-019-1175-2.

Johnson, Mark I., Carole A. Paley, Gareth Jones, Matthew R. Mulvey, and Priscilla G. Wittkopf. 2022. “Efficacy and Safety of Transcutaneous Electrical Nerve Stimulation (TENS) for Acute and Chronic Pain in Adults: A Systematic Review and Meta-Analysis of 381 Studies (the Meta-TENS Study).” *BMJ Open* 12 (2): e051073. https://doi.org/10.1136/bmjopen-2021-051073.

Kales, Helen C., Laura N. Gitlin, Barbara Stanislawski, Katherine Marx, Molly Turnwald, Daphne C. Watkins, and Constantine G. Lyketsos. 2017. “WeCareAdvisor™: The Development of a Caregiver-Focused, Web-Based Program to Assess and Manage Behavioral and Psychological Symptoms of Dementia.” *Alzheimer Disease and Associated Disorders* 31 (3): 263–70. https://doi.org/10.1097/WAD.0000000000000177.

Kapoor, Yamini, and Robin Orr. 2017. “Effect of Therapeutic Massage on Pain in Patients with Dementia.” *Dementia (London, England)* 16 (1): 119–25. https://doi.org/10.1177/1471301215583391.

Kolberg, Eirin, Gunnhild Johnsen Hjetland, Eirunn Thun, Ståle Pallesen, Inger Hilde Nordhus, Bettina S. Husebo, and Elisabeth Flo-Groeneboom. 2021. “The Effects of Bright Light Treatment on Affective Symptoms in People with Dementia: A 24-Week Cluster Randomized Controlled Trial.” *BMC Psychiatry* 21 (1): 377. https://doi.org/10.1186/s12888-021-03376-y.

Lai, Nai Ming, Sharon Mei Wern Chang, Siok Shen Ng, Fiona Stanaway, Shir Ley Tan, and Nathorn Chaiyakunapruk. 2019. “Animal-assisted Therapy for Dementia.” *The Cochrane Database of Systematic Reviews* 2019 (1): CD013243. https://doi.org/10.1002/14651858.CD013243.

Liao, Yo-Jen, Jyotsana Parajuli, Ying-Ling Jao, Lisa Kitko, and Diane Berish. 2021. “Non-Pharmacological Interventions for Pain in People with Dementia: A Systematic Review.” *International Journal of Nursing Studies* 124 (December): 104082. https://doi.org/10.1016/j.ijnurstu.2021.104082.

Liu, Yu-Hui, Yang Chen, Qing-Hua Wang, Ling-Ru Wang, Li Jiang, Ying Yang, Xian Chen, et al. 2022. "One-Year Trajectory of Cognitive Changes in Older Survivors of COVID-19 in Wuhan, China: A Longitudinal Cohort Study." *JAMA Neurology* 79 (5): 509–17. https://doi.org/10.1001/jamaneurol.2022.0461.

Lodha, Pragya. 2019. "Nonpharmacological Management of Dementia: A Review." *Indian Journal of Private Psychiatry* 13 (2): 62–70. https://doi.org/10.5005/jp-journals-10067-0038.

Lotan, Meir, and Christian Gold. 2009. "Meta-Analysis of the Effectiveness of Individual Intervention in the Controlled Multisensory Environment (Snoezelen) for Individuals with Intellectual Disability." *Journal of Intellectual & Developmental Disability* 34 (3): 207–15. https://doi.org/10.1080/13668250903080106.

Ma, Shi-Qi, Hai-Peng Huang, Meng-Qi Li, Bin Yu, Li-Ying Zhang, Ke Huang, Meng-Yuan Li, Lin Yao, and Hong-Feng Wang. 2021. "Effects of Acupuncture on Dementia: An Overview of Systematic Reviews." *European Journal of Integrative Medicine* 41 (January): 101256. https://doi.org/10.1016/j.eujim.2020.101256.

Margenfeld, Felix, Carina Klocke, and Stefanie Joos. 2019. "Manual Massage for Persons Living with Dementia: A Systematic Review and Meta-Analysis." *International Journal of Nursing Studies* 96 (August): 132–42. https://doi.org/10.1016/j.ijnurstu.2018.12.012.

Maseda, Ana, Nuria Cibeira, Laura Lorenzo-López, Isabel González-Abraldes, Ana Buján, Carmen de Labra, and José Carlos Millán-Calenti. 2018. "Multisensory Stimulation and Individualized Music Sessions on Older Adults with Severe Dementia: Effects on Mood, Behavior, and Biomedical Parameters." *Journal of Alzheimer's Disease: JAD* 63 (4): 1415–25. https://doi.org/10.3233/JAD-180109.

McKhann, Guy M., David S. Knopman, Howard Chertkow, Bradley T. Hyman, Clifford R. Jack, Claudia H. Kawas, William E. Klunk, et al. 2011. "The Diagnosis of Dementia Due to Alzheimer's Disease: Recommendations from the National Institute on Aging-Alzheimer's Association Workgroups on Diagnostic Guidelines for Alzheimer's Disease." *Alzheimer's & Dementia: The Journal of the Alzheimer's Association* 7 (3): 263–69. https://doi.org/10.1016/j.jalz.2011.03.005.

Meland, Beverly. 2009. "Effects of Reiki on Pain and Anxiety in the Elderly Diagnosed with Dementia: A Series of Case Reports." *Alternative Therapies in Health and Medicine* 15 (4): 56–57.

Mitchell, Susan L. 2015. "Advanced Dementia." *The New England Journal of Medicine* 373 (13): 1276–77. https://doi.org/10.1056/NEJMc1509349.

Momtaz, Reham Ibrahem. 2017. "Healing Gardens- A Review of Design Guidelines." *International Journal of Current Engineering and Technology* 7 (5): 1864–71.

Moniz Cook, Esme D., Katie Swift, Ian James, Reem Malouf, Marjolein De Vugt, and Frans Verhey. 2012. "Functional Analysis-Based Interventions for Challenging Behaviour in Dementia." *The Cochrane Database of Systematic Reviews*, no. 2 (February): CD006929. https://doi.org/10.1002/14651858.CD006929.pub2.

Moreno-Morales, Celia, Raul Calero, Pedro Moreno-Morales, and Cristina Pintado. 2020. "Music Therapy in the Treatment of Dementia: A Systematic Review and Meta-Analysis." *Frontiers in Medicine* 7 (May): 160. https://doi.org/10.3389/fmed.2020.00160.

Murroni, Veronica, Raffaele Cavalli, Andrea Basso, Erika Borella, Chiara Meneghetti, Andrea Melendugno, and Francesca Pazzaglia. 2021. "Effectiveness of Therapeutic Gardens for People with Dementia: A Systematic Review." *International Journal of Environmental Research and Public Health* 18 (18): 9595. https://doi.org/10.3390/ijerph18189595.

National Collaborating Centre for Mental Health (UK). 2007. *Dementia: A NICE-SCIE Guideline on Supporting People With Dementia and Their Carers in Health and Social Care*. National Institute for Health and Care Excellence: Guidelines. Leicester (UK): British Psychological Society (UK). http://www.ncbi.nlm.nih.gov/books/NBK55459/.

Navia, R. Osvaldo, and Lori Anne Constantine. 2022. "Palliative Care for Patients with Advanced Dementia." *Nursing* 52 (3): 19–26. https://doi.org/10.1097/01.NURSE.0000820024.83629.ee.

Neal, Martin, and Philip Barton Wright. 2003. "Validation Therapy for Dementia." *The Cochrane Database of Systematic Reviews*, no. 3: CD001394. https://doi.org/10.1002/14651858.CD001394.

Ojagbemi, Akin, and Nnenna Akin-Ojagbemi. 2019. "Exercise and Quality of Life in Dementia: A Systematic Review and Meta-Analysis of Randomized Controlled Trials." *Journal of Applied Gerontology* 38 (1): 27–48. https://doi.org/10.1177/0733464817693374.

O'Neil, Maya E., Michele Freeman, Vivian Christensen, Robin Telerant, Ashlee Addleman, and Devan Kansagara. 2011. *A Systematic Evidence Review of Non-Pharmacological Interventions for Behavioral Symptoms of Dementia*. VA Evidence-Based Synthesis Program Reports. Washington (DC): Department of Veterans Affairs (US). http://www.ncbi.nlm.nih.gov/books/NBK54971/.

Palmer, Jennifer A, Michelle Hilgeman, Tracy Balboni, Sara Paasche-Orlow, and Jennifer L Sullivan. 2022. "The Spiritual Experience of

Dementia From the Health Care Provider Perspective: Implications for Intervention." *The Gerontologist* 62 (4): 556–67. https://doi.org/10.1093/geront/gnab134.

Park, Sangki, Ahream Bak, Sujin Kim, Yunkwon Nam, Hyeon Soo Kim, Doo-Han Yoo, and Minho Moon. 2020. "Animal-Assisted and Pet-Robot Interventions for Ameliorating Behavioral and Psychological Symptoms of Dementia: A Systematic Review and Meta-Analysis." *Biomedicines* 8 (6): 150. https://doi.org/10.3390/biomedicines8060150.

Prins, Angela Joanna, Erik J. Anton Scherder, Annemieke van Straten, Yvonne Zwaagstra, and Maarten Valentijn Milders. 2020. "Sensory Stimulation for Nursing-Home Residents: Systematic Review and Meta-Analysis of Its Effects on Sleep Quality and Rest-Activity Rhythm in Dementia." *Dementia and Geriatric Cognitive Disorders* 49 (3): 219–34. https://doi.org/10.1159/000509433.

Pyne, Jeffrey D., and Adam M. Brickman. 2021. "The Impact of the COVID-19 Pandemic on Dementia Risk: Potential Pathways to Cognitive Decline." *Neuro-Degenerative Diseases* 21 (1–2): 1–23. https://doi.org/10.1159/000518581.

Saragih, Ita Daryanti, Santo Imanuel Tonapa, Ching-Teng Yao, Ice Septriani Saragih, and Bih-O. Lee. 2022. "Effects of Reminiscence Therapy in People with Dementia: A Systematic Review and Meta-Analysis." *Journal of Psychiatric and Mental Health Nursing* 29 (6): 883–903. https://doi.org/10.1111/jpm.12830.

Satija, Aanchal, and Sushma Bhatnagar. 2017. "Complementary Therapies for Symptom Management in Cancer Patients." *Indian Journal of Palliative Care* 23 (4): 468–79. https://doi.org/10.4103/IJPC.IJPC_100_17.

Sharew, Nigussie Tadesse. 2022. "The Effect of Multimodal Non-Pharmacological Interventions on Cognitive Function Improvement for People With Dementia: A Systematic Review." *Frontiers in Public Health* 10: 894930. https://doi.org/10.3389/fpubh.2022.894930.

Sikkes, Sietske A. M., Yi Tang, Roos J. Jutten, Linda M. P. Wesselman, Lyn S. Turkstra, Henry Brodaty, Linda Clare, et al. 2021. "Toward a Theory-Based Specification of Non-Pharmacological Treatments in Aging and Dementia: Focused Reviews and Methodological Recommendations." *Alzheimer's & Dementia: The Journal of the Alzheimer's Association* 17 (2): 255–70. https://doi.org/10.1002/alz.12188.

Smith, Bryce Carsone, and Mariana D'Amico. 2020. "Sensory-Based Interventions for Adults with Dementia and Alzheimer's Disease: A

Scoping Review." *Occupational Therapy in Health Care* 34 (3): 171–201. https://doi.org/10.1080/07380577.2019.1608488.

Strøm, Benedicte S., Siri Ytrehus, and Ellen-Karine Grov. 2016. "Sensory Stimulation for Persons with Dementia: A Review of the Literature." *Journal of Clinical Nursing* 25 (13–14): 1805–34. https://doi.org/10.1111/jocn.13169.

Tan, Jun Song Isaac, Ling Jie Cheng, Ee Yuee Chan, Ying Lau, and Siew Tiang Lau. 2022. "Light Therapy for Sleep Disturbances in Older Adults with Dementia: A Systematic Review, Meta-Analysis and Meta-Regression." *Sleep Medicine* 90 (February): 153–66. https://doi.org/10.1016/j.sleep.2022.01.013.

Thomas, Jeena Mary, and Duygu Sezgin. 2021. "Effectiveness of Reminiscence Therapy in Reducing Agitation and Depression and Improving Quality of Life and Cognition in Long-Term Care Residents with Dementia: A Systematic Review and Meta-Analysis." *Geriatric Nursing* 42 (6): 1497–1506. https://doi.org/10.1016/j.gerinurse.2021.10.014.

Woods, Diana Lynn, Cornelia Beck, and Karabi Sinha. 2009. "The Effect of Therapeutic Touch on Behavioral Symptoms and Cortisol in Persons with Dementia." *Forschende Komplementarmedizin* 16 (3): 181–89. https://doi.org/10.1159/000220479.

World Health Organization. 2022. "Dementia." https://www.who.int/news-room/fact-sheets/detail/dementia.

Yakimicki, Michelle L., Nancy E. Edwards, Elizabeth Richards, and Alan M. Beck. 2019. "Animal-Assisted Intervention and Dementia: A Systematic Review." *Clinical Nursing Research* 28 (1): 9–29. https://doi.org/10.1177/1054773818756987.

2

COGNITIVE IMPACT AFTER WHOLE BRAIN RADIOTHERAPY: CLINICAL COMPARISON WITH DEMENTIA

TIARA ANINDITHA, DIATRI NARI LASTRI, HENRY RIYANTO SOFYAN AND IRMA SAVITRI[1]

Introduction

The Burden of Cognitive Impairment

Cognitive ability is one of the essential functions of the human brain. This function is associated with structural and physiological abnormalities that can develop in dementia, such as arteriosclerosis in vascular dementia (VD) or neurofibrillary tangles from tau protein and beta-amyloid protein plaques in Alzheimer's dementia (AD).(Cortes-Canteli & Iadecola, 2020) Dementia is one of the primary causes of disability and dependency among older people and the seventh-most significant cause of death among all diseases.(World Health Organization (WHO), 2022) A study found that 58% of people with dementia live in lower middle-class countries, a number predicted to increase to 63% in 2030 and 71% in 2050.(Prince et al., 2013)

Neoplasm and its related therapies, such as radiotherapy and chemotherapy, have been associated with cognitive impairment, in addition to the common neurodegenerative causes.(Noh & Walbert, 2018) Brain tumors are classified as primary brain tumors and secondary or metastatic brain tumor. Compared to primary tumor, metastatic brain tumor patients are at greater risk of developing impaired cognitive function, whose proportion is 90% out of all metastatic brain tumor patients.*(Gerstenecker et al., 2014)* There are three reasons for this: Firstly, metastatic brain tumor patients have

[1] Mangunkusumo Hospital , Jakarta , Indonesia

systemic comorbidities from their primary tumor. Secondly, metastatic tumor lesions are usually multiple, with significant peritumoral edema. Thirdly, patients are at risk of developing complications due to their intracranial lesions or as a side-effect of their therapy, such as brain radiation. One of the clinical manifestations of metastatic brain tumor, and the focus of this study, is cognitive impairment, particularly memory.

The prevalence of cognitive impairment in metastatic brain tumor patients in the largest general hospital in Indonesia was 81.5% in 2019, with a significant difference between those with a history of radiation and those without brain radiation.(Maharani et al., 2015) In 2019, at the Central Cancer Hospital in Indonesia, Ardhini et al. found that patients with metastatic brain tumors already experience cognitive impairment before and after conventional whole-brain radiotherapy (WBRT).(Ardhini et al., 2019) The prognosis and treatment of cognitive impairment due to neurodegenerative causes is very different from neoplasm and its related therapy. The clinical diagnosis is quite challenging, and therefore special skills and knowledge are required in order to distinguish between the two.

Clinical Manifestations of Cognitive Impairment

The clinical presentation of cognitive impairment varies among individuals. It can manifest as memory loss, communication and language impairments, agnosia (inability to recognize objects), apraxia (inability to perform previously learned tasks), and impaired executive function, depending on the individual's clinical presentation of the disease (reasoning, judgment, and planning). Injuries to the cerebral cortex caused by synapse failure, inflammation, and changes in brain metabolism may lead to cognitive impairment. Dementia is an umbrella term used to describe a clinical syndrome of progressive cognitive decline. There are four common types of dementia: Alzheimer's disease, vascular dementia, Lewy body dementia, and frontotemporal dementia.(Duong, 2017)

Alzheimer's disease usually occurs with an insidious onset that is accompanied by a slow progressive decline of the patient's cognitive function. Devastating neuronal loss, changes in neurotransmitters such as decreased choline acetyltransferase activity and a decrease in cholinergic neurons, gliosis, and shrinkage of the hippocampus account for short-term memory loss, which is the most common and early manifestation. In later stages, executive function impairment occurs.(*Hippocampus and Its Involvement in Alzheimer's Disease: A Review - PMC*, n.d.)

Vascular dementia is caused by oxygen deprivation of neurons resulting from diseases that restrict or limit blood supply to the brain, such as stroke. Depending on the parts of the brain that are affected and the degree of blood vessel destruction, the symptoms might vary greatly. It has a sudden or gradual onset and is often correlated with cerebrovascular disease (stroke, lacunar infarcts) and atherosclerotic comorbidities (diabetes, hypertension, coronary heart disease). In the early stages, mild memory impairment may occur. In addition, there may also be possible gait difficulties and falls (depending on the extent of the stroke).(Duong, 2017)

Lewy body dementia is a type of dementia caused by abnormal Lewy body deposits (alpha-synuclein protein) inside of neurons. Patients generally experience fluctuating cognitive impairment with a variation of attention and alertness and recurrent complex visual hallucinations; it is also associated with Parkinsonism. Poor executive function and visual hallucinations often occur in the early stage and are manifested in deficits on tests designed to examine visual perception (pentagons, cubes, trails, clock faces). Meanwhile, in patients with frontotemporal dementia, personality changes (disinhibition) and behavioral disturbances (apathy, aggression, agitation with less memory impairment in the early stages) are manifested to a greater degree. The visuospatial function is typically unaffected, unlike Alzheimer's disease.

More than 90% of people with brain tumors reported cognitive deficits in at least one area, 78% of patients reported executive function abnormalities, and more than 60% of patients also reported memory and concentration problems. According to a previous study at cancer institute in Italy, cognitive abnormalities were observed in 46.25% of patients with brain tumors and 53.75% of those patients presented with multidomain impairment.(Abu-Hegazy & El-Hadaad, 2016)

This is also supported by the research of Primandari et al. at a general hospital in Indonesia, which found that the proportion of cognitive impairment in patients with metastatic brain tumors was 96.1%, with memory and executive function as the two most frequently disturbed domains.(Rima Anindita Primandari, 2016) Studies in patients with neuroepithelial tumors showed that patients with left frontal lobe lesions had lower cognitive test scores for attention, executive functions, and memory, whereas patients with right frontal lobe lesions scored significantly better in most of the subtests for memory.(Gempt et al., 2017)

The association cortices is the traditional name for the human parietal lobe. Perception, judgment, numerical cognition, integration, speech comprehension, and spatial awareness are a few of their important roles in processing sensory information. Accordingly, patients with lesions in the parietal lobe demonstrate a severe impairment in verbal-association abilities and have significantly lower test scores in the categories of attention and memory.(Culham & Kanwisher, 2001)

Comparison of the Clinical Manifestation of Brain Metastases and Dementia

There are differences in the clinical manifestations of cognitive impairment in post-WBRT patients and dementia patients. Patients with brain metastases tend to have more complex cognitive impairments, which are influenced by the lesion's location, size, and type, and usually affect memory and executive function. The clinical manifestations may occur or worsen following acute WBRT, subacute/early delayed WBRT, or even late-delayed WBRT. Patients with brain metastases are generally aged 50-60 years and still have the potential to experience dementia.(Saha et al., 2013) Thus, it is essential to distinguish patients with cognitive impairment after receiving WBRT treatment from patients with dementia. However, the incidence of memory impairment can be reduced or prevented by performing the hippocampal-sparing technique.

Clinical course and disease are essential in differentiating brain tumor disorders from degenerative dementia. In brain tumors, the clinical course is influenced by the patient's premorbid factors and tumor-related factors, such as tumor type, location, lateralization, grade, volume, biology, tumor stability, and clinical features. The clinical manifestations include seizures/epilepsy and brain edema, factors related to treatment (time of treatment in the course of the disease, surgery as a general effect, resection of tumor extension, complications during or following surgery, chemotherapy, radiotherapy, anti-seizure drugs, and corticosteroids). Other factors, such as the cognitive examination tools used and the time of examination relative to the course of the disease, may also influence the premorbid factors. Therefore, the progression of cognitive impairment in brain tumors can occur faster than in degenerative dementia. Cognitive impairment symptoms and increased intracranial pressure may accompany other physical and neurological clinical symptoms.

In patients with dementia, cognitive impairment generally occurs in relation to the neurodegeneration process, which mainly occurs in advanced age. There is a predominance of age as one of the distinguishing characteristics. In addition, clinical manifestations usually start with memory impairment. Initially, patients or their families report that they often forget things in their daily lives. Another differentiation from post-WBRT cognitive disorder is that once the degenerative condition has occurred, it cannot be prevented because it occurs with increasing age (degenerative process). However, unlike the WBRT mentioned earlier, efforts can be made to minimize the risk of cognitive impairment.

The Importance of Understanding and Managing Cognitive Impairment in General and Based on Its Etiology

Cognitive impairment has strong associations with quality of life.(*Cognitive Dysfunction and Health-Related Quality of Life among Older Chinese | Scientific Reports*, n.d.; Stites et al., 2018; Williams et al., 2017) Screening should be conducted before undergoing WBRT to assess whether patients have dementia, dementia risk factors, or are normal, as this would determine therapeutic approach, including pharmacological and non-pharmacological treatment. Neurocognitive function impairment, as one of the clinical manifestations of the tumor, is typically influenced not only by the underlying tumor's location but also by the size, type, and biology.(Schiff et al., 2018) Therefore, a neurocognitive examination will help to determine functional tumor lesions so that large, respectable lesions can be operated on to improve cognitive impairment.

Cognitive Impairment in Metastatic Brain Tumors

In general, metastatic cancer cells occur through a cascade of metastases. Tumor cells invade the surrounding tissue, intravasate (enter the bloodstream), attach to the capillaries of blood vessels, and then extravasate and proliferate at the site of metastases.(*Brain Metastasis as Complication of Systemic Cancers | Request PDF*, n.d.) Most brain metastases arise from the embolization of tumor cells through hematogenous spread. As a result, brain metastases are mainly discovered in locations where there are changes in the size of the diameter of blood vessels, from larger to smaller, such as the white-gray matter junction. In 80% of cases, lesions are found in the cerebral hemispheres, 15% in the cerebellum, and 5% in the brain stem.(*Brain Metastasis as Complication of Systemic Cancers | Request PDF*, n.d.) Understanding the pathophysiology of these brain metastases allows us to visualize the characteristics of the manifestations that can occur.

Metastatic brain tumors may cause cognitive impairment either directly or indirectly. The suppression of nearby structures directly impacts the expansion of the tumor mass. Meanwhile, an indirect impact is caused by edema or elevated intracranial pressure around the tumor (peritumoral). Language function, including verbal learning, memory, and speaking, is likely to be disrupted by tumors that affect the dominant hemisphere and frontotemporal region. Nonverbal communication, visual-spatial, and visual-perceptual abilities are more likely to be affected by nondominant hemisphere tumors.

Frontal lobe tumors commonly cause executive dysfunction and personality changes, while parietal lobe tumors usually cause spatial orientation problems. Tumors in the occipital lobes can cause visual-perceptive deficits. Patients with brain stem lesions and cerebellar tumors have also been reported to experience neurocognitive and mood disorders, providing evidence that the cerebellum plays a significant role in neural network systems that are relevant to higher cognitive function.

Cognitive function might be impacted by the disease and tumor-related therapies, such as WBRT. WBRT is the most frequently used and recommended therapy in brain metastases with multiple lesions, according to the National Comprehensive Cancer Network (NCCN).(National Comprehensive Cancer Network, 2017) Cognitive impairment due to WBRT is a complex and multifactorial process. Radiation induces damage to deoxyribonucleic acid (DNA), which may result in neuronal cell damage. In the past, cognitive impairment due to radiotherapy was considered a late effect of therapy due to microvascular and glial damage. However, current scientific evidence suggests that there are acute and subacute effects of head radiation due to injury to the neurogenic zone of the hippocampus. Therefore, radiation-induced neurotoxicity is divided into three stages: acute, early-delayed, and late-delayed reaction.(Schiff et al., 2018)

Rupture of the blood-brain barrier, inflammatory processes, vascular toxicity, and cerebral edema are thought to be the causes of the acute phase's symptoms. The acute phase usually develops within days to weeks of therapy and is characterized by subacute neurological impairment, increased fatigue, and deterioration of previous deficiencies.(Schiff et al., 2018) This condition may be reversible upon appropriate supportive care. Early-delayed neurotoxic symptoms may appear weeks to months later. Fatigue, inattentiveness, and short-term memory problems are the prominent symptoms.(Schiff et al., 2018) It is believed that radiation-induced temporary demyelination causes early-delayed neurotoxic effects. The majority of late-delayed side effects are irreversible and progressive and can manifest months to years after radiation. Memory, concentration problems, and executive dysfunction are all common complaints.(Schiff et al., 2018) Patients will experience progressive cognitive loss in more severe cases of late-delayed radiation toxicity.

The therapy modality for cognitive impairment in tumors is influenced by factors related to the disease. In several studies, memantine can be given as a preventive therapy for cognitive impairment in patients before and during WBRT. In degenerative dementia, until now, there has been no disease-modifying therapy. The existing pharmacological drugs are cognitive boosters that can slow the progression of the clinical course.

Treatment

From the point of view of pathophysiology, the management of cognitive impairment differs significantly between dementia and brain tumors. Tumor-related cognitive disorders can be operated on, with indications for systemic tumor control, a good score on the Karnofsky Performance Scale, and an approachable location. To avoid memory impairment, radiotherapy can be performed by avoiding the hippocampus (hippocampal sparing), based on the theory that the hippocampus is the center of memory. There is some evidence supporting the role of hippocampal sparing in WBRT in preserving the cognitive functions of metastatic brain tumor patients.(Gondi et al., 2010)

Methods for preventing side effects or reducing the severity of symptoms are included in therapeutic interventions. Some therapeutic approaches have demonstrated a possible clinical advantage in the management of adverse effects of cancer therapy on neurocognition. Psychostimulants such as methylphenidate and modafinil are effective treatments for cognitive impairment caused by cancer therapy.(Schiff et al., 2018) In brain tumor patients, donepezil has been proven to enhance mental acuity, disposition, and quality of life.(Schiff et al., 2018)

Considering the abundant scientific evidence describing the important role of neurogenic stem cell damage in post-WBRT cognitive dysfunction, radiation techniques have been developed to protect the hippocampus.(Dye et al., 2015; Kazda et al., 2014) This radiation is known by several terms, including hippocampal-avoidance or hippocampal-sparing radiotherapy. With this technique, the average dose received by neurogenic stem cells can be reduced by at least 80%, while maintaining dose homogeneity and adequate exposure of the rest of the brain parenchyma.(Apple et al., 2017) Treatment of patients with cognitive impairment is carried out holistically through multicomponent interventions and according to each patient's specific needs. The role of the caregiver becomes crucial for the patient because of the progression of the disease, which makes the patient increasingly dependent on help from other people in carrying out their daily activities. A previous study revealed that caregivers of dementia patients provide an average of 56 hours of assistance per week and spend significantly more time providing care when they are a spouse/partner of the care recipient and when the care recipient's functional status is worse or their dementia is more severe.(Bayly et al., 2019)

However, caregivers face various consequences due to the considerable stress involved in long-term care. Providing knowledge, skills, and psychosocial support is essential to prevent negative physical and mental effects among caregivers, including cardiovascular disease, stress-related disorders, burden, sleep problems, anxiety, and even depression, all of which affect the caregivers' role. To promote caregiving and improve the quality of life for caregivers and patients, caregivers need social and professional support. When informal caregivers and dementia patients are followed up on and accompanied by medical professionals, problems in physical and emotional health can be quickly identified, facilitating early intervention and referrals to specific facilities.(Frias et al., 2020)

Conclusions

Cognitive impairment can be caused by neurodegenerative conditions such as dementia or by non-degenerative conditions such as neoplasms and their related therapy. There are differences in the clinical manifestation of dementia compared to metastatic brain tumor patients who have undergone WBRT. In post-WBRT patients, cognitive impairment occurs after WBRT and can affect patients of all ages with brain tumors. Meanwhile, in patients with dementia, cognitive impairment occurs progressively, in relation to the neurodegeneration process. It mainly occurs in advanced age and usually starts with memory impairment. Understanding the difference between the two is important because cognitive impairment can affect patients' and caregivers' quality of life. The therapy provided comprises medical therapy as well as non-medical therapy. Interventions for caregivers are also needed because of the high stress levels involved in dealing with patients with cognitive impairment.

References

Abu-Hegazy, M., & El-Hadaad, H. A. (2016). *Neurocognitive Effects of Primary Brain Tumors. Neurooncology—Newer Developments*. Amit Agrawal. DOI: 10.5772/62924

Apple, D. M., Fonseca, R. S., & Kokovay, E. (2017). The role of adult neurogenesis in psychiatric and cognitive disorders. *Brain Research, 1655*, 270–276. https://doi.org/10.1016/j.brainres.2016.01.023

Ardhini, R., Aninditha, T., Andriani, R., & Sofyan, H. (2019). Cognitive function after whole brain radiotherapy in brain metastases in Cipto Mangunkusumo Hospital and Dharmais Cancer Hospital Jakarta. *16th Asian Society for Neurooncology Meeting.*

Bayly, M., Morgan, D., Kosteniuk, J., Elliot, V., Froehlich Chow, A., Peacock, S., McLean, A., & O'Connell, M. E. (2019). Protocol for a systematic review on interventions for caregivers of persons with mild cognitive impairment and early dementia: Does early stage intervention improve caregiver well-being and ability to provide care? *BMJ Open, 9*(5), e028441. https://doi.org/10.1136/bmjopen-2018-028441

Brain Metastasis as Complication of Systemic Cancers | Request PDF. (n.d.). Retrieved December 22, 2022, from https://www.researchgate.net/publication/319873625_Brain_Metastasis_as_Complication_of_Systemic_Cancers

Cognitive dysfunction and health-related quality of life among older Chinese | Scientific Reports. (n.d.). Retrieved December 26, 2022, from https://www.nature.com/articles/srep17301

Cortes-Canteli, M., & Iadecola, C. (2020). Alzheimer's Disease and Vascular Aging. *Journal of the American College of Cardiology, 75*(8), 942–951. https://doi.org/10.1016/j.jacc.2019.10.062

Culham, J. C., & Kanwisher, N. G. (2001). Neuroimaging of cognitive functions in human parietal cortex. *Current Opinion in Neurobiology, 11*(2), 157–163. https://doi.org/10.1016/S0959-4388(00)00191-4

Duong, S. (2017). Dementia. *Can Pharm J (Ott), 150*(2), 118–129. https://doi.org/10.1177/1715163517690745

Dye, N. B., Gondi, V., & Mehta, M. P. (2015). Strategies for preservation of memory function in patients with brain metastases. *Chinese Clinical Oncology*, *4*(2), 24. https://doi.org/10.3978/j.issn.2304-3865.2015.05.05

Frias, C. E., Cabrera, E., & Zabalegui, A. (2020). Informal Caregivers' Roles in Dementia: The Impact on Their Quality of Life. *Life*, *10*(11), Article 11. https://doi.org/10.3390/life10110251

Gempt, J., Lange, N., Bette, S., Foreman, S. C., Cammardella, J. H., Albertshauser, J., Gradtke, C., Buchmann, N., Ryang, Y.-M., Schmidt-Graf, F., Meyer, B., & Ringel, F. (2017). Factors influencing neurocognitive function in patients with neuroepithelial tumors. *Scientific Reports*, *7*(1), Article 1. https://doi.org/10.1038/s41598-017-17833-w

Gerstenecker, A., Nabors, L. B., Meneses, K., Fiveash, J. B., Marson, D. C., Cutter, G., Martin, R. C., Meyers, C. A., & Triebel, K. L. (2014). Cognition in patients with newly diagnosed brain metastasis: Profiles and implications. *Journal of Neuro-Oncology*, *120*(1), 179–185. https://doi.org/10.1007/s11060-014-1543-x

Gondi, V., Tolakanahalli, R., Mehta, M. P., Tewatia, D., & Rowley, H. (2010). Hippocampal-sparing whole-brain radiotherapy: A "how-to" technique using helical tomotherapy and linear accelerator-based intensity-modulated radiotherapy—PubMed. *Int J Radiat Oncol Biol Phys*, *78*(4), 1244–1252. https://doi.org/doi: 10.1016/j.ijrobp.2010.01.03

Hippocampus and its involvement in Alzheimer's disease: A review—PMC. (n.d.). Retrieved December 26, 2022, from https://www.ncbi.nlm.nih.gov/pmc/articles/PMC8807768/

Kazda, T., Jancalek, R., Pospisil, P., Sevela, O., Prochazka, T., Vrzal, M., Burkon, P., Slavik, M., Hynkova, L., Slampa, P., & Laack, N. N. (2014). Why and how to spare the hippocampus during brain radiotherapy: The developing role of hippocampal avoidance in cranial radiotherapy. *Radiation Oncology*, *9*(1), 139. https://doi.org/10.1186/1748-717X-9-139

Maharani, K., Larasari, A., Aninditha, T., & Ramli, Y. (2015). Gangguan kognitif pada tumor intrakranial primer dan metastasis. *Jurnal Kedokteran Indonesia*, *3(2)*, 107–114.

National Comprehensive Cancer Network. (2017). Central Nervous System Cancers. *United States*. https://www.nccn.org/professionals/physician_gls/default.aspx.

Noh, T., & Walbert, T. (2018). Brain metastasis: Clinical manifestations, symptom management, and palliative care. *Handbook of Clinical*

Neurology, *149*, 75–88. https://doi.org/10.1016/B978-0-12-811161-1.00006-2

Prince, M., Bryce, R., Albanese, E., Wimo, A., Ribeiro, W., & Ferri, C. P. (2013). The global prevalence of dementia: A systematic review and metaanalysis. *Alzheimer's & Dementia: The Journal of the Alzheimer's Association*, *9*(1), 63-75.e2. https://doi.org/10.1016/j.jalz.2012.11.007

Rima Anindita Primandari, A. (2016). *Gambaran gangguan fungsi kognitif pada tumor otak primer dan metastasis = Cognitive impairment profile in brain tumors*. Universitas Indonesia Library. https://lib.ui.ac.id

Saha, A., Ghosh, S. K., Roy, C., Choudhury, K. B., Chakrabarty, B., & Sarkar, R. (2013). Demographic and clinical profile of patients with brain metastases: A retrospective study. *Asian Journal of Neurosurgery*, *8*(3), 157–161. https://doi.org/10.4103/1793-5482.121688

Schiff, D., Arrillaga, I., & Wen, P. Y. (2018). *Cancer Neurology in Clinical Practice* (3rd ed.). Springer Nature.

Stites, S. D., Harkins, K., Rubright, J. D., & Karlawish, J. (2018). Relationships between Cognitive Complaints and Quality of Life in Older Adults with Mild Cognitive Impairment, Mild Alzheimer's Disease Dementia, and Normal Cognition. *Alzheimer Disease and Associated Disorders*, *32*(4), 276–283. https://doi.org/10.1097/WAD.0000000000000262

Williams, A. M., Lindholm, J., Cook, D., Siddiqui, F., Ghanem, T. A., & Chang, S. S. (2017). Association Between Cognitive Function and Quality of Life in Patients With Head and Neck Cancer. *JAMA Otolaryngology–Head & Neck Surgery*, *143*(12), 1228–1235. https://doi.org/10.1001/jamaoto.2017.2014

World Health Organization (WHO). (2022). *Dementia*. https://www.who.int/news-room/fact-sheets/detail/dementia

3

Phytotherapy for Patients with Dementia in Palliative Care: A Review

Adem Akcakaya[1] and Emrah Yucesan[2]

Abstract

The incidence of many neurological diseases, especially dementia, is increasing these days due to the aging of the population worldwide. This situation has extended the care duration required by the elderly population due to the disease and is stimulating the evaluation of different treatment alternatives. Although the patients are those primarily affected by dementia, the relatives who take care of the patient and the health workers who are responsible for the maintenance of the patients are also indirectly affected. Palliative care services are being continuously developed and updated in direct proportion to the long-term hospitalization of patients. In this context, the importance of palliative care for dementia patients is increasing, and the medical treatments being applied during this maintenance are crucial. Although routine drug treatment is applied to patients, the application of herbal-based treatments is becoming widespread, particularly today. These herbal approaches, called phytotherapy, have the opportunity to be applied in developed countries (US and EU). The most common applications of these herbal treatments in the context of our subject are Alzheimer's disease accompanied by dementia. Herbal medicines with a potential for clinical application are those with a mechanism of action similar to

---

[1] Department of General Surgery, Faculty of Medicine, Bezmialem Vakif University, Istanbul, Turkey, and Head of Palliative Care Unit, Faculty of Medicine, Bezmialem Vakif University, Istanbul, Turkey

[2] Department of Neurogenetics, Institute of Neurological Sciences, Istanbul University-Cerrahpasa, Istanbul, Turkey

acetylcholinesterase inhibitor drugs. In the present review, the applications of phytotherapy applications in dementia patients who need palliative care, scientific results, and possible alternative herbal medicine applications in the future are discussed.

Keywords: Palliative care, phytotherapy, dementia, acetylcholinesterase inhibitors, complementary and alternative therapies, NMDA receptor antagonist

In the history of philosophy, many thinkers, such as Plato, Aristotle, Cicero, and Seneca, wrote about the value of old age and its benefits for society (1). This conception may be valid for aging individuals who are healthy, but it is a known fact that many diseases occur with old age. Aging is the greatest risk factor for most diseases, including several cancers and cardiovascular and neurodegenerative diseases (2). Here, the neurodegenerative disease dementia will be evaluated. Dementia is a chronic, progressive, and irreversible neurodegenerative disease. Advanced dementia is characterized by profound cognitive deterioration and a lack of communication with others, and it is comorbid with several other neurological and psychiatric conditions (3). The clinical findings of dementia are highly heterogeneous among affected individuals and may include cognitive deficit, memory impairment and memory loss over time, loss of communication skills and language disorders, agnosia, and apraxia (4). Therefore, dementia is directly related to the quality of daily life both for the patients and their relatives (5).

There are approximately 47 million patients with dementia worldwide (6). According to a study published in 2017, the number of individuals diagnosed as having dementia worldwide will reach 75.6 million in 2030, and this number will be 135.5 million in 2050 (7). These numbers may differ between human populations. For instance, according to a meta-analysis of articles on "dementia" published between 1985 and 2019, the prevalence of dementia in Europe and North America was higher than in Asia, Africa, and South America (8). The individual lifetime cost of care for a person with diagnosed dementia is about $200,000 more than a person without dementia (9). There are many pathological conditions that cause dementia, with Alzheimer's disease (AD) being the most common cause; at least two-thirds of patients with dementia in people aged 65 or older have been diagnosed as having AD (10). Apart from AD, which develops due to aging, there are also various types of dementia that differ in clinical diagnosis? and etiopathogenesis. These are vascular dementia (usually correlated with cerebrovascular disease and atherosclerotic comorbidities, i.e., diabetes, hypertension, coronary heart disease), Lewy body dementia (associated with Parkinsonism), and frontotemporal dementia (clumps of abnormal protein forming inside the brain cells) (4,5). Although the mechanisms of their occurrence are different, their clinical presentations are similar and all of them cause dementia.

Taking these aforementioned points into consideration, it is understood that dementia treatment should be approached in a holistic way that combines different disciplines. This holistic approach is a process in which many factors are actively involved throughout the patient's entire disease process and is called palliative care (5). Generally, palliative care focuses solely on patients with cancer who need care. However, in recent years, the palliative care approach has also been used for dementia, as it requires lifelong care (11). People with dementia can live for a long time, but it is hard to say precisely how long a patient with advanced dementia will live (3). It is known that more than 95% of patients with dementia require 24-hour care either in hospital, for a while, or a nursing home until the end of life. For this purpose, several multidisciplinary guidelines have been jointly developed by medical and palliative care staff, as well as health care providers (physicians and nurses), especially those working in the psychiatry unit. In the later stages of dementia, various manifestations such as behavioral problems, pain, dyspnea, anorexia, and cachexia can be given as examples of worsening conditions (11). As a result of these situations, the patient may die due to many different reasons related to old age, despite the palliative care (12).

Treatment approaches for dementia can be grouped under two main headings: One is a non-pharmacological approach including cognitive stimulation, physical activity, increased social activity with others, healthy diet, adequate sleep, personel hygiene, effective communication, and psychological health; the other one is a pharmacological approach involving, for instance, acetylcholinesterase inhibitors, NMDA receptor antagonists, and combination drugs (6). In brief, non-pharmacological approaches are based on studies such as the randomized clinical trials that examined different populations in different geographical regions and which reported that cognitive activity is related to positive results in elderly people with dementia. As an example, reading activity and playing brain-activating games like chess may help protect cognitive skills (13, 14). Physical activities may directly improve cardiovascular disease via regulating blood pressure, and thus cognitive impairment may decrease indirectly (15). In addition, there are studies in the literature demonstrating the positive effects of social interaction on dementia (16). All these treatment options should be evaluated from a palliative care perspective.

Various complementary therapies, which have been developing with increasing momentum, have been added to the different palliative care approaches, especially in recent years (17). The benefits and efficacy of complementary therapies have been discussed in different studies in the literature. When the clinical conditions of patients in need of palliative care are evaluated, such discussions are almost inevitable. Considering the benefits and harms among patients in need of palliative care, these complementary therapies can be considered at least as supplements. Complementary therapy in palliative care is sometimes named 'alternative therapy', or called a combination of complementary and alternative therapies (CAM) (18, 19). Aromatherapy massage, acupuncture, breathing exercises, meditation, and reflexology can be given as examples for such therapies (20, 21). These therapies are increasingly used in the clinic, and their importance for enhancing the quality of life of patients who need palliative care will further increase in the future.

Phytotherapy, which is one of the alternative-complementary approaches in the treatment of dementia, has wide application areas, from urological diseases, diabetes, microbial resistance, gastrointestinal system diseases, cardiovascular diseases, and diabetic retinopathy to attention deficit and hyperactivity disorder (22-27). Although phytotherapy lost its prevalence for a while, especially in Western countries, it again became an area of interest, especially in the last quarter of the 20th century (28). To give a short definition, phytotherapy is a field of medicine that uses plants for treating patients with a specific disease. The term phytotherapy is also known as herbalism, especially in Western societies.

There are many studies in the literature on the necessity of palliative care in the elderly population, where dementia frequency is the highest (29, 30). Some of these researches take into account the neurological status of the elderly population and evaluate it in terms of a palliative care approach (31). It is often not possible to completely cure neurological diseases with conventional medical methods. Therefore, in neurological conditions, CAM therapies are considered supportive approaches, even though their effects have not been conclusively demonstrated (32). Although some of the patients with dementia respond positively to treatment, the CAM approach may be preferred, especially in dementia caused by AD (33).

Within the CAM approach, there are many scientific articles reporting the application of phytotherapy in dementia and the positive results obtained. For instance, known for its antioxidant and neuroprotective effects, *Ginkgo biloba* has been successfully applied to patients with AD. In Europe, especially in books written in ancient times, plants such as *Salvia officinalis* (sage) and *Melissa officinalis* (lemon balm) were known to have an activating effect on memory (33). In various subsequent studies, the use of *Ginkgo biloba* as a phytotherapy approach has been shown to have positive results in patients with dementia (34, 35). In a review article published by Wightman (2017), the effects of five different herbs (*Ginkgo biloba, Melissa officinalis, Salvia lavandulaefolia, Salvia officinalis* and ginseng) on dementia were examined and similar positive results were obtained (36). In a literature review published in 2022 of studies in which phytotherapeutic approaches were applied in the relief of different symptoms seen after Covid-19—including irreversible dementia—it was mentioned that phytotherapy provided relief for these symptoms. In that study, *Valeriana officinalis, Melissa officinalis, Passiflora incarnata, Piper methysticum, Humulus lupulus, Ballota nigra, Hypericum perforatum, Rhodiola rosea, Lavandula officinalis, Paullinia cupana, Ginkgo biloba, Murraya koenigii, Crataegus monogyna and oxyacantha, Hedera helix, Polygala senega, Pelargonium sidoides, Lichen islandicus, Plantago lanceolata* and their compounds (valeranon, valtrate, apigenin, citronellal, isovitexin, isoorientin, methysticin, humulone, farnesene, acteoside, hypericin, hyperforin, biapigenin, rosavidin, salidroside, linalool acetate, linalool, caffeine, ginkgolide, bilobalide, mihanimbine, epicatechin, hederacoside C, α-hederine, presegenin, umckalin, 6,7,8-trixydroxybenzopyranone disulfate, fumaroprotocetric acid, protolichesteric acid, aucubin, acteoside) were evaluated. In the conclusion of the article, the authors reported that these herbs reduced neurological (including dementia), respiratory, and cardiovascular symptoms after Covid-19 (37).

While various studies on the scientific competence of herbal products used for phytotherapy have been published, studies on the legal status of these products are continuing, especially in the European Union and the United States (38, 39). The main reason for the continued legal studies is that the effects of the herbs used in phytotherapy applications are not clearly known, except for the ones given as an example above and the ones whose effectiveness has been proven. Therefore, it is necessary to determine whether they are drugs or supplements and adjust the attitudes of governments toward this situation accordingly. In the literature, there are different studies on phytotherapy applications, explaining their benefits and harms and suggesting how they should be used or not used (40-43). These studies focus on the possible side effects of herbs with clinical applications in terms of phytotherapy. In this context, controlled clinical studies are needed to clarify the clinical importance of drug-herb interactions. This is crucial because herbs and drugs can interact in the same way that drug/drug interactions occur (44).

The herbs mentioned above generally show their effects with a similar mechanism of action as several known drugs. There are various drugs approved by the FDA that are used specifically in the treatment of AD, and these drugs can be used for all stages of dementia, from mild to moderate, to severe. Among these drugs, acetylcholinesterase inhibitors (AChEIs) can be used in all stages of dementia. Many studies have shown that these drugs have positive effects on the health of patients with dementia (45, 46). As known, AChEIs have been shown to provide a significant improvement in cognition in patients with AD. However, despite this finding, not all patients respond equally to these drugs, and for some responders, this effect may be of a limited duration. Therefore, studies on the development of different AChEIs continue (47).

Prior to discussing how AChEIs work, we briefly mentioned acetylcholine (Ach) and its impact on the brain. Reduced levels of Ach in the brain are recognized as a direct contributor to cognitive decline because they result from the inhibition of acetylcholinesterases, which play a crucial role in breaking down Ach. The goal is to prevent this decline in Ach levels within the brain." (48).

Currently, three AChEIs (donepezil, galantamine, and rivastigmine) have been approved for the treatment of dementia due to AD. AChEIs are used therapeutically not only in AD but also in vascular dementia (49). In a meta-analysis of 1773 articles from three different databases (Moreta et al. 2021), the overall effect of AChEIs on cognitive capacity was evaluated. According to the results of this review, AChEIs were generally inefficient in stimulating? cognitive improvement in patients with mild and moderate AD. Despite this, donepezil (10 mg/day) was stated to be the most effective treatment. The authors concluded that the data suggesting that AChEI stabilizes or slows cognitive deterioration and improves global status were insufficient. In another meta-analysis examining the effect of AChEIs in vascular dementia (Battle et al. 2021), studies from ten different databases that compared varying doses of three drugs with placebo groups were examined. The analysis found that donepezil (10 mg/day) and galantamine

(16 to 24 mg/da) may improve cognition and that with low certainty, rivastigmine (3 to 12 mg/day) may have a small positive effect on cognition. In the same paper, adverse events were reported, such as nausea, vomiting, diarrhea, dizziness, headache, and hypertension (49).

It has been stated in many studies in the literature that some plants used in phytotherapy application take advantage of the known mechanism of AChEIs. The plant named *Huperzia serrata* can be given as an example for such studies. Huperzine A (HupA), an alkaloid isolated from *Huperzia serrata*, is a specific and reversible acetylcholinesterase inhibitor that is able to cross the blood brain barrier more efficiently than donepezil and rivastigmine. In addition, it is both neuroprotective and antagonistic to NMDA receptors. HupA significantly improves memory deficits in patients with AD and vascular dementia (51). After this study was published in 2006, similar studies on the effect of HupA in rodents were published, and it was concluded that HupA ameliorated cognitive deficit via modulating BDNF, oxidative stress, inflammation, and apoptosis (52, 53).

Today, there are many plants known to have acetylcholinesterase inhibitory effects. An article published in 2013 provided a list of these herbs: *Buxaceae, Amaryllidaceae, Lycopodiaceae, Lamiaceae, Chenopodiaceae, Papaveraceae, Apocynaceae*, and *Labiatae* species (54). In a study published in the same year, 128 articles (2006-2012 first quarter) were reviewed and plants showing a similar mechanism of action of AChEIs were evaluated. Among other things, the review notes that the natural products obtained from *Huperzia* spp. and *Galanthus* spp. not only increase cognitive function, but also accelerate studies on the detection of secondary metabolites derived from them (55). In 2018, dos Santos et al. published a study in which 54 plant species from 29 families and 36 isolated compounds were classified and discussed according to their anti-AChE pharmacological potency. The IC_{50} and toxicological properties of the plants were also evaluated in this study, which reported that the aforementioned herbs positively affected the treatment of dementia (56). In a study published in 2021, Ahmed et al. discussed different medicinal herbs, their extracts, and phytocompounds that can be used as AChEIs in the treatment of AD. In this very detailed article, the analyzed plants were evaluated one by one in terms of their chemical structures, pharmacodynamics, and pharmacokinetic properties. Researchers examined these plants in terms of acetylcholinesterase inhibitory effects, according to their extracts (methanol-alkaloidal-methanol/chloroform), and phyto-compounds. For this purpose, 45 pyhto-compounds, 7 alkaloidals, 9 methanols/chloroforms, and 16 methanols exhibiting acetylcholinesterase inhibitory effects were evaluated. The authors concluded that medicinal herbs and bioactive phytoconstituents (AChEIs-like) have enormous potential in the treatment of AD. The authors of the article noted that studies on AChEIs' natural compounds should lead to the formulation of low-cost and efficacious herbal drugs that could be beneficial for every patient with dementia (57).

While similar researches are ongoing, other studies are attempting to clarify the molecular mechanisms of the aforementioned herbs. For example, in a study examining *Allium sativum, Areca catechu, Camellia sinensis, Curcuma longa, Lobelia chinensis, Nelumbo nucifera, Portulaca oleracea, Uncaria rhynchophylla*, and *Zingiber officinale*, scientists used molecular docking simulation. For this purpose, the 2D structures of the compounds in the herb samples were retrieved from the National Center for Biotechnology Information (NCBI) PubChem database. According to the results, alkaloidal extracts from *Nelumbo nucifera, Uncaria rhynchophylla*, and *Portulaca oleracea* exhibited the most significant effect against AChE. In the same study, they noted that *Areca catechu* showed the poorest AChE inhibition (58). Another study evaluated 19 different honeys (Szwajgier et al. 2022) and found an AChE inhibitory effect of honey, with thyme honey exhibiting a maximum efficiency of AChE inhibition (21.17% inhibition) (59). Although all these phytotherapy studies include different plants and extracts, the common mechanism in all of them is inhibition of acetylcholinesterase. As their efficiency differs, it is yet to be determined which natural products provide the most benefit with the least cost, and research continues in this regard with the aim of obtaining synthetic derivatives.

The NMDA (N-methyl-D-aspartate) antagonists are another alternative drug for the treatment of dementia. As known, the N-methyl-D-aspartate receptor (also known as the NMDA receptor), is a glutamate receptor and ion channel localized in neurons. The NMDA receptor is a protein which allows the passage of ions through the cell membrane, and it is crucial for controlling synaptic plasticity and regulating learning and memory. The most effective agent in this group is memantine (molecular formula: $C_{12}H_{21}N$). It was approved in the European Union, mainly in Germany, and also in the United States. Preclinical and clinical evidence for the effectiveness and neuroprotective features of memantine has been shown (60). It is known that glutamate excitotoxicity (NMDA-receptor-mediated) is a major risk factor for Aβ-induced neuronal death, and NMDA receptor activation has been detected in AD related to synaptic dysfunction (61). Therefore, NMDA receptors are promising targets for preventing the progression of neurodegeneration. As reported in the literature, the following are examples of herbs that act on the NMDA receptor: *Rhizoma Curcumae Longae, Radix Achyranthis Bidentatae, Herba Lycopodii Serrati, Radix Notoginseng, Radix Polygalae, Semen Zizyphi Spinosae, Radix et Rhizoma Valerianae, Ramulus Uncariae cum Uncis, Rhizoma Gastrodiae, Semen Cassiae, Rhizoma Acori, Radix Glycyrrhizae, Radix Ginseng, Folium Ginkgo,* and *Radix Scrophulariae* (62). Another extract associated with NMDA receptor activity is curcumin, obtained from the Curcuma longa plant. The molecular mechanism of curcumin, which produces its effect through NMDA, has been studied in detail and its direct effects on the brain have been examined (63, 64). In a study of a transgenic mouse model of AD that directly examined curcumin's effect on dementia, it was shown to reduce oxidative damage in the brain (65). Finally, although differing from the explanations above, it has been reported that omega-3 fatty acids and vitamin E also have positive effects on dementia (66, 67).

In summary, the discussion of the use of phytotherapy continues among today's scientific community and clinical practice through mutual feedback. Of course, these discussions should be based on the prioritization of scientific methods and approaches and especially the experimental model. As with every drug, herbs used for phytotherapy can also have side effects, and these can only be determined by scientific methods. That said, the scientific developments on this subject are quite exciting and fruitful. We can assume that phytotherapy applications, whose positive and negative features were presented here, will increase in the future, especially in diseases such as dementia that require palliative care, after being approved by clinical trials.

References

1. Blasimme A, Boniolo G, Nathan MJ. Rethinking ageing: introduction. Hist Philos Life Sci. 2021 Aug 6;43(3):95.
2. Wahl D, Solon-Biet SM, Cogger VC, Fontana L, Simpson SJ, Le Couteur DG, et al. Aging, lifestyle and dementia. Neurobiol Dis. 2019 Oct;130:104481.
3. Murphy E, Froggatt K, Connolly S, O'Shea E, Sampson EL, Casey D, et al. Palliative care interventions in advanced dementia. Cochrane Database Syst Rev. 2016 Dec 2;12:CD011513.
4. Duong S, Patel T, Chang F. Dementia: What pharmacists need to know. Can Pharm J CPJ Rev Pharm Can RPC. 2017 Apr;150(2):118–29.
5. Sampson EL. Palliative care for people with dementia. Br Med Bull. 2010;96:159–74.

6. Arvanitakis Z, Shah RC, Bennett DA. Diagnosis and Management of Dementia: Review. JAMA. 2019 Oct 22;322(16):1589–99.
7. Lo AT, Karuza J, Berall A, Perri GA. Prevalence of Dementia in a Geriatric Palliative Care Unit. Am J Hosp Palliat Care. 2018 May;35(5):799–803.
8. Cao Q, Tan CC, Xu W, Hu H, Cao XP, Dong Q, et al. The Prevalence of Dementia: A Systematic Review and Meta-Analysis. J Alzheimers Dis JAD. 2020;73(3):1157–66.
9. Emmady PD, Tadi P. Dementia. In: StatPearls [Internet]. Treasure Island (FL): StatPearls Publishing; 2022 [cited 2022 Oct 9]. Available from: http://www.ncbi.nlm.nih.gov/books/NBK557444/
10. Kumar A, Sidhu J, Goyal A, Tsao JW. Alzheimer Disease. In: StatPearls [Internet]. Treasure Island (FL): StatPearls Publishing; 2022 [cited 2022 Oct 9]. Available from: http://www.ncbi.nlm.nih.gov/books/NBK499922/
11. Stewart JT, Schultz SK. Palliative Care for Dementia. Psychiatr Clin North Am. 2018 Mar;41(1):141–51.
12. Shuster JL. Palliative care for advanced dementia. Clin Geriatr Med. 2000 May;16(2):373–86.
13. Cheng ST, Chow PK, Song YQ, Yu ECS, Chan ACM, Lee TMC, et al. Mental and physical activities delay cognitive decline in older persons with dementia. Am J Geriatr Psychiatry Off J Am Assoc Geriatr Psychiatry. 2014 Jan;22(1):63–74.
14. Rebok GW, Ball K, Guey LT, Jones RN, Kim HY, King JW, et al. Ten-year effects of the advanced cognitive training for independent and vital elderly cognitive training trial on cognition and everyday functioning in older adults. J Am Geriatr Soc. 2014 Jan;62(1):16–24.
15. Moniruzzaman M, Kadota A, Akash MS, Pruitt PJ, Miura K, Albin R, et al. Effects of physical activities on dementia-related biomarkers: A systematic review of randomized controlled trials. Alzheimers Dement N Y N. 2020;6(1):e12109.
16. Duffner LA, Deckers K, Cadar D, Steptoe A, de Vugt M, Köhler S. The role of cognitive and social leisure activities in dementia risk: assessing longitudinal associations of modifiable and non-modifiable risk factors. Epidemiol Psychiatr Sci. 2022 Jan 11;31:e5.
17. Hemming L, Maher D. Complementary therapies in palliative care: a summary of current evidence. Br J Community Nurs. 2005 Oct;10(10):448–52.
18. Lewis CR, de Vedia A, Reuer B, Schwan R, Tourin C. Integrating complementary and alternative medicine (CAM) into standard hospice and palliative care. Am J Hosp Palliat Care. 2003 Jun;20(3):221–8.

19. Zeng YS, Wang C, Ward KE, Hume AL. Complementary and Alternative Medicine in Hospice and Palliative Care: A Systematic Review. J Pain Symptom Manage. 2018 Nov;56(5):781-794.e4.
20. Konstantinou A, Alexakis LC. Managing terminal restlessness, anxiety, and distress during the dying process with Yintang (EX-HN 3) point acupuncture or acupressure: a case series of 19 palliative care patients from a hospital in Germany. Pan Afr Med J. 2022;42:99.
21. Kreye G, Wasl M, Dietz A, Klaffel D, Groselji-Strele A, Eberhard K, et al. Aromatherapy in Palliative Care: A Single-Institute Retrospective Analysis Evaluating the Effect of Lemon Oil Pads against Nausea and Vomiting in Advanced Cancer Patients. Cancers. 2022 Apr 24;14(9):2131.
22. Kim SW. Phytotherapy: emerging therapeutic option in urologic disease. Transl Androl Urol. 2012 Sep;1(3):181–91.
23. Governa P, Baini G, Borgonetti V, Cettolin G, Giachetti D, Magnano AR, et al. Phytotherapy in the Management of Diabetes: A Review. Mol Basel Switz. 2018 Jan 4;23(1):E105.
24. Enioutina EY, Teng L, Fateeva TV, Brown JCS, Job KM, Bortnikova VV, et al. Phytotherapy as an alternative to conventional antimicrobials: combating microbial resistance. Expert Rev Clin Pharmacol. 2017 Nov;10(11):1203–14.
25. Kelber O, Bauer R, Kubelka W. Phytotherapy in Functional Gastrointestinal Disorders. Dig Dis Basel Switz. 2017;35 Suppl 1:36–42.
26. Zhang HW, Zhang H, Grant SJ, Wan X, Li G. Single herbal medicine for diabetic retinopathy. Cochrane Database Syst Rev. 2018 Dec 19;12:CD007939.
27. Dutta T, Anand U, Mitra SS, Ghorai M, Jha NK, Shaikh NK, et al. Phytotherapy for Attention Deficit Hyperactivity Disorder (ADHD): A Systematic Review and Meta-analysis. Front Pharmacol. 2022;13:827411.
28. Tyler VE. Herbal medicine: from the past to the future. Public Health Nutr. 2000 Dec;3(4A):447–52.
29. Leong M, Smith TJ, Rowland-Seymour A. Complementary and integrative medicine for older adults in palliative care. Clin Geriatr Med. 2015 May;31(2):177–91.
30. Kogan M, Cheng S, Rao S, DeMocker S, Koroma Nelson M. Integrative Medicine for Geriatric and Palliative Care. Med Clin North Am. 2017 Sep;101(5):1005–29.

31. Wells RE, Baute V, Wahbeh H. Complementary and Integrative Medicine for Neurologic Conditions. Med Clin North Am. 2017 Sep;101(5):881–93.
32. Wells RE, Phillips RS, Schachter SC, McCarthy EP. Complementary and alternative medicine use among US adults with common neurological conditions. J Neurol. 2010 Nov;257(11):1822–31.
33. Perry EK, Pickering AT, Wang WW, Houghton PJ, Perry NS. Medicinal plants and Alzheimer's disease: from ethnobotany to phytotherapy. J Pharm Pharmacol. 1999 May;51(5):527–34.
34. Wang BS, Wang H, Song YY, Qi H, Rong ZX, Wang BS, et al. Effectiveness of standardized ginkgo biloba extract on cognitive symptoms of dementia with a six-month treatment: a bivariate random effect meta-analysis. Pharmacopsychiatry. 2010 May;43(3):86–91.
35. Yuan Q, Wang CW, Shi J, Lin ZX. Effects of Ginkgo biloba on dementia: An overview of systematic reviews. J Ethnopharmacol. 2017 Jan 4;195:1–9.
36. Wightman EL. Potential benefits of phytochemicals against Alzheimer's disease. Proc Nutr Soc. 2017 May;76(2):106–12.
37. Nawrot J, Gornowicz-Porowska J, Budzianowski J, Nowak G, Schroeder G, Kurczewska J. Medicinal Herbs in the Relief of Neurological, Cardiovascular, and Respiratory Symptoms after COVID-19 Infection A Literature Review. Cells. 2022 Jun 11;11(12):1897.
38. Tang TY, Li FZ, Afseth J. Review of the regulations for clinical research in herbal medicines in USA. Chin J Integr Med. 2014 Dec;20(12):883–93.
39. Bilia AR, Costa M do C. Medicinal plants and their preparations in the European market: Why has the harmonization failed? The cases of St. John's wort, valerian, ginkgo, ginseng, and green tea. Phytomedicine Int J Phytother Phytopharm. 2021 Jan;81:153421.
40. Posadzki P, Watson LK, Ernst E. Adverse effects of herbal medicines: an overview of systematic reviews. Clin Med Lond Engl. 2013 Feb;13(1):7–12.
41. Dwivedi S, Chopra D. Adverse effects of herbal medicine. Clin Med Lond Engl. 2013 Aug;13(4):417–8.
42. Laccourreye O, Werner A, Laccourreye L, Bonfils P. Benefits, pitfalls and risks of phytotherapy in clinical practice in otorhinolaryngology. Eur Ann Otorhinolaryngol Head Neck Dis. 2017 Apr;134(2):95–9.
43. Pinn G. Adverse effects associated with herbal medicine. Aust Fam Physician. 2001 Nov;30(11):1070–5.
44. Koni AA, Nazzal MA, Suwan BA, Sobuh SS, Abuhazeem NT, Salman AN, et al. A comprehensive evaluation of potentially significant drug-

drug, drug-herb, and drug-food interactions among cancer patients receiving anticancer drugs. BMC Cancer. 2022 May 14;22(1):547.
45. Knight R, Khondoker M, Magill N, Stewart R, Landau S. A Systematic Review and Meta-Analysis of the Effectiveness of Acetylcholinesterase Inhibitors and Memantine in Treating the Cognitive Symptoms of Dementia. Dement Geriatr Cogn Disord. 2018;45(3–4):131–51.
46. Mohammad D, Chan P, Bradley J, Lanctôt K, Herrmann N. Acetylcholinesterase inhibitors for treating dementia symptoms - a safety evaluation. Expert Opin Drug Saf. 2017 Sep;16(9):1009–19.
47. Small DH. Acetylcholinesterase inhibitors for the treatment of dementia in Alzheimer's disease: do we need new inhibitors? Expert Opin Emerg Drugs. 2005 Nov;10(4):817–25.
48. Marucci G, Buccioni M, Ben DD, Lambertucci C, Volpini R, Amenta F. Efficacy of acetylcholinesterase inhibitors in Alzheimer's disease. Neuropharmacology. 2021 Jun 1;190:108352.
49. Battle CE, Abdul-Rahim AH, Shenkin SD, Hewitt J, Quinn TJ. Cholinesterase inhibitors for vascular dementia and other vascular cognitive impairments: a network meta-analysis. Cochrane Database Syst Rev. 2021 Feb 22;2:CD013306.
50. Moreta MPG, Burgos-Alonso N, Torrecilla M, Marco-Contelles J, Bruzos-Cidón C. Efficacy of Acetylcholinesterase Inhibitors on Cognitive Function in Alzheimer's Disease. Review of Reviews. Biomedicines. 2021 Nov 15;9(11):1689.
51. Wang R, Yan H, Tang X can. Progress in studies of huperzine A, a natural cholinesterase inhibitor from Chinese herbal medicine. Acta Pharmacol Sin. 2006 Jan;27(1):1–26.
52. Mao XY, Cao DF, Li X, Yin JY, Wang ZB, Zhang Y, et al. Huperzine A ameliorates cognitive deficits in streptozotocin-induced diabetic rats. Int J Mol Sci. 2014 May 5;15(5):7667–83.
53. Cai Y, Huang P, Xie Y. Effects of huperzine A on hippocampal inflammatory response and neurotrophic factors in aged rats after anesthesia. Acta Cir Bras. 2020;34(12):e201901205.
54. Ahmed F, Ghalib RM, Sasikala P, Ahmed KKM. Cholinesterase inhibitors from botanicals. Pharmacogn Rev. 2013 Jul;7(14):121–30.
55. Murray AP, Faraoni MB, Castro MJ, Alza NP, Cavallaro V. Natural AChE Inhibitors from Plants and their Contribution to Alzheimer's Disease Therapy. Curr Neuropharmacol. 2013 Jul;11(4):388–413.
56. Dos Santos TC, Gomes TM, Pinto BAS, Camara AL, Paes AM de A. Naturally Occurring Acetylcholinesterase Inhibitors and Their Potential Use for Alzheimer's Disease Therapy. Front Pharmacol. 2018;9:1192.

57. Ahmed S, Khan ST, Zargaham MK, Khan AU, Khan S, Hussain A, et al. Potential therapeutic natural products against Alzheimer's disease with Reference of Acetylcholinesterase. Biomed Pharmacother Biomedecine Pharmacother. 2021 Jul;139:111609.
58. Chen YX, Li GZ, Zhang B, Xia ZY, Zhang M. Molecular evaluation of herbal compounds as potent inhibitors of acetylcholinesterase for the treatment of Alzheimer's disease. Mol Med Rep. 2016 Jul;14(1):446–52.
59. Szwajgier D, Baranowska-Wójcik E, Winiarska-Mieczan A, Gajowniczek-Ałasa D. Honeys as Possible Sources of Cholinesterase Inhibitors. Nutrients. 2022 Jul 20;14(14):2969.
60. Sonkusare SK, Kaul CL, Ramarao P. Dementia of Alzheimer's disease and other neurodegenerative disorders--memantine, a new hope. Pharmacol Res. 2005 Jan;51(1):1–17.
61. Kodis EJ, Choi S, Swanson E, Ferreira G, Bloom GS. N-methyl-D-aspartate receptor-mediated calcium influx connects amyloid-β oligomers to ectopic neuronal cell cycle reentry in Alzheimer's disease. Alzheimers Dement J Alzheimers Assoc. 2018 Oct;14(10):1302–12.
62. Liang W, Lam WP, Tang HC, Leung PC, Yew DT. Current Evidence of Chinese Herbal Constituents with Effects on NMDA Receptor Blockade. Pharm Basel Switz. 2013 Aug 21;6(8):1039–54.
63. Matteucci A, Frank C, Domenici MR, Balduzzi M, Paradisi S, Carnovale-Scalzo G, et al. Curcumin treatment protects rat retinal neurons against excitotoxicity: effect on N-methyl-D: -aspartate-induced intracellular Ca(2+) increase. Exp Brain Res. 2005 Dec;167(4):641–8.
64. Mallozzi C, Parravano M, Gaddini L, Villa M, Pricci F, Malchiodi-Albedi F, et al. Curcumin Modulates the NMDA Receptor Subunit Composition Through a Mechanism Involving CaMKII and Ser/Thr Protein Phosphatases. Cell Mol Neurobiol. 2018 Aug;38(6):1315–20.
65. Lim GP, Chu T, Yang F, Beech W, Frautschy SA, Cole GM. The curry spice curcumin reduces oxidative damage and amyloid pathology in an Alzheimer transgenic mouse. J Neurosci Off J Soc Neurosci. 2001 Nov 1;21(21):8370–7.
66. Burckhardt M, Herke M, Wustmann T, Watzke S, Langer G, Fink A. Omega-3 fatty acids for the treatment of dementia. Cochrane Database Syst Rev. 2016 Apr 11;4:CD009002.
67. Farina N, Llewellyn D, Isaac MGEKN, Tabet N. Vitamin E for Alzheimer's dementia and mild cognitive impairment. Cochrane Database Syst Rev. 2017 Apr 18;4:CD002854.

4

BEHAVIORAL AND PSYCHOLOGICAL SYMPTOMS IN END-OF-LIFE DEMENTIA

DARLON JAN, MD[1] AND KYE KIM, MD[2]

Abstract

Care of the dementia patient continues to be challenging. Especially, end-of-life care in dementia presents unique challenges to both patients and their caregivers. In this stage, caregivers often feel overwhelmed and burdened by physical care and concurrent medical conditions. In addition, commonly accompanied behavioral and psychological symptoms complicate the patient's end-of-life care. Dementia is a progressive terminal illness with high variability, which often requires individualized approach to meet the needs for different individuals. Consequently, there are variations in the approach to care for these patients, though some general trends are available to guide care during this final stage of dementia. Overall, close communication between involved parties and education on the expectations and possible presentations will help alleviate the distress. As the disease is terminal, minimizing distress for individuals and caregivers is a priority and numerous advances in both pharmacology and non-pharmacology are ongoing. While several options are available, much remains to be done and improved upon for care in end-of-life dementia.

Keywords: Dementia, end-of-life care, behavioral and psychological symptoms, pharmacological interventions, non-pharmacological interventions

[1] Resident Physician, Department of Psychiatry and Behavioral Medicine, Virginia Tech Carilion School of Medicine, Roanoke, VA, USA

[2] Professor, Department of Psychiatry and Behavioral Medicine, Virginia Tech Carilion School of Medicine, Roanoke, VA, USA

Overview

Dementia, a progressive condition with deterioration in multiple domains in cognitive functions, is anticipated to rise in prevalence with the increase in the older population. In 2016 it was already the 3rd largest contributor of global neurological disability-adjusted life years behind stroke and migraines (Feigin and Vos 2019). Alzheimer's Disease (AD), the single most common cause of dementia was already the 6th leading cause of death in the United States in 2013 in addition to its other extensive costs to individuals, families, and societies (Kimchi and Lyketsos 2015). It is estimated that medical and caregiver costs from AD exceed $500 billion dollars in 2020 alone, projected to rise to $1.6 trillion dollars by 2050, of which 75% are expected to be paid through Medicare or Medicaid. Per capital cost for people with AD are expected to reach $92,060 by 2030 with compared to $24,783 for those without AD or dementia. In particular, the costs for the last year of life in people living with dementia among the highest with much of costs from out-of-pocket spending and informal caregiving. Additionally, some ethnic groups are noted to have higher prevalence and incidences of dementia, resulting in healthcare disparities and more adverse outcomes for both the patient and their caregivers (Aranda, et al. 2021) (Kelley, et al. 2020).

Dementia presents numerous care demands on caregivers. As a prolonged and progressive decline in function, many dementia patients are cared at home with family, especially early on. Studies note that even with transitions to care facilities or institutions caregivers experienced increased feelings of burden and depression (Eisenmann, et al. 2020) (Cheng 2017). Beyond physical limitations associated with decreased activities of daily living (ADLs) and instrumental activities of daily living (IADLs) challenges to relationships have been noted, especially with behavioral and psychological symptoms associated with dementia. These challenging symptoms include hallucinations, agitation, aggression, and many others that are highly distressing to caregivers. Dementia patients also have numerous medical comorbidities, which further contribute to further distress towards caregivers (Trinh, Lee and Kim 2019) (Cheng 2017).

There is a variety of end-of life (EoL) definitions regarding dementia. In some studies, EoL in dementia is defined through cuff off scores from validated tools. Others utilize descriptions or prognosis of less than 6 months survival, or a combination of the above. Often a general pattern shared is that severe dementia/severe cognitive impairment and complete dependency with ADLs are commonly used to define EoL dementia (Browne, et al. 2021). Overall severe dementia is noted for loss of functional abilities and several scales generally correlate with atrophy of the hippocampus and other pathological changes in brain structures. This tends to occur around 7-14 years into the disease. Some examples of characteristics associated with severe dementia include inability to dress or bath properly, progressively worsening speech function starting with limitations of speech to half-a dozen words (short phrases) to a single word, to ultimately the loss of the ability to smile or hold the head up. Eventually, speech utilization for communication is often limited to just "yes", "no", and other similar one-word phrases for communication. Severe dementia generally begins with a loss of ADLs with incontinence concerns and progress towards incipient nonverbal, incipient non-ambulatory, and eventually immobility (Reisberg, et al. 2006) (Gauthier 2006). Estimates suggest a quarter of dementia patients will progress to the advance stage. While the duration of EoL and advanced dementia varies greatly between individuals, this stage can last up to 2-3 years in some cases with numerous associated medication and environmental burdens to patients and caregivers (Eisenmann, et al. 2020) (Trinh, Lee and Kim 2019). In addition to rigidity, because of lack of mobility and contractures, studies suggest that in the terminal stage, nearly all patients will have some infantile reflex (sucking, grasp, rooting) present with up to 75% with the Babinski reflex in some studies (Reisberg, et al. 2006). Additionally, pain is a major symptom during EoL care with some studies noted it as the most common symptom. These changes, coupled with the numerous behavioral and neuropsychiatric symptoms create a great deal of distress for patients, their loved ones, and caregivers (Sampson, et al. 2018) (Hendriks, et al. 2014). While the decrease in communicative abilities pose a challenge to the management of pain, recognition of discomfort can be identified through nonverbal cues such as countenance changes (Trinh, Lee and Kim 2019) (Eisenmann, et al. 2020).

Pathophysiological Changes

Dementia is characterized by numerous pathophysiological changes affecting the neurochemical and structural environment within the brain. The scope of these changes and the research into them is beyond the scope of this chapter and thus only a brief synopsis will be discussed. New advances are constantly being discovered and identified, as are new treatments and developments. A progressive decline in cholinergic function is noted in most dementias and particularly noted between the transition from moderate to severe dementia. Some variations have been noted between different types of dementia, with studies having suggest increase loss of neocortical cholinergic neurons in Lewy body dementia compared to AD. Studies have noted similar losses between choline acetyltransferases and nicotinic acetylcholine receptors in similar brain areas in Lewy body dementia and AD. Muscarinic cholinergic receptors are also noted to be decreased, though past studies have been less clear on whether or not a correlation is present between dementia severity and muscarinic receptors as opposed to choline acetyltransferases and nicotinic receptors (Sharp, Fancis and Ballard 2006) (Hampel, et al. 2018). There is also evidence of decreased serotonergic changes in various types of dementia is several studies (Sharp, Fancis and Ballard 2006). Serotoninergic changes have been studied for their roles in the management of neuropsychiatric symptoms associated with dementia (Li, et al. 2021).

Behavioral and Psychological Symptoms of Dementia

As a result of the pathophysiological changes, behavioral and psychological symptoms of dementia (BPSD) are common features of severe dementia. These often include agitation, anxiety, depression and mood lability, apathy, delusions/hallucinations, sleep/appetite disturbances, irritability, and disinhibition. As BPSD affect both the patient and their caregivers, oftentimes the BPSD are just as or even more concerning/burdensome compared to cognitive changes to caregivers and patients (Byrne, Collins and Burns 2006) (Burhan, Hirsch and Marlatt 2018). Several scales, such as the Neuropsychiatric Inventory, the Cohen-Mansfield Agitation Inventory, the Behavioral Pathology in AD, the Neurobehavioral Rating Scale, and others can be used to screen for BPSD symptoms. Agitation, as an example, is divided into physical aggressive or nonaggressive and verbal aggressive or nonaggressive in the Cohen-Mansfield Agitation Inventory. Overall, many severe dementia patients have some BPSD, with some studies suggesting up to 87-90% of AD patients presenting with some form of BPSD. Some of the most common BPSD in AD include apathy, depression, aggression/agitation, though an association between different BPSD and the stage of dementia has been noted. Delusion and aggression tended to be higher towards terminal/EoL stages, though aggression/agitation is to be common throughout all stages. The etiology of these BPSD is often multifactorial from non-disease elements such as psychosocial factors to neurochemical and structural changes. These BPSD can be the result of unmet needs or decreased stress thresholds because of decrease executive skills/function and loss of functioning with ADLs and IADLs in severe dementia. Aggression is generally associated with the hypothalamus, prefrontal cortex, and limbic system. Additionally serotonergic receptor polymorphisms have been associated with aggression and some other BPSD in AD, with studies noting an association between acetylcholine, dopamine, and glutamine in some BPSD in AD. Consequently, biopsychosocial-spiritual model should be utilized in approaching BPSD in EoL dementia (Byrne, Collins and Burns 2006) (Burhan, Hirsch and Marlatt 2018).

As AD is generally the most common and most studied dementia, BPSD in AD tends to be the most studied. Studies in BPSD in vascular dementia suggest apathy, depression, and irritability are the most common behavioral symptoms. Interestingly nursing home settings noted appetite changes as a major BPSD in vascular dementia. Consistent with disease hallmarks, Parkinson's disease dementia and Lewy body dementia tended to have higher rates of delusions/hallucinations, agitation, and irritation compared to AD or vascular dementia. Similarly consistent with disease hallmarks, frontotemporal dementia tended to be noted with less mood symptoms and more disinhibition, apathy, and aberrant motor behaviors (Burhan, Hirsch and Marlatt 2018). Dementia related psychosis is noted to be particularly frustrating to caregivers and is highly variable with individual fluctuations (Aarsland 2020).

Depression is a common BPSD with dementia and is noted to generally become more pronounced with ongoing progression of dementia. Depressive symptoms such as sleep and appetite disturbance can overlap with other BPSD in severe dementia, making recognition of depression in EoL dementia difficult at times. More atypical features of depression such as apathy, withdrawal, or food refusal are symptoms to consider/monitor when assessing for depression with severe dementia (Bielinski and Lawlor 2006). It should be noted that while BPSD are a major concern with dementia and severe dementia, the terminal stage of severe dementia is marked by a decline in BPSD symptoms. BPSD tend to peak during the moderate and early stages of severe dementia. Delusions are particularly noteworthy as these delusions tend not to be fixed in severe dementia. As noted above, cognition remains present, though comparable to early childhood in severe dementia and a similar level of delusions/fantasies associated with early childhood can be analogized towards the delusions in severe dementia (Reisberg, et al. 2006).

Management of BPSD

Management of EoL dementia needs to address the cognitive and functional impairments as well as the behavioral symptoms and burdens on the patient and caregivers previously mentioned. Treatment of the BPSD is primarily achieved through either non-pharmacological or behavioral treatments, and pharmacological methods, with behavioral treatments often considered first line, though the efficacy of non-pharmacological treatments is often limited regarding. Additionally, management of EoL dementia often needs to be coordinated with the caregivers, who may not be professional staff, who may be more comfortable with pharmacological treatment options. Pharmacological options such as N-methyl-D-aspartate (NDMA) receptor antagonists and acetylcholinesterase inhibitors (AChEI) can still be utilized as with mild or moderate dementia, though the BPSD symptoms may require neuroleptics, antidepressants, anxiolytics, and antiepileptics (Porsteinsson and Tariot 2006) (Woodwad and Feldman 2006) (Deyn 2006) (Magierski, et al. 2020).

Memantine operates as moderate affinity, noncompetitive NMDA receptor antagonist. NMDA receptors are a class of ionotropic glutamate receptor, which can enhance the production of pathologic forms of tau and Aβ, further enhancing the neurotoxic effects of glutamate through neuronal calcium overload and other causes/sequela. While glutamate can enhance cognitive function and physiological stimulation of NDMA, which are believed to play a role in memory encoding and storage and are found in high concentrations in the neocortex and hippocampus, overstimulation of NMDA is thought to lead to neuronal injury. Memantine is not displaced as easily displaced as Mg^{2+} with prolonged moderate depolarization and thus does not result in the calcium influx. Additionally, memantine has been shown to have some efficacy with management of agitation/anti-psychotic effects, which may be due to its blocking of 5-HT_3 receptors (Porsteinsson and Tariot 2006) (Scuteri, et al. 2021).

Acetylcholinesterase inhibitors, such as donepezil, rivastigmine, and galantamine, increase acetylcholine concentration within the brain, with the rationale of addressing cholinergic deficits correlating with cognitive deficits found particularly in AD, though also in vascular dementia and Lewy body dementia (DLB). These agents have been shown to be effective in milder dementias with cognitive stability/cognition benefits, though the benefits in severe dementia are more debated. Studies in the past generally indicate some benefit in the previously aforementioned scales (Woodwad and Feldman 2006). These benefits can be temporary for a six-to-nine-month period, with some discussion on value of continuing these medications on a long-term basis. Discontinuation can result in rapid cognitive decline and some authors have recommended switching from one anticholinergic agent to another in cases of intolerance. Donepezil is a reversible cholinesterase inhibitor with high selectivity for neuronal AChE. Rivastigmine is a slowly reversible inhibitor to both neuronal AChE and butyryl-cholinesterase and may have some more specificity for the hippocampus, amygdala, and cerebral cortex. Galantamine is a competitive reversible cholinesterase inhibitor with some effects at nicotinic receptors. Though some differences are present between the agents, all three agents are approved for mild to moderate AD with donepezil and the patch formulation of rivastigmine approved for severe AD. It has been recommended to add memantine to the cholinesterase inhibitors in cases of severe AD. Additionally these agents have been shown to have benefit in severe dementia associated with DLB and Parkinson's disease dementia (PDD). Evidence of anticholinergic value in frontotemporal dementia is more lacking. At this time due to a lack of clear clinical data, tolerability, ease of use, cost, and experience are the main factors determining agent of choice (Kimchi and Lyketsos 2015) (Woodwad and Feldman 2006).

While improvement or maintenance of cognition function often is the primary concern with mild/moderate dementia, in EoL dementia, the focus often shifts to BPSD. Agitation, psychosis, and wandering are common reasons for caregiver burden and subsequent residential admissions. Unfortunately, randomized controlled trials on BPSD symptoms in dementia are generally sparse and few drugs are indicated for treatment of the neuropsychiatric symptoms, resulting in most treatments being off label, though clinically justified (Magierski, et al. 2020). Commonly studied medication class include typical and atypical antipsychotics, antidepressants, anticonvulsants/mood stabilizers, and benzodiazepines. Management of BPSD symptoms should always consider the potential of severe adverse effects. As an example, citalopram has been shown to be effective for agitation management, but also carries the risk of QTc prolongation, particularly in the geriatric population. Overall, a historical trend of anti-psychotic use for BPSD is present with several studies/reviews noting concern for overuse of antipsychotics. Use of antipsychotics is appropriate in some cases, especially if psychotic symptoms are present (Scuteri, et al. 2021) (Deyn 2006). However, use of antipsychotics is associated higher risks of cerebrovascular and cardiovascular effects, and thus may increase mortality compared to other psychotropic options such as antidepressants or anticonvulsants. The CATIE-AD trial noted that risperidone and olanzapine had the most benefit for agitation and psychosis, though no improvement in cognition and functioning were noted. Additionally, though atypical antipsychotics are noted for decrease risks of extrapyramidal side effects (EPS) compared to typical antipsychotic agents, DLB patients are highly susceptible to this side effects. Clozapine was noted to have less EPS risks for DLB patients. Similarly, clozapine and quetiapine were noted to have less risks with exacerbating Parkinsonian symptoms with PDD. Ultimately, use of antipsychotics in EoL dementia will depend on a risk versus benefit analysis, especially as BPSD with severe dementia patients are often associated with distress and possible danger to the patient. Additionally, studies have suggested that pain and symptom management medications may be underutilized during EoL situations (Hendriks, et al. 2014) (Jansen, et al. 2017). Currently drug algorithms and meta-analyses have identified risperidone, aripiprazole, or quetiapine as overall early options with acceptable safety for management of BPSD, particularly for agitation/aggression and psychosis (Kimchi and Lyketsos 2015) (Magierski, et al. 2020) (Scuteri, et al. 2021) (Deyn 2006) (Tampi and Jeste 2022).

Treatment of BPSD symptoms of depression and apathy are more challenging. While selective serotonin receptor inhibitors (SSRIs) and serotonin and norepinephrine reuptake inhibitors (SNRIs) are the primary recommendations for depression in dementia, some meta-analysis note little evidence of efficacy in their use for depression with dementia. While the evidence of the benefit of SSRIs and antidepressants in the management of agitation and depression is not pronounced and antidepressants can be associated with known side effects, some studies suggest a similar level of benefit as with commonly use antipsychotics with less of a mortality risk in some cases. Overall treatment of depression in dementia has primarily been focused on AD and recommendations are to utilize the same treatment approaches as depression associated with AD with depression associated with other dementias. (Kimchi and Lyketsos 2015) (Magierski, et al. 2020). Some studies have suggested a risk of apathy with anti-depressant use and apathy treatment in AD has generally demonstrated mixed results or no efficacy with cholinesterase inhibitors, NMDA antagonists, antidepressants, antipsychotics, psychostimulants, or other drugs. Some benefit was noted with Agomelatine in FTD and studies in the 1970s with methylphenidate, follow up later in the 2010s, suggested some slight benefit with apathy, though risks of adverse effects from weight loss and anxiety counterbalance some of the benefits for apathy treatment (Scuteri, et al. 2021) (Li, et al. 2021).

Several new pharmacological options are being studied to help with alleviating the distress from the BPSD. Recently studies have looked at brexpiprazole, dextromethorphan, lumateperone, ketamine, and many other medications (Magierski, et al. 2020) (Scuteri, et al. 2021). Recent studies into the possible benefits of cannabis on management of BPSD symptoms have noted promise in moderate and severe cases especially for agitation. Some case reports identified some possible benefit for cannabinoids for sleep disturbances and abnormal sexual behavior, though there is limited evidence. Dronabinol and nabilone have the most evidence, both of which have generally mild side effects (Stella, et al. 2021). Pharmacological interventions are summarized in Table 1.

Table 1 Pharmacological Interventions

Medication	Class	Recommended Dosages in Geriatric Patients
Donepezil	Acetylcholinesterase inhibitors	5-10 mg Daily
Rivastigmine	Acetylcholinesterase inhibitors	3-12 mg Daily
Galantamine	Acetylcholinesterase inhibitors	8-24 mg Daily
Memantine	Non-competitive NMDA receptor antagonist	5-20 mg Daily
Risperidone	Atypical antipsychotics	0.25-2 mg Daily
Olanzapine	Atypical antipsychotics	2.5-10 mg Daily
Quetiapine	Atypical antipsychotics	12.5-300 mg Daily
Aripiprazole	Atypical antipsychotics	5-15 mg Daily
Brexpiprazole	Atypical antipsychotics	0.5-2 mg Daily
Pimavanserin	Atypical antipsychotics	34 mg DAily
Lumateperone	Atypical antipsychotics	Not studied in geriatric population, adult dosage is 42 mg Daily
Sertraline	Selective serotonin reuptake inhibitor	25-100 mg Daily
Citalopram	Selective serotonin reuptake inhibitor	10-20 mg Daily

Escitalopram	Selective serotonin reuptake inhibitor	5-10 mg Daily
Mirtazapine	Selective serotonin reuptake inhibitor	15-30 mg Daily
Fluvoxamine	Selective serotonin reuptake inhibitor	25-200 mg Daily
Vilazodone	Selective serotonin reuptake inhibitor/5-HT_{1A} receptor partial agonist	10-40 mg Daily
Venlafaxine	Serotonin and Norepinephrine reuptake inhibitor	75-225 mg Daily
Desvenlafaxine	Serotonin and Norepinephrine reuptake inhibitor	50 mg Daily
Duloxetine	Serotonin and Norepinephrine reuptake inhibitor	30-120 mg Daily
Bupropion Sustained Release	Dopamine/Norepinephrine-Reuptake Inhibitor	150-300 mg total Daily dose
Nortriptyline	Tricyclic antidepressant	10-100 mg Daily
Desipraimine	Tricyclic antidepressant	10-150 mg Daily

Non-pharmacological interventions for BPSD fall into general categories of sensory stimulation, cognitive and emotional approaches, behavioral management, caregiver/patient education, animal assisted, and multicomponent (Magierski, et al. 2020). Overall, there are less adverse effects associated with non-pharmacological options and they have been shown to be beneficial in numerous studies and meta-analyses. A key aspect of non-pharmacological interventions depends on the identification of stressors and needs for the patient. With progressive impairment of cognitive functions, communication often becomes a challenge and these unmet needs, be it insecurity, anxiety, pain, or others, can manifest as the BPSD. The "DICE" approach is a mnemonic for Describe, Investigate, Create, and Evaluate; and has been shown to be effective for management of BPSD. The first step is to accurately characterize the issue in detail and then to identify sources/causes. This involves a holistic consideration of the patient, caregiver, environment, etc. Afterwards a treatment plan addressing the causes is created and evaluated (Kimchi and Lyketsos 2015) (Kales, Gitlin and Lyketsos 2014) (Tampi and Jeste 2022).

Some examples of sensory stimulation include aromatherapy, Snoezelen, music, or bright light therapy. These are generally nonverbal interventions aimed at adjusting the environment to reduce stressors and cognitive demands. For example, bright light therapy helps with circadian rhythm and sundowning (Khachiyants, et al. 2011). Aromatherapy stimulates smell to relax and reduce agitation an aggression, whereas music utilizes sounds for a similar effect. Snoezelen therapy utilizes a multi-sensory approach through sight, smell, sound, and touch. Additionally, adjustments of the environment, through reduction of potentially disruptive or agitating events such as loud sounds, routine changes, complex directions, and other cognitively taxing and potentially distressing events help to limit the BPSD (Overshott and Burns 2006) (Khachiyants, et al. 2011) (Magierski, et al. 2020).

Behaviorally focused educational programs can help caregivers understand the causes of distress and thus aid in communication with the patient and in limiting the distressing factors that eventually manifest as BPSD. These tend to be more direct interventions as they aim to change the lifestyle or interactions with the patient directly to help address their needs. Therapies such as validation therapy, validation of feelings distressing the patient, or activities such as animal or humor therapy have also been found to decrease distress and reduce the need for agitation management medications. Overall avoiding a lack of activity has also been noted to contribute to decreased agitation and interventions should be approached in a multifaceted manner given the wide ranges of causes that could be associated with distress within this population (Overshott and Burns 2006) (Kimchi and Lyketsos 2015) (Khachiyants, et al. 2011) (Eisenmann, et al. 2020) (Magierski, et al. 2020). Table 2 provides an overview of nonpharmacological interventions described in the chapter.

Table 2 Nonpharmacological Interventions

Nonverbal Interventions	Sensory Stimulations: • Snoezelen Therapy • Music Therapy • Bright Light Therapy • Aromatherapy • Exercise Therapy • Touch Therapy • Environmental adjustments – horticulture, etc. Behavioral Management • Routine activities and schedules • Behavioral reinforcement strategies

Verbal Interventions	Behavioral and Education Programs • Care Giver Education • Cognitive Behavioral Therapies • Behavioral reinforcement strategies • Communication training • Habit training Cognitive and Emotional Approaches • Reminisce Therapy • Validation Therapy • Simulated Presence Therapy • Cognitive Stimulation (word games, puzzles, discussions, etc.)

Caregiver Education

A major challenge with the progression of dementia is that as the disease progresses, the patient is progressively becomes less able to participate in decision making for his/her care. Consequently, caregivers are placed in a role of assuming much of the decision making and responsibilities for decisions as the severity of the disease progresses. A major aspect is EoL care and EoL decision making (Zarit and Gaugler 2006) (Eisenmann, et al. 2020). Increasing EoL care is taking place within specific institutions such as nursing homes or hospitals as opposed to home and some studies have suggested that 20% of American will die within a nursing home or hospital (Trinh, Lee and Kim 2019). Notwithstanding challenges to long term care facilities due to resource availability as the population ages, studies suggest that the decision of placement places undue burden and stress of caregivers (Zarit and Gaugler 2006) (Eisenmann, et al. 2020).

The establishment of advanced care planning is noted to help with good quality EoL care and helps to limit stressors on both caregivers and help with caregivers adhering to the wishes of the patient. Advance directives, living wills, and power of attorney can help future caregivers with answering the existential decisions necessary as the terminal stage approaches. Having these discussions while the patient still has capacity also helps identify the values and perceptions of the patient and helps prepare caregivers and patients for future expectations and possibilities, such as feeding tubes or resuscitation (Zarit and Gaugler 2006) (Eisenmann, et al. 2020). Studies have shown that about a fifth of caregivers feel adequately aware and educated about EoL situations and expectations (Eisenmann, et al. 2020). In situations without prior preparations, providers should help caregiver identify possible future concerns, such as artificial feeding, possibilities of numerous hospitalizations from infections and other medical conditions, etc. Education to caregivers on the BPSD will also help preserve/help with sense of declining relationships and help with management of the BPSD symptoms and stressors (Trinh, Lee and Kim 2019) (Feast, et al. 2016). Studies into programs in caregiver education have noted overall benefit reported by caregivers (Evertson, et al. 2021) (Possin, et al. 2019).

One of the challenges noted with advanced care planning and palliative care planning for dementia is the lack of recognition that the disease is terminal. Additionally, understanding of the limited EoL care options is not often well communicated to caregivers (Eisenmann, et al. 2020) (Zarit and Gaugler 2006). Some studies evaluating the knowledge of caregivers and family members note discrepancies in recognizing different support needs for racial/ethnic minorities and sexual differences. Cultural sensitivities were also identified as an area of improvement. The heterogeneity of different programs has made comparisons between education programs more limited and while utilization of validated instruments to measure knowledge would benefit, this was not noted to be present in some studies (Resciniti, et al. 2020) (Eisenmann, et al. 2020). Though several educational options are available, it should be emphasized that there is no consensus on palliative care in dementia, and thus educations on the expectations and involvement of the family and caregivers is vital to the provision of care (Trinh, Lee and Kim 2019) (Zarit and Gaugler 2006) (Eisenmann, et al. 2020).

Summary

EoL care in dementia presents several challenges to both individuals and their caregivers and is increasingly important as dementia becomes more prevalent with our aging population both for care and resource management. Multiple barriers and challenges are present, with loved ones often overwhelmed and burden by both physical and medical responsibilities associated as well as emotional distress from both the progressive nature of the illness and the numerous BPSD associated with it. Dementia is a progressive terminal illness and is highly variable and individualized in the needs for different individuals. Consequently, there are variations in the approach to care for these patients, though some general trends are available to guide care during this final stage of dementia. While a great deal of research and developments have occurred in the study and management of dementia overall, the complexity and variability associated with it continues to challenge the provision of available care as well as the best approaches to care. Overall, close communication between involved parties and education on the expectations and possible presentations will help alleviate the distress. As the disease is terminal, limiting distress for individuals and caregivers is a priority and numerous advances in both pharmacology and non-pharmacology are ongoing. While several options are available, much remains to be done/improved upon for care in severe dementia.

References

Aarsland, Dag. 2020. "Epidemiology and Pathophysiology of Dementia related Psychosis." *Jounral of Clinical Psychiatry* 81.

Aranda, Maria P, Ian N Kremer, Ladson Hinton, Julie Zissimopoulos, Rachel A Whitmer, Cynthia Huling Hummel, Laura Trejo, and Canee Fabius. 2021. "Impact of Dementia: Health Disparities, Population Trends, Care Interventions, and Economic Costs." *Journal of American Geriatric Society* 1774-1783.

Association, American Psychiatric. 2022. "Neurocognitive Disorders." In *Diagnostic and Statistical Manual of mental Disorders (5th Ed.., text rev.)*, by American Psychiatric Association. American Psychiatric Association.

Bielinski, Kate, and Brian Lawlor. 2006. "Depression in Severe Dementia." In *Severe Dementia*, by Alistair Burns and Bengt Winblad, 63-74. Chicester: John Wiley & Sons, Ltd.

Browne, Bria, Nuriye Kupeli, Kristen J Moore, Elizabeth L Sampson, and Nathan Davies. 2021. "Defining end of life in dementia: A systemic Review." *Palliative Medicine* 1733-1746.

Burhan, Amer M, Calvin H Hirsch, and Nicole E Marlatt. 2018. "Neuropsychiatric Symptoms of Major or Mild Neurocognitive Disorders." In *Geriatric Psychiatry A Case-Based Textbook*, by Ana Hategan, James A. Bourgeois, Calvin H. Hirsch and Caroline Giroux, 467-494. Cham: Springer International Publishing Group.

Byrne, E Jane, Deborah Collins, and Alistair Burns. 2006. "Behavioral and Psychological Symptoms of Dementia-Agitation." In *Severe Dementia*, by Alistair Burns and Bengt Winblad, 51-61. Chicester: John Wiley & Sons, Ltd.

Cheng, Sheung-Tak. 2017. "Dementia Caregiver Burden: A research Update and critical analysis." *Current Psychiatry Reports.*

Compta, Yarosalu, and Tamas Revesz. 2021. "Neuropathological and Biomarker Findings in Parkinson's Disease and Alzheimer's Disease:

From Protein Aggregates to Synatptic Dysfunction." *Journal of Parkinson's Disease* 107-121.

Cope, Thomas E, Jeremy D Isaacs, and Michael D Kopelman. 2020. "Memory Disorders and Dementias." In *Oxford Textbook of Neuropsychiatry*, by Niruj Agrawal, Rafey Faruqui and Mayur Bodani, 277-308. Oxford: Oxford University Press.

Deyn, Peter Paul De. 2006. "Drug Treatment: Treatment of Behavioral and Psychological Symptoms of Dementia with Neuroleptics." In *Severe Dementia*, by Alistair Burns and Bengt Winblad, 151-162. Chicester: John Wiley & Sons, Ltd.

Eisenmann, Yvonne, Heidrun Golla, Holger Schmidt', Raymond Voltz, and Kalus Maria Perrar. 2020. "Palliative Care in Advanced Dementia." *FRotiers in Psychiatry.*

Evertson, Leslie Chang, Lee A Jennings, David B Reugen, Kassandra E Zaila, Nadia Akram, Tahmineh Romero, and Zaldy S TAn. 2021. "Caregiver outcomes of a dementia care program." *Geriatric Nusring* 447-459.

Farrer, L A, L A Cupples, J L Haines, B Hyman, W A Kukull, R Mayeux, M A Pericak-VAnce, N Risch, and C M van Duijn. 1997. "Effects of age, sex, and ethincity on the association between apolipoprotein E genotype and Alzheimer disease. A meta-analysis. APOE and Alzheimer Disease MEta Analysis Consortium." *JAMA* 1349-56.

Feast, Alexandra, Martin Orrell, Georginia Charlesworth, Nina Melunsky, Fiaona Poland, and Esme Moniz-Cook. 2016. "Behavioral and Psychological symptoms in dementia and the challenges for family carers: systematic review." *The British Journal of Psychiatry: the Journal of mental science* 429-434.

Feigin, Valery L, and Theo Vos. 2019. "Global, regional, and national burden of neurological disorders, 1990-2016: a systematic analysis for global burden of disease study 2016. ." *Lancet Neurology* 459-480.

Gauthier, Serge. 2006. "Clinical Features of Severe Dementia: Function." In *Severe Dementia*, by Alistair Burns and Bengt Winblad, 117-121. Chicester: John Wiley & Sons, Ltd.

Hampel, Harald, M-Marsel Mesulam, A Claudio Cuello, MArtin R Farlow, Ezio Ciacobini, George T Grossberg, ara S Khachaturian, et al. 2018. "The Cholingerig System in the Pathophysiology and treatment of Alzheimer's disease." *Grain* 1917-1933.

Hendriks, Simone A, Martin Smallbrugge, Cees M P M Hertogh, and Jenny T van der Steen. 2014. "Dying with dementia: Symptoms, treatments, and quality of life in the last week of life." *Journal of Pain and symptom Management* 710-720.

Jansen, Bannin De Witt, Kevin Brazil, Peter Passmore, Hilary Buchanan, Dorren Maxwell, Sonja J Mcllfactrick, Sharon M Morgan, Max Watson, and Carole Parsons. 2017. "Nurses' experiences of pain management for people with advanced dementia approaching the end of life: a qualitative study." *Journal of clinical nursing* 1234-1244.

Kales, Helan C, Laura N Gitlin, and Constantine G. Lyketsos. 2014. "Managemetn of Neuropsychiatric Symptoms of Dementia in Clinical Settings: Recommnedations from a Multipdisciplinary Expert Panel." *Journal of American Geriatric Society* 762-769.

Kelley, Amy S, Kathleen McGarry, Evan Bollens-Lund, Omari-Khalid Rahman, Mohammed Husain, Katelyn B Ferreira, and Jonathan S Skinner. 2020. "Residential Setting and the Cumulative Financial Burden of Dementia in the 7 Years before Death." *Journal of American Geriatric Society* 1319-1324.

Khachiyants, Nina, David Trinkle, Sang Joon Son, and Kye Y. Kim. 2011. "Sundown Syndrome in Persons with Dementia: An Update." *Psychiatry Investigations* 275-287.

Kimchi, Eitan Z., and Constantine C Lyketsos. 2015. "Dementia and Mild Neurocognitive Disorders." In *Textbook of Geriatric Psychiatry*, by David C. Steffens, Dan G. Blazer and Mugdha E Thakur, 177-242. Washington DC: American Psychiatric Publishing.

Li, Hui-Hua, Ziao-Yan Yao, Sheng Tao, Xue Sun, Pan-Pan Li, Xi-Xin Li, Zhu-Li Liu, and Chao Ren. 2021. "Serotonin 2 Receptors, Agomelatine, and Behavioral and Psychological Symptoms of Dementia in Alzheimer's Disease." *Behavorial Neurology.*

Magierski, Radoslaw, Tomasz Sobow, Emilia Schwertner, and Dorota Religa. 2020. "Pharmacotherapy of Behavioral and Psychological Symptoms of Dementia: State of the Art and Future Progress." *Frontiers in Pharmacology* 1-15.

Overshott, Ross, and Alistair Burns. 2006. "Non-pharmacological Treatemtn of Severe Dementia: An Overview." In *Severe Dementia*, by Alistair Burns and B Winblad, 163-175. Chicester: John Wiley & Sons, LTD.

Porsteinsson, Anton P, and Pierre N Tariot. 2006. "Drug Treatment: Memantine." In *Severe Dementia*, by Alistair Burns and Bengt Winblad, 125-130. Chicester: John Wiley & Sons, Ltd.

Possin, Katherine L, Jennifer J Marrilees, Sarah Dulaney, Stephen J Bonasera, Winston Chiong, Kirby Lee, Sarah M Hooper, et al. 2019. "Effect of Collaborative Dementia Care via Telephone and Internet on Quality of Life, Caregiver Well being, and health care use: The Care

Ecosystem Randomized Clinical Trial." *JAMA Internal Medicine* 1658-1667.

Reisberg, Barry, Jerzy Wegiel, Emile FRanssen, Sridhar Kadiyala, Stefanie Auer, Liduin Souren, Marwan Sabbagh, and James Golomb. 2006. "Clinical Features of Severe Dementia: Staging." In *Severe Dementia*, by Alistair Burns and Bengt Winblad, 83-115. Chicester: John Wiley & Sons, Ltd.

Resciniti, Nicholas V, Weizhou Tang, Masroora Tabassum, Joseph Lee Pearson, Sharon Melinda Spencer, Matthew C Lohman, Diane K Ehlers, et al. 2020. "Knowledge evaluation instrucments for dementia caregiver education programs: A scoping review." *Geriatrics and gerontology international* 397-413.

Sampson, Elizabeth L, Bridget Candy, Sarah Davis, Anna Buylova Gola, Jane Harrington, Michael King, Nuriye Kupeli, et al. 2018. "Living and dying with advanced dementia: A prospective cohort study of symptoms, service use and care at the end of life." *Palliative Medicine* 668-681.

Scuteri, Damiana, Maria Tiziana Corasaniti, Paolo Tonin, Pierluigi Nicotera, and Giacinto Bagetta. 2021. "New Trends in Pharmacological control of neuropsychiatric symptoms of dementia." *Current Opinion in Pharmacology* 69-76.

Sharp, Sally I, Paul T. Fancis, and Clive G. Ballard. 2006. "Cholinergic and Serotonergic Systems in Severe Dementia." In *Severe Dementia*, by Alister Burns and Bengt Winblad, 21-31. Chicester: John Wiley & Sons, Ltd.

Stella, Florindo, Leandro C Lane Valiengo, Vanessa J R de Paula, Carlos Augusto de Mendonca Lima, and Orestes V Forlenza. 2021. "Medical Cannabinoids for treatment of neuropsychiatric symptoms in dementia: a systemic review." *Trends in Psychiatry and Psychotherapy* 243-255.

Tampi, Rajesh R, and Dilip V Jeste. 2022. "Dementia is more than memory loss: Neuropsychiatric symptoms of dementia and their nonpharmacological and pharmacological management." *The American Journal of Psychiatry* 528-543.

Tiwari, Sneham, Venkata Atluri, Ajeet Kaushik, Adriana Yndart, and Madhavan Nair. 2019. "Alzheimer's disease: pathogenesis, diagnostics, and thearpeutics." *International Journal of Nanomedicine* 5541-5554.

Trinh, Eric, Andrew Lee, and Kye Y. Kim. 2019. "End-of-Life Care of Persons with Alzheimer Disease: An Update for Clinicians." *Alzheimer's/Dementia and Neuromuscular Disorders.*

Uddin, Md Sahab, Md Tanvir Kabir, Maroua Jalouli, Md Ataur Rahman, Philippe Jeandet, Tapan Behl, Athanasios Alexiou, et al. 2022.

"Neuroinflammatory signaling in the pathogenesis of Alzheimer's Disease." *Current neurophramacology* 126-146.
Woodwad, Michael, and Howard H Feldman. 2006. "Drug Treatment: Cholinesterase Inhibitors." In *Severe Dementia*, by Alistair Burns and Bengt Winblad, 131-150. Chicester: John Wiley & Sons, Ltd.
Zarit, Steven H., and Joseph E Gaugler. 2006. "Care by Families for Late Stage Dementia." In *Severe Dementia*, by A Burns and B Winblad, 185-191. Chicester: John Wiley & Sons, Ltd.

5

WHEN NIGHT FALLS: SUNDOWNING IN PATIENTS WITH DEMENTIA, AN UPDATED REVIEW

IVY AKID MD/MPH[1]

Abstract

This updated review on the topic of sundowning in patients with dementia aims to provide a comprehensive review on the definition for sundowning and management for palliation. The term sundowning refers to a combination of neuropsychiatric symptoms which tend to occur in elderly patients later in the evening around when the sun is normally setting. Common symptoms include confusion, aggression, anxiety, agitation, mood swings and even visual or auditory hallucinations. No exact etiology of sundowning has been elucidated. The biggest differentiator between delirium and sundowning is the timing of when the symptoms occur. The best treatments for sundowning are non-pharmacologic and include re-orientation, avoiding naps in the day, keeping the room dark at night and addressing behavioral modifications such as treating pain and constipation, redirecting the patient and preventing confusion. If agitation becomes severe, atypical antipsychotics are recommended. Additionally, a case example is provided and cultural differences are discussed.

Keywords: sundowning, dementia, sleep disturbance, agitation, palliation, re-orientation, melatonin

---

[1] Johns Hopkins Hospital, Johns Hopkins School of Medicine, Assistant Professor of Medicine, Assistant Program Director, HPM Fellowship

Sundowning, also known as sundown syndrome, is a combination of neuropsychiatric symptoms occurring in elderly patients in the evening around the time of sunset[1]. Sundowning appears to be common for individuals with dementia, with prevalence rates reported as high as 66%, and is often a reason for institutionalization[2]. Sundowning is not a formal psychiatric diagnosis which is found in Diagnostic and Statistical Manual of Mental Disorders fifth edition[3]; however, it is a well known grouping of symptoms[4]. Well known sundowning symptoms include confusion, anxiety, aggression, agitation, disorientation, wandering, pacing, resistance to redirection, yelling, screaming, mood swings, suspiciousness, an abnormally demanding attitude, and even visual or auditory hallucinations. What distinguishes sundowning symptoms from the disruptive symptoms of other disorders such as Alzheimer's dementia, delirium, sleep disturbances or Parkinson's disease is the time of day during which these disruptive symptoms occur[1].

Etiology of Sundowning

No exact etiology for sundowning has been determined. Researchers have attempted to explain the etiology of sundowning in three major groups of studies: psychological, physiological, and environmental[5]. One thought on the etiology of sundowning is that it is created by inadequate exposure to light during the day, and this is the basis behind light therapy for patients with dementia[1]. Duckett[5] (1993) suggested that the elderly with dementia frequently have visual problems such as macular degeneration. They were thus more sensitive to the varying amount of light in hospitals, and these subtle differences would not be apparent to healthy eyes. This was the reasoning behind modifying ambient light in hospitals in order to match "light readings obtained from the day and evening hours"[5]. In their hypotheses for the pathogenesis of sundowning, some researchers believe it to be a cyclical disturbance of circadian rhythm in patients with cognitive impairment. Many researchers have looked into sundowning as a common non-specific symptom seen with many different types of dementia, and it was thought that in this way, sundowning represented physiological manifestations of interference with the normal circadian rhythm[1]. In another study, researchers postulated that Alzheimer's dementia leads to deterioration of the suprachiasmatic nucleus in the hypothalamus, which is critical in regulating the sleep wake cycles by releasing alert signals during the day and sleep-inducing signals at night[1]. The suprachiasmatic nucleus acts as a conductor of circadian rhythm and critically affects multiple physiological functions in the body, including heart rate, core body temperature and hormonal secretions[6]. One possible mechanism in how the suprachiasmatic nucleus is damaged with age is through the formation of senile plaque, which may explain how patients develop the signs of sundowning during disturbed sleep, confusion and agitation[1]. Another key player of regulating circadian rhythm is melatonin, which is synthesized by the pineal gland during times of darkness or sleep[7]. Researchers have found in postmortem studies that deceased patients with Alzheimer's disease had decreased levels of melatonin in their cerebrospinal fluid[8]. Decreased melatonin levels lead to a dysregulation of the circadian rhythm and were found to decrease the neuroprotective effect of the suprachiasmatic nucleus[9]. This neuroprotective effect of melatonin is the basis behind the use of melatonin in patients with Alzheimer's disease[7].

Studies have shown that nearly 50% of patients with dementia have notable sleep- wake disturbances. Research has shown that disturbances in the quality and total duration of sleep increases as people age[1]. Around 29% of patients over 65 have problems maintaining sleep while around 36% have problems with sleep initiation[10]. While recent evidence indicates a relationship between sleep disturbances and the development of behavioral disruptions in demented patients in the late afternoon and early evening, the exact nature of the relationship as well as any causality has not been proven. Similarly, while evidence shows an increased incidence of assorted sleep disruptions in patients with dementia, the exact nature of the relationship between these sleep problems and sundowning has not been directly studied. Some other studies have suggested that sleep fragmentation is a key component causing sundowning in patients. Another study found that in demented nursing home patients, any awakenings after the time of sunset triggered agitated behavior more frequently, regardless of whether the awakenings were spontaneous or caused by nursing care[11].

There also exist changes in sleep with dementia including more frequent sleep disruption and arousals during the night, decreased total sleep time, lower sleep efficiency, decreased time in stages 3 and 4 (slow wave sleep) and more time spent in stage 1 of sleep[12]. While these are expected changes that occur with age they are more pronounced in older patients with dementia. Additionally, dementia patients may exhibit more daytime sleepiness and nighttime wakefulness[12]. There is a link between the physiological changes to sleep with cognitive changes appearing with sundowning. However, due to a dearth of evidence the mechanism is unknown. It is arguably difficult to enroll patients with delirium in studies, as they cannot self-enroll. Often, a caregiver who may be experiencing burnout must advocate for this research.

Clinical Presentation

Sundowning presents in patients developing neuropsychiatric symptoms in the late afternoon, evening, or night which resolve by the morning, and redevelop again the following evening. Unfortunately, even though clinical observations of sundowning are numerous, no consensus definition has been provided, and disagreement occurs regarding many aspects of the syndrome. Clinically, it presents as delirium and may even mimic delirium or depression. Delirium is described as confusion, agitation, or altered mentation which may be acute, reversible and due to one or multiple stimuli. Delirium similarly presents a fluctuating course with periods of altered mentation and lucidity[1].

The diagnosis of sundowning is clinical and based on signs and symptoms and often a diagnosis of exclusion. Additionally, common medical problems such as sleep disorders, pain, paresthesia, cough, dyspnea, and gastroesophageal reflux disease can exacerbate sundowning. Furthermore, medications such as diuretics, cholinesterase inhibitors, antidepressants, anti parkinson's, and antihypertensives and substances such as alcohol may impair sleep and in turn affect sundowning patterns[1].

How to Differentiate Sundowning from Delirium

There are subtle differences between delirium and sundowning. The biggest difference will be that delirium has an acute onset that fluctuates throughout the day and may last from hours to days; on the other hand, sundowning will have a consistent pattern of symptoms which begin and peak in the late afternoon, evening, or night which resolve in the morning but then recur in the evenings[1]. Delirium is defined as a fluctuating course, generally with an inciting, reversible cause. Hence, an astute clinician will ascertain a good history from the caregiver and conduct a thorough physical exam. If there is a chance to reverse an acute process, workup and interventions are warranted. This also depends on the goals of the person and their surrogate decision makers. Doctors should factor the prognosis of the patient, quality of life, and risks vs. benefits when considering aggressive interventions or further workup.

Additionally, diagnoses are not mutually exclusive, and patients who are sundowning may also be delirious. In fact, some researchers believe that dementia may be a necessary, but not a sufficient condition for sundowning. Thus, not every demented patient will sundown, but almost every patient who sundowns has dementia, and many of these patients have episodes of delirium when they are sundowning[13].

Different Cultural Beliefs Affecting Treatment Plan

Across different cultures, people do and do not talk about disease, particularly ones that concern mental health. Lack of communication often leads patients' and their families to suffer in silence and feel neglected. Additionally, in such cultures it is the norm to institutionalize persons with dementia. Other cultures have been known to normalize signs of dementia as "just normal aging" in an attempt to maintain normalcy when patients begin having cognitive impairments and disruptive behaviors and sundowning patterns. When patients in these cultures have been institutionalized they are often thought to be possessed by a spirit as a means to explain away their actions.

Brazil provides a good example of how culture interacts with dementia. "In Brazil, people with dementia frequently value family caregivers' wishes as their own…. To express wishes while depending on others is not compatible with their sense of dignity.[14] Meanwhile in Western countries, "The autonomy centered model reflects the values of people; however, choices and wishes are usually affected by relationships[15]."

Case Example

Ms. Y is an 87-year-old female who was brought to her provider at an outpatient clinic by her daughter, L. L shares that Ms. Y has been sleeping most of the day and awake at night. L appears exhausted as her mother is agitated at night, calling her names, which is atypical behavior. Additionally, Ms. Y has had increased accidents at night, often unable to make it to the restroom. She drops things and is perceived as more "clumsy." For this reason, daughter L bought her mother a dog, hoping it would lift her spirits.

Ms. Y is of Jewish descent, and she emigrated later in life from Russia. She fondly speaks of her Jewish heritage and keepsakes. She recalls childhood memories, particularly during the revolution and the Cold War. Often during the evenings, she loses her English tongue and speaks only in Russian. She shares stories on each of her pieces of jewelry and pendants, her husband's paintings and holds on tightly to her possessions. At nighttime, she exhibits paranoia and is often accusatory to those around her, believing that people are stealing her things. She calls her caregiver a rat and becomes agitated if her belongings are misplaced. She revisits trauma faced as a marginalized Jewish person in Russia and recalls when her father was arrested.

She regularly attends swimming lessons at the YMCA in the evenings. Twice, she has wandered away from her evening class, lost in the neighborhood streets and brought home by the local police. She is less agitated when around people with whom she feels safe; they can often reorient her by explaining other people's actions. They also remind her of her disease. Her daughter L asks, "Do you remember, mom, that you have a condition?" There is no shame in Judaism in discussing highly personal matters. Culturally, people often speak openly of illness and even death. The doctor has spoken with daughter L and normalized the behaviors that come with dementia. The doctor has also educated her on disease expectations and management. With age, there may be a reaction of anxiety or depression to the loss of independence and autonomy, particularly for someone who has been independent and values their independence highly. Red flags to monitor are safety; if Ms. Y puts herself in jeopardy or inadvertently causes harm to someone else. Ms. Y lost her ability to drive a year ago, which was a devastating loss of independence for her. Her wandering and cognitive impairment is a threat to her safety, and she will need adequate support. Daughter L has the choice of institutionalizing her mother, which will provide twenty-four-hour nursing care. However, financial resources are needed to cover room and board, as in non-socialized medicine areas, insurance does not cover these costs. The other option is to hire a skilled nurse or private caregiver to stay in the home. The number of hours required is determined by the needs of the patient and the flexibility of family.

Daughter L does not need to hire a twenty-four-hour hired caregiver, as she works remotely from home only during the day. She feels she can hire someone for eight hours overnight for respite. Additionally, there are daycare services in the local aging community. L has provided her mother with a Life Alert button on a necklace, so Ms. Y can call for help anytime.

How to Prepare for Advanced Dementia and Sundowning

In the geriatric outpatient setting, it is important to document a durable power of attorney and the wishes of the patient early in their disease, especially if there are any known family histories of dementia or early signs of mild cognitive impairment. Often, dementia patients are vulnerable both financially and legally. Losing capacity will be inevitable, and thus it is important to develop rapport with the patient while capacity is intact. Capacity is often a spectrum, and patients with advanced dementia may still be able to name surrogate decision makers, even though they may lack complex decision-making capacity. If they are able to complete an advanced directive naming a decision maker or complete questions about wishes on different circumstances of terminal illness to the end of life, that may help providers with difficult decisions when the time comes. Although it is an uncomfortable conversation, it helps to prepare for the worst and not take away hope as some may be averse to discussing such difficult topics.

It is important to bring in medication bottles to regular appointments so that providers may see what patients are taking at home. This is helpful in understanding any potential polypharmacy and compliance with medications. It also helps doctors educate on the indications and side effects of medications and bring up any potential medications which may exacerbate or lead to sundowning.

The Montreal Cognitive Assessment[16] screens for cognitive impairment domains within the visuospatial function, executive function, language, memory and recall, abstraction, and orientation[16]. This screening tool is valid and can offer a picture of the progress of cognitive impairment if assessed on multiple visits [16]. This is particularly helpful in understanding the rate of the disease trajectory and anticipating sundowning symptoms. Sundowning generally presents in moderate to late stages of dementia, however it can also occur in people with mild cognitive impairment as well. The severity and intensity of symptoms as well as the longer duration and frequency of sundowning correlate with the severity of the disease. The Montreal Cognitive Assessment[16] screen can also pinpoint memory and recall impairment, which is often associated more with sundowning[16].

Prognostication tools such as the Eastern Cooperative Oncology Group[17] scale, the palliative performance scale, and Functional Assessment Staging Tool[18] can help determine prognosis. Eprognosis.org has further data on determining life expectancy [19]. Determination of prognosis not only helps to begin conversations and educate on disease expectations and management but also helps to solidify the goals of the patient and their loved ones. It may assist providers in discussing a palliative referral. Furthermore, resources such as hospice may also need to be explored depending on the severity of the disease.

Patients with dementia are unable to express that they are ill or have physical discomfort; thus they often express their physical symptoms through aggression, screaming, yelling or refusing to eat[1]. A popular mnemonic for evaluating dementia-related behavioral problems is "S-M-A-R-T" Safety—Medical work-up—Assessment of competency—Rest/Review of causes of behavioral abnormalities—Trial of medications[20].

How We Can Palliate (Addressing Psychological/ Emotional, Physical, and Spiritual Impact)

According to the medical literature, the most useful treatments for sundowning in patients with dementia include behavior modifications as well as environmental interventions—particularly bright light therapy—along with melatonin, antipsychotic medications and acetylcholinesterase inhibitors[1].

Behavioral Modifications and Environmental Interventions

Examples of behavioral modifications and environmental interventions useful in treating sundowning include: light therapy, aroma therapy, music therapy, simulated presence therapy, caregiver education, multisensory stimulation, adherence to a stable daily routine, minimizing unnecessary noise, managing a patients' mood symptoms (depression, sadness, feelings of guilt, feelings of grief, feelings of worthlessness, feelings of anxiety and frustration) and offering simple instructions for meals and bathing[1]. A beneficial behavioral plan helps to keep patients mentally occupied during the day with a structured daily schedule including lots of opportunities for physical exercise and then following with a sleep hygiene routine at night [21]. Other behavioral modifications such as addressing pain, constipation, dyskinesias, reassurance, redirection, distraction, and meeting the patient's physical needs are all tools that can help prevent confusion, agitation and the behavioral disturbances associated with sundowning[22]. A frequently missed environmental or behavioral modification is limiting the patient's television viewing. The frightening and violent events depicted on television may stress and disturb the patient as they may believe that the events are happening to them, and this may exacerbate the symptoms of sundowning.

Re-orientation

Reorientation may be provided by caregivers or nurses. Familiarity is important during sundowning and periods of confusion, particularly because neurologically a part of memory is affected, but often long-term memory is preserved. Cues such as watches or calendars and clocks hung on the wall may help. In one study, researchers investigated family videos and found that the audio and familiarity of voices alone helped mitigate the symptoms of sundowning. The robotic doll "Paro" provides a constant companion and comfort despite changes in the environment.

Bright Light Therapy

One study found that placing a full-spectrum fluorescent lamp (2500-5000 lux) about one meter from a patient with a history of sundowning in the morning and within the patient's visual field and leaving it to run for a few hours may lead to changes in the circadian rhythm, making patients less agitated and confused[23]. Another study found that bright light therapy (10,000 lux bright light) had a positive effect on improving motor restlessness in patients with dementia[24]. Ta-Wei (2022) conducted nine studies on bright light therapy in London. Bright light is defined as > 1000 lux within the blue to green light spectrum[13]. It is hypothesized that inadequate lighting in facilities contributes to sundowning. Sundowning was noted to occur in darker spaces, even in the 1940s[1]. Studies saw that higher light exposure during the day correlated with less disrupted rest-activity rhythms, higher intra-daily rest-activity rhythm variability and longer sleep duration. Additionally, low light may correlate with visual hallucinations [25]. Typically with aging, the light used for image forming is usually reduced due to degenerative changes affecting light transmission in the eye and retinal ganglion cell loss [26]. Of note, the Charles Bonnet syndrome is an eye condition in which people have visual hallucinations. Low light worsens this [27]. In terms of sun- downing, non-image forming functions may contribute to behavioral and psychological symptoms of dementia (BPSD) through disrupted circadian rhythms while image forming functions of the eye through light may contribute through impairing vision, increasing misperceptions and difficulty identifying objects and, possibly, visual hallucinations. Natural light can reduce depression [13].

Melatonin

Several researchers have looked at the use of melatonin in dementia and found that it was helpful in reducing nocturnal activity, decreasing sleep latency, improving the quality of sleep and reducing sundowning behavior[28]. However, another literature review found that melatonin's effect on daytime functioning and sleep quality was inconclusive[28]. Based on multiple literature reviews and independent studies, no conclusive data was found regarding the effectiveness of melatonin treatment in demented patients who have sundowning[1].

Antipsychotic Medications

German researchers found that >40% of neuropsychiatrists and family physicians considered antipsychotic medications the drugs of choice when treating sundowning in elderly demented patients[29]. They carry side effects including the onset of diabetes, weight gain, gait disturbances with falls, cardiac effects, stroke, dysphagia, urinary retention, constipation, and increased cognitive impairment[1]. Multiple studies noted that atypical antipsychotics are useful when treating sundowning as they are better tolerated than typical antipsychotics with a better side-effect profile and that in addition to treating sundowning and confusion they also can treat delusions, paranoid ideations, and hallucinations[1].

Acetylcholinesterase Inhibitors

Acetylcholinesterase inhibitors are the standard treatment for Alzheimer's disease. However, no clear evidence exists for their use in treating behavioral symptoms such as sundowning. In fact, some studies show that donepezil actually worsens nocturnal agitation because it induces insomnia and/or nightmares[30]. However, another study showed that donepezil shortened sleep latency and increased sleep efficiency when it was given once a day in the morning [31]. Currently, no clear recommendations exist for treating sundowning with Acetylcholinesterase inhibitors[1].

Music

In *Nature Based Videos*, Robert Rados[32] looked at mitigating sundowning using brief six-minute nature videos with classical music and music-only in nursing home residents[32]. There is not much data on non-pharmacotherapies. However, music therapy has been extensively studied as a non-pharmaco measure. In fact, short duration measures have been proven to work[32]. There are defined music therapy programs for patients with dementia. However, passive listening with pre-recorded songs have also been shown to be beneficial[33]. Pastoral music was shown to lift patients' moods[34]. Rados's[32] study used pastoral nature photographs "as predominantly rural and natural scenes with grasslands, rivers, and minimal human influence[34]." Nature is thought to bring about psychological positivity. Nature and music combined had strong effects both subjectively on patients and as observed by staff. The use of music only was statistically nonsignificant. The study had a moderate to large effect clinically. The use of images and music together stopped aggressive behavior, resolved or mitigated hallucinations, and stopped the throwing of things, with patients visibly calmer. Residents showed changes in vitals signs and appeared less tachycardic. It optimized restorative benefits. Nature emoted positivity, psychological healing properties and a sense of renewal[32].

Sleep

It is crucial to have uninterrupted sleep with a calm, comfortable and low light environment and appropriately screen for sleep disorders. Providers may encourage documenting sleep-in logs. They may ask screening questions for sleep such as "Is the person satisfied with his or her sleep? Does sleep or fatigue interfere with daytime activities? Does a partner complain of behaviors during sleep such as snoring, interrupted breathing, or movements?" Polysomnography may screen for sleep apnea, narcolepsy, periodic limb movement disorder, violent behaviors during sleep, and other sleep disorders, including circadian rhythm disturbances.

Pharmacotherapy to Restore Circadian Rhythm

According to Mcleery's[35] systematic review of medications to improve sleep in dementia patients, it is widely known that the disruption of circadian rhythms can increase agitation and sundowning behaviors. According to Mcleery[35]:

> "There is some evidence that sleep itself may contribute to keeping in step with the circadian pacemaker. Hence, interventions to improve sleep at night may also improve circadian timing and potentially minimize other circadian symptoms such as sundowning, which is a phenomenon of increased motor activity and agitation in the late afternoon or evening." [35]

Perhaps disruptive sleep patterns seen early on in even mild to moderate dementia can accelerate the progression of disease and the appearance of sundowning at early stages[35]. Thus, it is crucial for clinicians to treat insomnia, initiate behavioral modifications if warranted, and offer pharmacotherapy to help sleep. Mcleery's[35] review looked at nine studies and medications: melatonin, trazodone, ramelteon, and orexin antagonists. Some off-the-label medications such as quetiapine or olanzapine are used in practice to help dementia patients with sleep, and also carry dual effects for agitation. However, these medications are linked with higher mortality, and carry a high risk of anticholinergic side effects. This may lead to worsened cognition, increased falls, caregiver burden, and institutionalization[37]. Overall, the study found melatonin to be ineffective. Similarly, ramelteon was no better than placebo[35]. Neither drug caused harm. It also found that 50mg of trazodone nightly for two weeks improved sleep efficacy and total time asleep, but not necessarily the frequency of awakenings. No major adverse effects occurred with these medications at that dosage. Patients taking orexin antagonists slept longer, spending less time awake, with more sleep benefits overall [35].

Emotional Impact and Caregiver Burden

The emotional impact can be burdensome for caregivers, as their loved ones may forget who they are. Patients generally forget and are unaware of their delirium and experience short-term memory loss. Emotionally, they may feel agitated and overwhelmed, they may be aware that their body is changing from loss of autonomy, loss of control. This at times is the hardest emotional burden.

Different Settings for Placement

Providers may discuss with patients caregivers the appropriate setting for protecting the patient's safety. It is crucial to understand the global functionality of the patient and whether the appropriate resources are available in the current setting they are in—for example, if they are having multiple falls at night going to the bathroom, perhaps they need twenty-four-hour supervision. Twenty-four-hour caregiving is generally recommended when people are at risk of harm from themselves, or in an unsafe setting or when there is a skilled nursing care need and these needs are out of the caregiver's scope/capacity. Families and loved ones have other responsibilities in their daily lives—going to work and childcare. In the U.S., due to a non-socialized medical system, private duty caregivers are out of pocket and often expensive. Does the patient then need to be institutionalized? There are different levels of care at assisted living facilities, depending on different degrees of need, functional status, and nursing overhead, it can be challenging to find the appropriate placement. For this reason, it is recommended to have an interdisciplinary team including a social worker help support a family and provide resources.

Sedation for Severe Agitation in Hospice Patients

Depending on life expectancy and the goals of the patient, when cognitive impairment is aggressive and intense, which is difficult to control even in the institutionalized setting, families may elect to enroll in hospice. Patients in this cohort generally have poor quality of life at baseline from their dementia and a prognosis of less than six months to live. Patients do not want to burden their caregivers, nor be a financial burden to their loved ones. If the agitation seen in sundowning is extreme, hospice teams may elect to sedate or utilize anti-psychotics to attempt to manage symptoms. Furthermore, the diurnal pattern for expected symptoms can be incredibly difficult for the families to see and expect daily. In this case, such medications that may cause more hypoactive delirium are appropriate.

Spirituality

Spirituality may be an important element in processing terminal disease, such as dementia. Some cultures equate demonic behavior or spirits transitioning through the body with the cognitive and behavioral changes seen[15]. Spirituality is important throughout illness as some patients value faith or organized religion. Religious communities may offer a strong support system. They may also provide Last Rites or Sacrament of the Sick in advanced stages of disease.

Summary: Sundown syndrome is a combination of neuropsychiatric symptoms occurring in elderly patients in the evening [1]. It is distinct from delirium where delirium presents with fluctuating course with an inciting and reversible cause. Sundowning is mostly prevalent in patients with dementia who are institutionalized. This may be from modifiable and non-modifiable factors. Sleep regulation plays a strong role in its presentation. Re-orientation with bright light and music therapy have moderate evidence for positive impact on sundowning. Pharmaco-measures such as melatonin and Z drugs have little or insufficient evidence for impact. On the occasion where agitation becomes severe, atypical antipsychotics may be the preferred choice for methods of controlling sundowning. There is significant cultural influence which impacts re-orientation, open discussion of illness, and impacts placement and socio-economic costs.

Bibliography

1. Khachiyants, Nina, David Trinkle, Sang Joon Son, and Kye Y. Kim. "Sundown Syndrome in Persons with Dementia: An Update." *Psychiatry Investigation* 8, no. 4 (2011): 275. https://doi.org/10.4306/pi.2011.8.4.275.
2. Canevelli, Marco, Martina Valletta, Alessandro Trebbastoni, Giuseppe Sarli, Fabrizia D'Antonio, Leonardo Tariciotti, Carlo de Lena, and Giuseppe Bruno. "Sundowning in Dementia: Clinical Relevance, Pathophysiological Determinants, and Therapeutic Approaches." *Frontiers in Medicine* 3 (December 27, ducke2016). https://doi.org/10.3389/fmed.2016.00073.
3. *DSM-5: Diagnostic and Statistical Manual of Mental Disorders, 5th Edition*. Generic Tyzek, 2023.
4. Cameron, D. Ewen. "Studies in Senile Nocturnal Delirium." *The Psychiatric Quarterly* 15, no. 1 (January 1941): 47–53. https://doi.org/10.1007/bf01613953.
5. Duckett, Stephane. "Managing the Sundowning Patient." *Journal of Rehabilitation* 59, no. 1 (December 31, 1992): 24. https://www.questia.com/library/journal/1G1-13839730/managing-the-sundowning-patient.
6. Wu, Ying-Hui, and Dick F. Swaab. "The Human Pineal Gland and Melatonin in Aging and Alzheimer's Disease." *Journal of Pineal Research* 38, no. 3 (April 2005): 145–52. https://doi.org/10.1111/j.1600-079x.2004.00196.x.
7. Huitrón-Reséndiz, Salvador, Manuel Sánchez-Alavez, Roger Gallegos, Greta Berg, Elena Crawford, Jeannie L Giacchino, Dora Games, Steven J Henriksen, and José R Criado. "Age-Independent and Age-Related Deficits in Visuospatial Learning, Sleep–Wake States, Thermoregulation and Motor Activity in PDAPP Mice." *Brain Research* 928, no. 1–2 (February 2002): 126–37. https://doi.org/10.1016/s0006-8993(01)03373-x.
8. Liu, R.-Y. "Decreased Melatonin Levels in Postmortem Cerebrospinal Fluid in Relation to Aging, Alzheimer's Disease, and Apolipoprotein E-4/4 Genotype." *Journal of Clinical Endocrinology &Amp; Metabolism* 84, no. 1 (January 1, 1999): 323–27. https://doi.org/10.1210/jc.84.1.323.

9. REITER, RUSSEL J., DUN XIAN TAN, LUCIEN C. MANCHESTER, and MAMDOUH R. EL-SAWI. "Melatonin Reduces Oxidant Damage and Promotes Mitochondrial Respiration." *Annals of the New York Academy of Sciences* 959, no. 1 (April 2002): 238–50. https://doi.org/10.1111/j.1749-6632.2002.tb02096.x.
10. Foley, Daniel J., Andrew A. Monjan, S. Lori Brown, Eleanor M. Simonsick, Robert B. Wallace, and Dan G. Blazer. "Sleep Complaints Among Elderly Persons: An Epidemiologic Study of Three Communities." *Sleep* 18, no. 6 (August 1995): 425–32. https://doi.org/10.1093/sleep/18.6.425.
11. Bliwise, Donald L., Jennifer S. Carroll, Kathryn A. Lee, Jamie C. Nekich, and William C. Dement. "Sleep and 'Sundowning' in Nursing Home Patients with Dementia." *Psychiatry Research* 48, no. 3 (September 1993): 277–92. https://doi.org/10.1016/0165-1781(93)90078-u.
12. Pacala, James T, and James T Sullivan. *Geriatrics Review Syllabus: A Core Curriculum in Geriatric Medicine.* Paperback. American Geriatrics Society, 2010.
13. Guu, Ta-Wei, Dag Aarsland, and Dominic ffytche. "Light, Sleep-wake Rhythm, and Behavioural and Psychological Symptoms of Dementia in Care Home Patients: Revisiting the Sundowning Syndrome." *International Journal of Geriatric Psychiatry* 37, no. 5 (April 26, 2022). https://doi.org/10.1002/gps.5712.
14. Nishimura, Mayumi, Karen Harrison Dening, Elizabeth L. Sampson, Edison Iglesias de Oliveira Vidal, Wilson Correia de Abreu, Sharon Kaasalainen, Yvonne Eisenmann, et al. "Cross-Cultural Conceptualization of a Good End of Life with Dementia: A Qualitative Study." *BMC Palliative Care* 21, no. 1 (June 8, 2022). https://doi.org/10.1186/s12904-022-00982-9.
15. Malarney, Shaun Kingsley. *Culture, Ritual, and Revolution in Vietnam (Anthropology of Asia Series) (Anthropology in Asia)*. Univ of Hawaii Pr, 2022.
16. MoCA – Cognitive Assessment. "MoCA - Cognitive Assessment," December 12, 2022. https://mocacognition.com/.
17. ECOG-ACRIN Cancer Research Group. "ECOG Performance Status Scale," December 29, 2022. https://ecog-acrin.org/resources/ecog-performance-status/.
18. Compassus. "Functional Assessment Staging Tool (FAST Scale) for Dementia," June 17, 2022. https://www.compassus.com/healthcare-professionals/determining-eligibility/functional-assessment-staging-tool-fast-scale-for-dementia.

19. "EPrognosis Time to Benefit." Accessed December 22, 2022. https://eprognosis.ucsf.edu/time_to_benefit.php.
20. Rabheru, Kiran. "Take a S-M-A-R-T Approach: Unpredictable Course of Dementia Symptoms Can Be Managed." *Canadian Family Physician* 49 (2003): 389.
21. Schulz, Richard, Steven H. Belle, Sara J. Czaja, Laura N. Gitlin, Stephen R. Wisniewski, and Marcia G. Ory. "Introduction to the Special Section on Resources for Enhancing Alzheimer's Caregiver Health (REACH)." *Psychology and Aging* 18, no. 3 (2003): 357–60. https://doi.org/10.1037/0882-7974.18.3.357.
22. Bachman, David, and Peter Rabins. "'Sundowning' and Other Temporally Associated Agitation States in Dementia Patients." *Annual Review of Medicine* 57, no. 1 (February 1, 2006): 499–511. https://doi.org/10.1146/annurev.med.57.071604.141451.
23. McGonigal-Kenney, Meghan L, and Debra L Schutte. "Evidence-Based Guideline." *Journal of Gerontological Nursing* 32, no. 2 (February 2006): 9–9. https://doi.org/10.3928/0098-9134-20060201-05.
24. Haffmans, P. M. Judith, Rob C. Sival, Stefan A. P. Lucius, Quirine Cats, and Lies Van Gelder. "Bright Light Therapy and Melatonin in Motor Restless Behaviour in Dementia: A Placebo-Controlled Study." *International Journal of Geriatric Psychiatry* 16, no. 1 (December 31, 2000): 106–10. https://doi.org/10.1002/1099-1166(200101)16:1.
25. Juda, Myriam, Teresa Liu-Ambrose, Fabio Feldman, Cristian Suvagau, and Ralph E. Mistlberger. "Light in the Senior Home: Effects of Dynamic and Individual Light Exposure on Sleep, Cognition, and Well-Being." *Clocks &Amp; Sleep* 2, no. 4 (December 14, 2020): 557–76. https://doi.org/10.3390/clockssleep2040040.
26. Turner, Patricia L., Eus J.W. Van Someren, and Martin A. Mainster. "The Role of Environmental Light in Sleep and Health: Effects of Ocular Aging and Cataract Surgery." *Sleep Medicine Reviews* 14, no. 4 (August 2010): 269–80. https://doi.org/10.1016/j.smrv.2009.11.002.
27. Teunisse, Robert J., Frans G. Zitman, and Dick C.M. Raes. "Clinical Evaluation of 14 Patients with the Charles Bonnet Syndrome (Isolated Visual Hallucinations)." *Comprehensive Psychiatry* 35, no. 1 (January 1994): 70–75. https://doi.org/10.1016/0010-440x(94)90172-4.
28. Jonghe, A. de, J. C. Korevaar, B. C. van Munster, and S. E. de Rooij. "Effectiveness of Melatonin Treatment on Circadian Rhythm Disturbances in Dementia. Are There Implications for Delirium? A Systematic Review." *International Journal of Geriatric Psychiatry* 25, no. 12 (November 18, 2010): 1201–8. https://doi.org/10.1002/gps.2454.

29. Stoppe, Gabriela, Hagen Sandholzer, Jürgen Staedt, Silke Winter, Jörg Kiefer, and Eckart Rüther. "Sleep Disturbances in the Demented Elderly: Treatment in Ambulatory Care." *Sleep* 18, no. 10 (December 1995): 844–48. https://doi.org/10.1093/sleep/18.10.844.
30. Rogers, Sharon L. "Donepezil Improves Cognition and Global Function in Alzheimer Disease<Subtitle>A 15-Week, Double-Blind, Placebo-Controlled Study</Subtitle>" *Archives of Internal Medicine* 158, no. 9 (May 11, 1998): 1021. https://doi.org/10.1001/archinte.158.9.1021.
31. Mizuno, Soichi, Atsuko Kameda, Takuji Inagaki, And Jun Horiguchi. "Effects of Donepezil on Alzheimer's Disease: The Relationship between Cognitive Function and Rapid Eye Movement Sleep." *Psychiatry and Clinical Neurosciences* 58, no. 6 (December 2004): 660–65. https://doi.org/10.1111/j.1440-1819.2004.01317.x.
32. Rados, Robert, Jun Kim, Shintaro Kono, and Jennifer Horton. "Nature-Based Video with Music for Individuals Experiencing an Episode of Sundown Syndrome." *Journal of Long-Term Care* 0, no. 2021 (September 29, 2021): 294. https://doi.org/10.31389/jltc.69.
33. Vink, Annemieke, and Suzanne Hanser. "Music-Based Therapeutic Interventions for People with Dementia: A Mini-Review." *Medicines* 5, no. 4 (October 8, 2018): 109. https://doi.org/10.3390/medicines5040109.
34. Kim, Jun, Namyun Kil, Stephen Holland, and Wendi K. Middleton. "The Effect of Visual and Auditory Coherence on Perceptions of Tranquility after Simulated Nature Experiences." *Ecopsychology* 9, no. 3 (September 2017): 182–89. https://doi.org/10.1089/eco.2016.0046.
35. McCleery, Jenny, and Ann L Sharpley. "Pharmacotherapies for Sleep Disturbances in Dementia." *Cochrane Database of Systematic Reviews* 2020, no. 11 (November 15, 2020). https://doi.org/10.1002/14651858.cd009178.pub4.
36. Buxton, Orfeu M., Georges Copinschi, Anne Van Onderbergen, Theodore G. Karrison, and Eve Van Cauter. "A Benzodiazepine Hypnotic Facilitates Adaptation of Circadian Rhythms and Sleep-Wake Homeostasis to an Eight Hour Delay Shift Simulating Westward Jet Lag." *Sleep* 23, no. 7 (October 1, 2000): 1–13. https://doi.org/10.1093/sleep/23.7.1g.
37. Schneider, Lon S., Karen Dagerman, and Philip S. Insel. "Efficacy and Adverse Effects of Atypical Antipsychotics for Dementia: Meta-Analysis of Randomized, Placebo-Controlled Trials." *The American Journal of Geriatric Psychiatry* 14, no. 3 (March 2006): 191–210. https://doi.org/10.1097/01.jgp.0000200589.01396.6d.

38. Asayama, Kentaro, Hiroshi Yamadera, Takao Ito, Hideaki Suzuki, Yoshihisa Kudo, and Shunkichi Endo. "Double Blind Study of Melatonin Effects on the Sleep-Wake Rhythm, Cognitive and Non-Cognitive Functions in Alzheimer Type Dementia." *Journal of Nippon Medical School* 70, no. 4 (2003): 334–41. https://doi.org/10.1272/jnms.70.334.
39. Azermai, Majda, Mirko Petrovic, Monique M. Elseviers, Jolyce Bourgeois, Luc M. Van Bortel, and Robert H. Vander Stichele. "Sybuxtstematic Appraisal of Dementia Guidelines for the Management of Behavioural and Psychological Symptoms." *Ageing Research Reviews* 11, no. 1 (January 2012): 78–86. https://doi.org/10.1016/j.arr.2011.07.002.
40. Chung, Joohyun, Seong-In Choi, and Jun Kim. "Experience of Media Presentations for the Alleviation of Agitation and Emotional Distress among Dementia Patients in a Long-Term Nursing Facility." *Dementia* 15, no. 5 (July 26, 2016): 1021–33. https://doi.org/10.1177/1471301214550660.
41. Evans, Simon Chester, Julie Barrett, Neil Mapes, June Hennell, Teresa Atkinson, Jennifer Bray, Claire Garabedian, and Chris Russell. "Connections with Nature for People Living with Dementia." *Working With Older People* 23, no. 3 (August 29, 2019): 142–51. https://doi.org/10.1108/wwop-01-2019-0003.
42. Javadpour, Ali, Laaya Ahmadzadeh, and Mohammad Jafar Bahredar. "An Educative Support Group for Female Family Caregivers: Impact on Caregivers Psychological Distress and Patient's Neuropsychiatry Symptoms." *International Journal of Geriatric Psychiatry* 24, no. 5 (May 2009): 469–71. https://doi.org/10.1002/gps.2138.
43. Kim, Pavel, C. Louis, S. Muralee, and Rajesh R Tampi. "Sundowning Syndrome in the Older Patient." *Clinical Geriatrics* 13 (April 2005): 32–36.
44. Martin, Jennifer, Matthew Marler, Tamar Shochat, and Sonia Ancoli-Israel. "CIRCADIAN RHYTHMS OF AGITATION IN INSTITUTIONALIZED PATIENTS WITH ALZHEIMER'S DISEASE." *Chronobiology International* 17, no. 3 (January 2000): 405–18. https://doi.org/10.1081/cbi-100101054.
45. Milev, Roumen V., Tracey Kellar, Marilyn McLean, Vicky Mileva, Veb Luthra, Shiela Thompson, and Linda Peever. "Multisensory Stimulation for Elderly With Dementia: A 24-Week Single-Blind Randomized Controlled Pilot Study." *American Journal of Alzheimer's Disease &Amp; Other Dementiasr* 23, no. 4 (March 28, 2008): 372–76. https://doi.org/10.1177/1533317508316681.

46. Monti, Jaime M., and Daniel P. Cardinali. "A Critical Assessment of the Melatonin Effect on Sleep in Humans." *Neurosignals* 9, no. 6 (2000): 328–39. https://doi.org/10.1159/000014656.
47. Nguyen, Quynh-anh, and Carol Paton. "The Use of Aromatherapy to Treat Behavioural Problems in Dementia." *International Journal of Geriatric Psychiatry* 23, no. 4 (2008): 337–46. https://doi.org/10.1002/gps.1886.
48. Olde Rikkert, M. G. M., and A.-S. P. Rigaud. "Melatonin in Elderly Patients with Insomnia." *Zeitschrift Für Gerontologie Und Geriatrie* 34, no. 6 (December 1, 2001): 491–97. https://doi.org/10.1007/s003910170025.
49. Reus, Victor I., Laura J. Fochtmann, A. Evan Eyler, Donald M. Hilty, Marcela Horvitz-Lennon, Michael D. Jibson, Oscar L. Lopez, et al. "The American Psychiatric Association Practice Guideline on the Use of Antipsychotics to Treat Agitation or Psychosis in Patients With Dementia." *American Journal of Psychiatry* 173, no. 5 (May 2016): 543–46. https://doi.org/10.1176/appi.ajp.2015.173501.
50. Riemersma-van der Lek, Rixt F. "Effect of Bright Light and Melatonin on Cognitive and Noncognitive Function in Elderly Residents of Group Care Facilities." *JAMA* 299, no. 22 (June 11, 2008): 2642. https://doi.org/10.1001/jama.299.22.2642.
51. Swaab, D.F., E. Fliers, and T.S. Partiman. "The Suprachiasmatic Nucleus of the Human Brain in Relation to Sex, Age and Senile Dementia." *Brain Research* 342, no. 1 (September 1985): 37–44. https://doi.org/10.1016/0006-8993(85)91350-2.
52. Todd, William D. "Potential Pathways for Circadian Dysfunction and Sundowning-Related Behavioral Aggression in Alzheimer's Disease and Related Dementias." *Frontiers in Neuroscience* 14 (September 3, 2020). https://doi.org/10.3389/fnins.2020.00910.
53. Van Gelder, R N. "Blue Light and the Circadian Clock." *British Journal of Ophthalmology* 88, no. 10 (October 1, 2004): 1353–1353. https://doi.org/10.1136/bjo.2004.042861/045120.
54. Vink, Annemiek C, Manon S Bruinsma, and Rob JPM Scholten. "Music Therapy for People with Dementia." Edited by Annemiek C Vink. *Cochrane Database of Systematic Reviews*, October 20, 2003. https://doi.org/10.1002/14651858.cd003477.pub2.
55. Zetteler, Jessica. "Effectiveness of Simulated Presence Therapy for Individuals with Dementia: A Systematic Review and Meta-Analysis." *Aging &Amp; Mental Health* 12, no. 6 (November 2008): 779–85. https://doi.org/10.1080/13607860802380631.

6

ON THE MANAGEMENT OF OPTIMAL DEMENTIA CARE IN THE UNITED STATES – A NURSE PERSPECTIVE

MIRANDA MEUNIER, BSN, MSN[1]

Abstract

In the Unites States, 6 million individuals are living with dementia. By 2050, that number is expected to reach 13 million. The lack of disease-modifying interventions combined with rising prevalence and substantial financial considerations have led to Alzheimer's Disease and Related Dementias (ADRD) to be considered one of the top public health priorities in the nation. Dementia not only affects those diagnosed with the disease, but also their families and friends. Family members and caregivers struggle with substantial emotional, physical, and financial stress caring for their loved ones with ADRD as the disease progresses. Management of dementia is more focused on risk reduction and social interventions instead of traditional medical interventions. Ideally, dementia care is focused on person-centered interventions focused on maintaining cognitive and functional abilities and meeting the patient where they are in a proactive vs. reactionary way. Given the lack of medical treatment options for dementia and the evitable functional and cognitive decline associated with the disease, supporting and encouraging a more palliative approach to care as dementia progresses should be the standard of care.

Keywords: Dementia, Palliative Care, Caregiver, Diagnosis, Management, Community-based

---

[1] Nurse Practitioner, Billings Clinic Geriatrics Department

Like most adults who reach their mid-80s, my maternal grandmother began noticing cognitive and functional decline. Although never diagnosed officially with dementia, she began showing early signs of the disease. Alzheimer's disease and related dementias (ADRD) are irreversible, progressive brain diseases that slowly destroy brain function by causing severe damage to neurons which leads to cognitive decline behavioral disorders, and functional deficits. However, the progression is often slow and uncertain.

In the Unites States, 6 million individuals are living with dementia. Most of those individuals are over the age of 75. By 2050, that number is expected to reach 13 million, fueled by the surge of aging baby boomers. By 2030, all baby boomers will be 65 or older and by 2060, nearly 25% of the population of the United States will be over 65. As population growth in general, however, is stagnating in the US, this higher concentration of older adults will put a higher strain on working-age adults to fund social programs such as Social Security, Medicaid, and Medicare on which older population will rely. The lack of disease-modifying interventions combined with rising prevalence and substantial financial considerations have led to ADRD considered one of the top public health priorities in the nation.

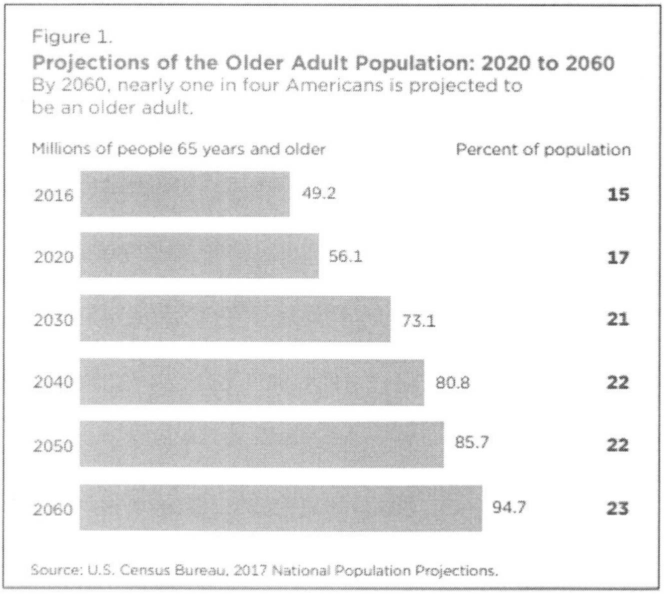

Figure 6-1: Projections of the Older Adult Population in the United States. (US Census Bureau 2020)

Costs

Much of the dementia disease process is spent in a state of disability and dependence. Research has shown individuals with dementia have more inconsistency in outpatient medical care, higher rates of preventable emergency department visits and hospitalizations, and a large number of unorganized care transitions when compared to their peers who do not have dementia (Odenheimer et al. 2014, 559). They also have significantly higher use of assisted living, skilled nursing, and long-term care facilities. In 2022, it is estimated dementia-related care costs will reach $321 billion in the US (Alzheimer's Association 2022).

In their 2016 Fact and Figures report, the Alzheimer's Association did a special report on caregivers. They found caregivers can spend in excess of $5000 annually in out-of-pocket costs to cover the care costs associated with dementia, making it the chronic disease with the highest out-of-pocket expenses. Given inflation, this number is likely higher. Many caregivers cut back on basic necessities including food and medical care for themselves and other family members to cover the high out-of-pocket costs of dementia care. The same Alzheimer's Association survey reported that 28% of caregivers responded they ate less or were hungry because they did not have enough money to afford decent meals. The excessive costs of dementia care contribute to food and housing insecurity for many families.

Caregivers

Dementia not only affects those diagnosed with the disease, but also their families and friends. Family members and caregivers struggle with substantial emotional, physical, and financial stress caring for their loved ones with ADRD as the disease progresses. Caregivers include family members, friends, or paid professional who provide care to a person with dementia. Eventually the neuronal damage extends to the part of the brain responsible for basic functions such as walking and swallowing. Disease progression occurs in a continuum, as outlined in Figure 2. However, the timeline of the continuum varies. Studies have shown that individuals generally live 4-8 years after diagnosis of dementia, although can live for as many as 20 years.

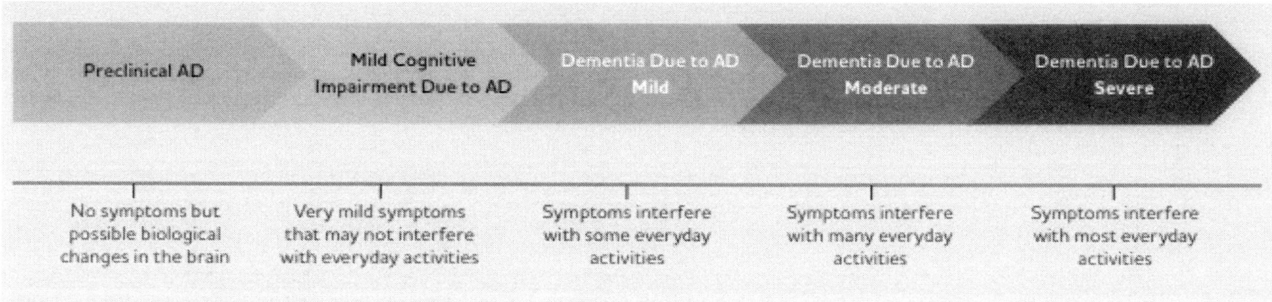

Figure 6-2: Continuum of Alzheimer's disease. (Alzheimer's Association 2022)

Because of the stigma associated with dementia, extended family members and friends may be uncomfortable discussing the disease or interacting with an individual once the diagnosis has been made. As the disease progresses, the affected individual often withdraws from activities they used to enjoy and may even withdraw from spending time with cherished friends and family. This is very isolating for both individuals with dementia as well as their caregivers (Reinhard et al. 2015). It is our societal responsibility to ensure individuals with dementia and their caregivers remain engaged in our communities and feel welcome.

As the individual with dementia continue to decline in cognitive and functional abilities, caregiver responsibilities increase, as does the potential for increased financial and emotional stress, the risk for depression, and poor health outcomes for both the individual with dementia as well as their caregiver. Typical caregiver tasks are outlined in Figure 3. By providing psychosocial and resource support to caregivers, facility placement of an individual with dementia can be delayed by as much as 1.5 years (Pinquart and Sorenson 2006, 584; Family Caregiver Alliance 2016)

- Bathing, dressing, grooming
- Walking assistance
- Household chores
- Meal preparation
- Managing finances
- Managing behavior symptoms
- Arranging for paid caregivers
- Overseeing medication management with sometimes complex regimens
- Providing transportation
- Shopping
- Companionship
- Medical/nursing tasks

Figure 6-3: Caregiving Tasks

The burden of caregiving can be reduced by enrolling in respite services such as adult day care and in-home care that give the caregiver a break from the responsibilities. Case management, support groups, and training programs can also be effective (Alzheimer's Association 2016).

I, too, am a caregiver. My husband Nathan was diagnosed with myotonic dystrophy at age 29, when our son was just a few months old. Although the pathologic pathways of myotonic dystrophy and Alzheimer's disease differ and the symptoms of the diseases vary, the shock of hearing the diagnosis of a progressive, degenerative condition for your loved one is crushing. Over the 10+ years since his diagnosis, I have seen my husband's subtle and not-so-subtle changes. He has shrunk both physically and metaphorically. His world is much smaller than it used to be, based on both his functional decline and worsened apathy. He is now becoming more unsteady, and I worry how much longer he will be able to walk, let alone work. I worry about his medical needs in the future and if we will be able to afford the care he may require. I worry about his inevitable early passing and the toll it will have on myself and my children. I often feel lonely and isolated. I grieve the loss of the future life we planned, and the loss of the man I married. I hope I will be strong enough to honor his wishes of not pursuing life sustaining treatment. Nancy Reagan famously named Alzheimer's disease "the long goodbye" which is so appropriate for most progressive, terminal conditions.

Diagnosis

Despite all that is known about ADRD, it remains difficult to get a definitive diagnosis. Only half of Medicare beneficiaries who have billing records of an ADRD diagnosis are told they have this diagnosis. ADRD is most often diagnosed by an individual's primary care provider (PCP). However, most PCPs do not feel comfortable addressing, diagnosing, and/or managing dementia. Even for those that receive a diagnosis, very few individuals and their families receive education about the disease or information about how to care for someone with dementia. Barriers for diagnosis and education include (Alzheimer's Association 2022):

- Perceived lack of clear diagnostic guidelines and reliable screening tools
- Complexity and variability of dementia
- Fear of emotional distress
- Futility of diagnosis for a virtually untreatable disease
- Individual or caregiver wishes not to pursue workup
- Lack of knowledge
- Stigma associated with dementia
- Time constraints

There is a lack of knowledge surrounding dementia in all levels of healthcare providers. As Atul Gawande states in his best-seller Being Mortal, the purpose of medical school is to educate on treating disease and saving lives, not tending to "unfixable" problems such as dementia. As Americans, we are conditioned to put our healthcare needs in the hands of practitioners "valued more for their technical prowess than for their understanding of human needs." (Gawande 2014, 128) There is also a dearth of healthcare providers dedicated to the care of older adults. The American Geriatrics Society recommends one geriatrician for every 300 older adults. BY 2030, in the US there is projected to be only one geriatrician for nearly 4,000 older adults. Access to dementia specialists is highly dependent on residency as well with much less availability in rural areas. Direct care workers including nurses and personal care aides are also in high demand. The COVID pandemic has made staffing challenges even more critical as many of these direct care workers have left the healthcare profession entirely.

Despite barriers and attitudes towards diagnosing ADRD, early diagnosis is a prerequisite for improving dementia care as it promotes autonomy and allows the individual to be involved in decision making regarding their future care. By having an earlier diagnosis, individuals with dementia may be eligible to be a participant in more research studies. Early diagnosis will also be critical for effective use of newly emerging treatments, based on the theory that treatments will be most successful in earlier stages of the disease. Primary care providers make the majority of dementia diagnoses. Figure 4 details the recommended process for cognitive assessment.

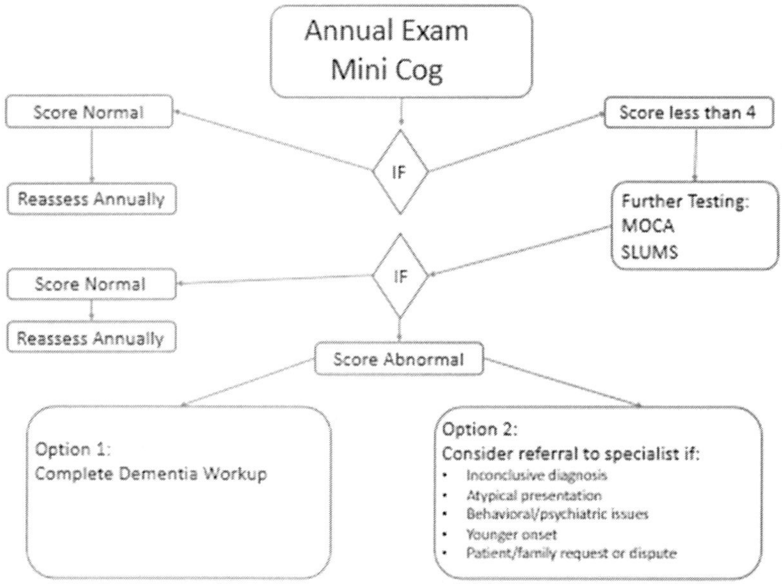

Figure 6-4: Cognitive Assessment Process. Adapted from ActOnAlz.org.

The are several risks associated with a lack of diagnosis including increased healthcare utilization, poor advanced care planning, and potential exploitation of vulnerable adults. Financial exploitation and/or poor financial decisions due to cognitive impairment can lead to significant downstream outcomes, even homelessness. Based on research by Margot Kushel out of the University of California San Francisco, the homeless population over the age of 50 in 1990 was 11%. Today that number is 50% (Brown et al. 2016).

Management

1 in 3 Americans dies with dementia, more than breast cancer and prostate cancer combined. Of the most common causes of death in the US, ADRD are the only ones that cannot be prevented, cured, or effectively treated. Although great strides have been made in dementia research in the last decade, there is still not a true disease-modifying treatment available. Therefore, management of dementia is more focused on risk reduction and social interventions instead of traditional medical interventions.

As I nurse practitioner, I am trained to focus on health promotion and disease prevention. For dementia, that process should begin in an individual's 30s or 40s. Research has shown that the pathways for neuronal damage leading to dementia symptoms begin as many as 20 years before the symptoms are expressed. Brain health is heart health so methods of improving cardiovascular health will also help to improve brain health and reduce risks of stroke and dementia including diet and exercise. There is a growing theory of inflammation as a trigger of the cascading causing neuronal damage. Therefore, an anti-inflammatory diet such as the Mediterranean diet might be better yet in risk reduction. Higher levels of education and social engagement have found to be protective factors in shielding the expression of dementia symptoms and may be a risk reduction tool as well.

There are nonpharmacologic methods of treating the disease which focus on effective management of underlying conditions, caregiver training, care coordination among healthcare professionals, and social engagement in meaningful activities. A proper treatment plan should also include end of life wishes and discussions on palliative and supportive care early in the disease process. Person-centered dementia care requires a broader lens than the traditional medical focus on how a disease affects only the patient. Instead, the focus is extended to family, caregivers, and support networks (Grand, Caspar, and McDonald 2011, 134-139).

- Optimize function and quality of life
- Manage chronic disease
- Promote positive mental health
- Assess safety and driving
- Optimize medication therapy including deprescribing as appropriate
- Facilitate advanced care planning discussions
- Assess caregiver needs, enhancing their well-being, skill, and comfort in caring for their loved one

Figure 6-5: Goals of Dementia Care
Adapted from Actonalz.org and Odenheimer 2014

Individuals with dementia can have extensive needs including cognitive, physical, social, financial, and emotional issues. Goals of dementia care are outlined in Figure 5. Ideally, dementia care is focused on person-centered interventions focused on maintaining cognitive and functional abilities and meeting the patient where they are in a proactive vs. reactionary way (Grand, Caspar, and McDonald 2011, 139). Because no single health specialty or discipline has the expertise to handle the complexity of these domains, meeting these goals requires a multidisciplinary approach, led by a dementia navigator as outlined in Figure 6. A dementia navigator is someone trained to help link individuals with dementia to information, support, and local resources in an effort to improve care and reduce costs. The multidisciplinary team follows the individual and their caregiver(s) across the continuum of the disease. (Montana Alzheimer's Disease/Dementia Workgroup 2016)

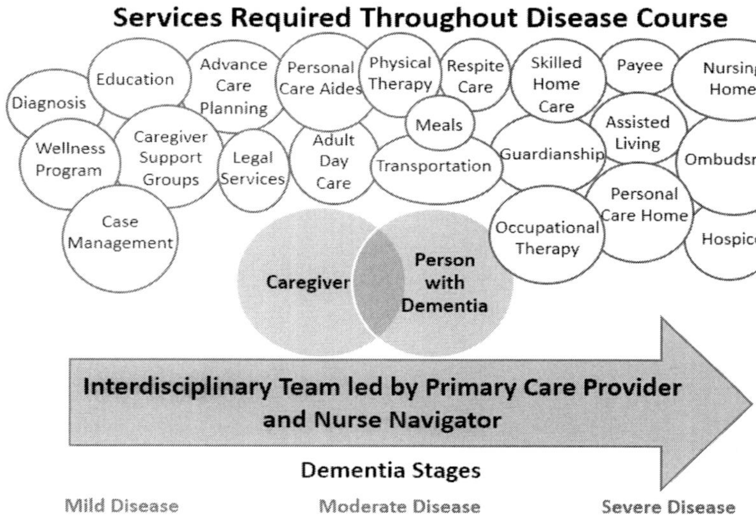

Figure 6-6: Continuity of Care. (Montana Alzheimer's Disease/Dementia Workgroup 2016)

As mentioned previously, advanced care planning and discussion of supportive and palliative care early in the disease process is vital to allow the individual with dementia the ability to participate in these decisions as much as possible. Advanced care planning may require the involvement of an attorney and/or financial advisor. Attorneys can aid in completing certain forms including power of attorney (POA), trusts, and wills. Financial advisors can help identify ways to help prepare for coming care-related costs by suggesting how to manage finances wisely, discovering other potential financial resources and tax deductions, and avoiding poor investment decisions. Figure 7 shows other considerations in legal and financial planning.

- Planning for health care and long-term care needs including estimates of costs for the entire disease course
- Planning for fiscal management including real estate properties to help cover future health care and living expenses
- Completing POA paperwork to name person able to make decisions in the name of the individual with dementia when they no longer have the capacity to do so

Figure 6-7: Legal and Financial Planning Considerations

Along with person-centered care, many communities are also moving to a community approach. One of the biggest determinants of health is where an individual lives and receives care. In 2009, the World Bank said, "place is the most important correlate of a person's welfare" (World Bank 2009). Individuals living in rural areas are at higher risk of poor outcomes due to the lack of healthcare facilities in general, but especially the lack of specialized care. One example of trying to turn the dial for those living with dementia is dementia-friendly communities.

The goal of dementia-friendly communities is to ensure individuals with dementia are empowered to feel comfortable and confident contributing and participating in community activities that are meaningful to them. Community barriers often exist which prohibit this goal including stigma and lack of understanding about the dementia, as well as lack of appropriate activities for affected individuals. However, the dementia-friendly community model has been shown to reduce health care costs, improve quality of life, and increase community integration for the participants (Alzheimer's Society 2018)

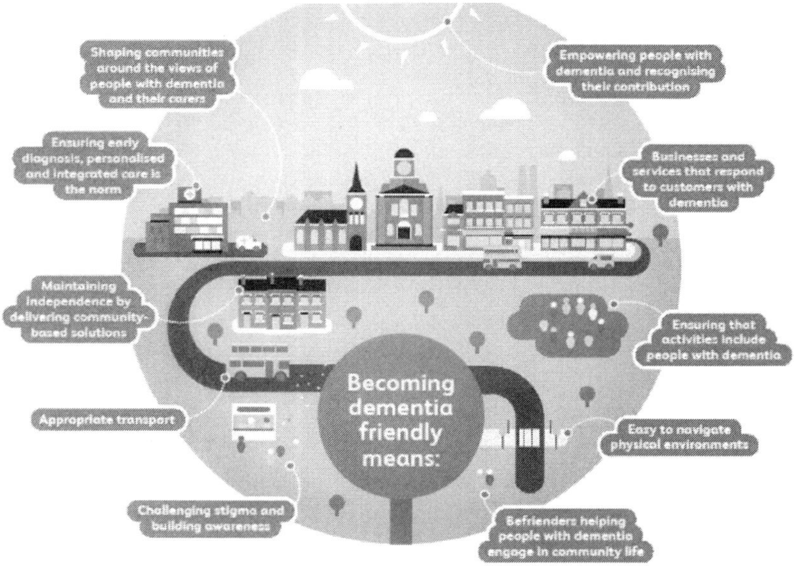

Figure 6-8: Conceptual Model of a Dementia-Friendly Community. (Act on Alzheimer's, n.d.)

After graduating with my nursing degree from St. Olaf College in Minnesota in 2002, I took my first nursing position at Overlake Hospital in Bellevue, Washington, on an ortho/med surg overflow unit. It was on this unit I began to question the way our health system treated older adults. We often cared for post-operative patients following some type of surgical repair of a fracture sustained because of a fall. Once they reached their inpatient goals, they were discharged, many to a rehabilitation facility for further strengthening before ultimately returning home. I saw many of the same patients returning to our unit and wondering why more was not being done to keep them out of the hospital. With each admission, they were down a peg or two before inevitably being admitted to a facility for long term care. As an inpatient nurse, however, I felt there was little I could do to stop this trend.

I therefore decided to go back to obtain a master's degree to become a nurse practitioner. Given my concerns with the care older adults in my community were receiving, I decided to focus on a geriatric specialty. At the time, Duke University had a partnership with the John A. Hartford Foundation to offer full scholarships to nurses pursuing advanced degrees focused on the care of the elderly. The Foundation's vision is "a nation where all older adults receive high-value evidenced-based health care, are treated with respect and dignity, and have their goals and preferences honored." I applied for and was awarded one of these scholarships.

Luckily, after finishing my graduate degree, a position for a nurse practitioner was open in the geriatrics department at Billings Clinic in Billings, Montana. Having grown up in Montana, I was unexpectedly thrilled at the opportunity to return home. At the time, the organization was just launching a Program of All-inclusive Care of the Elderly (PACE) program and I would serve as the primary provider at the site.

PACE honors the vision of the Hartford Foundation and is the gold standard for comprehensive care of older adults at the community level. PACE aims to keep older adults in their home communities and avoid institutionalization using a multidisciplinary, person-centered, and coordinated approach to care. To do that, these programs offer a wide range of services centered around a PACE clinic site. Services include adult day programs, medical visits, nursing care, social service consultation, transportation, and pharmacy support. PACE uses a capitated payment program where all patient care related costs come out of a bucket of money provided by Medicaid and Medicare, or private pay. Once that bucket is spent, the sponsoring organization is responsible for the remaining costs. This gives clear incentives to the healthcare team to keep individuals out of high-cost locations such as the emergency department, hospital, and nursing home. (Center for Consumer Engagement in Health Innovation 2018) PACE helps to balance an individual's desire to remain in the community while promoting health and safety which helps to honor a sense of self and a life of worth and purpose.

Palliative Care

The need for palliative care discussions earlier in the disease process is a recommendation not just for dementia but all care for older adults. One of the biggest health issues of our time is how to balance the amazing medical interventions available to treat serious conditions and potentially prolong life, with the understanding that all humans as we age are naturally on a downhill trend. When is it appropriate to say enough is enough? As Atul Gwande laments in his 2014 book, in this era of healthcare technology in a society that values health and youth, the gradual natural declines of aging are viewed as an embarrassment and weakness instead of the new normal and expected state of affairs as one ages. This philosophy is magnified when an individual also has dementia and the cognitive and functional decline happens more quickly.

The National Consensus Project on Palliative Care (Family Caregiver Alliance 2016) defines palliative care as

> "both a philosophy of care and an organized, highly structured system for delivering care. The goal of palliative care is to prevent and relieve suffering and to support the best possible quality of life for patients and their families, regardless of the stage of the disease or the need for other therapies. Palliative care expands traditional disease-model medical treatments to include the goals of enhancing quality of life for patients and family members, helping with decision making, and providing opportunities for personal growth. Palliative care can be rendered along with life-prolonging treatment or as the main focus of care."

A care model under the palliative care umbrella is hospice care. Hospice is often mistakenly thought of as only to be used at the very end of life. However, hospice is more of a change in focusing on invasive medical treatments in an effort to gain more time, to truly focusing on the now. The goal of hospice is to allow individuals with terminal illness to be as present and comfortable in their remaining days as possible, able to concentrate on what is truly important to them instead of focusing on the next medical intervention or appointment. When crisis happens, instead of fear in not knowing how to handle symptoms and thus going to the emergency room, there are comfort medications provided by hospice and staff on call 24-7 that can also be a source of comfort.

- Alleviating pain or discomfort
- Combating fatigue and loss of appetite
- Improving anxiety, depression, and sleep problems
- Treating nausea and constipation
- Alleviating fears related to living with a serious health condition

Figure 6-9: Focus of Palliative Care

Given the lack of medical treatment options for dementia and the evitable functional and cognitive decline associated with the disease, supporting and encouraging a more palliative approach to care as dementia progresses should be the standard of care. In the end stage of the disease process, most individuals would choose comfort and companionship over an endless stream of medical interventions. This allows our loved ones to die in peace, which produces peace within us as well.

References

Act on Alzheimer's. n.d. "Provider Practice Tools." Accessed October 24,2022. https://actonalz.org/provider-practice-tools.

Alzheimer's Association. 2016. "2016 Alzheimer's Disease Facts and Figures." Accessed October 24, 2022. https://www.alz.org/media/documents/alzheimers-facts-and-figures.pdf.

Alzheimer's Association. 2022. "2022 Alzheimer's Disease Facts and Figures." Accessed October 24, 2022. https://www.alz.org/media/documents/alzheimers-facts-and-figures.pdf.

Alzheimer's Society. 2013. "Building Dementia-friendly Communities: A priority for Everyone." Accessed October 24, 2022. https://dementiapartnerships.com/resource/building-dementia-friendly-communities.

Brown, Rebecca, Leah Goodman, David Guzeman, Lina Tieu, Claudia Ponath, and Margot Kushel. 2016. "Pathways to Homelessness among Older Homeless Adults: Results from the HOPE HOME Study." *PLoS ONE* 11 (5): e0155065. https://doi.org/10.1371/journal.pone.0155065.

Center for Consumer Engagement in Health Innovation. 2018. "Care that Works: Program of All-Inclusive Care for the Elderly (PACE)." Accessed October 24,2022. https://www.healthinnovation.org/resources/publications/care-that-works-pace.

Family Caregiver Alliance. 2016. "Understanding Palliative/Supportive Care: What Every Caregiver Should Know." Accessed October 24, 2022. https://www.caregiver.org/resource/understanding-palliativesupportive-care-what-every-caregiver-should-know/.

Gawande, Atul. 2014. *Being Mortal. Medicine and What Matters in the End.* New York: Macmillian Publishing.

Grand, Jacob, Sienna Caspar, and Stuart McDonald. 2011. "Clinical Features and Multidisciplinary Approaches to Dementia Care." *Journal of Multidisciplinary Healthcare* 4: 125-147. https://doi.org/10.2147/JMDH.S17773.

Montana Alzheimer's Disease/Dementia Workgroup. 2016. "The Montana Alzheimer's and Dementia State Plan: Addressing the Current and Future Needs of Individuals and Families with Alzheimer's Disease and Related Dementias". Accessed October 24, 2022. https://mtalzplan.org/state-plan.

Odenheimer Germaine, Soo Borson, Amy Sanders, Rebecca Swain-Eng, Helen Kyonen, Samantha Tierney, Laura Gitlin, et al. 2004. "Quality Improvement in Neurology: Dementia Management Quality Measures." *Journal of American Geriatrics Society* 62(3): 558-61.

Pinquart Martin, Silvia Sorensen. 2016. "Helping Caregivers of Persons with Dementia: Which Interventions Work and How Large are their Effects?" *International Psychogeriatric* 18(4): 577-95.

Reinhard, Susan, Lynn Feinberg, Rita Choula, and Ari Houser. 2015. "Valuing the Invaluable: 2015 Update." Accessed October 24, 2022. https://www.aarp.org/content/dam/aarp/ppi/2015/valuing-the-invaluable-2015-update-undeniable-progress.pdf

US Census Bureau. 2020. "Demographic Turning Points for the United States: Population Projections for 2020-2060." Accessed October 24, 2022. https://www.census.gov/content/dam/Census/library/publications/2020/demo/p25-1144.pdf

World Bank. 2007. "Reaching the Poor and Vulnerable: Targeting Strategies for Social Funds and other Community-driven Programs." Accessed October 24, 2022. https://web.worldbank.org/archive/website01536/WEB/IMAGES/0711.PDF

7

DEMENTIA IN PATIENTS WITH CANCER: COMPLEXITY, CHALLENGES, AND THE NEED FOR FURTHER RESEARCH

AMINAH JATOI, M.D.[1]

As large segments of the world population grow older – in effect, reach the age of 65 years and beyond – the quandary of learning how best to treat patients who have both dementia and cancer becomes more pressing. A diagnosis of cancer, perhaps more so than other serious illness, when superimposed upon dementia, creates unique challenges for concurrently managing these two very serious diagnoses. Yet, when one considers the growing frequency of the convergence of these two illnesses, particularly in the context of a growing population of older individuals, the available research in this area appears relatively paltry. Furthermore, even younger patients can develop dementia and, of course, younger patients are also diagnosed with cancer. Learning to manage all patients with these two diagnoses is a task that cuts across the spectrum of age and that requires further clinical and research effort.

The challenge and importance of managing cancer and dementia together is underscored by the observation that, in patients with cancer, dementia is associated with poorer survival relative to that observed in the general cancer population. To what extent are these patients' lives shortened? Libert and others provide a preliminary answer to this question. These investigators studied 357 consecutive patients (≥65 years old) with breast, prostate, or colorectal cancer. All were surgical candidates, and all were recruited to the research in a prospective manner [1]. The Montreal Cognitive Assessment was used to assess cognition and a variety of other

[1] Dr. Jatoi is the Betty J. Foust, M.D. and Parents' Professor of Oncology, Department of Oncology, Mayo Clinic, Rochester, Minnesota 55905 USA

baseline variables known to influence cancer survival. One hundred sixty-three patients (46%) had cognitive impairment. This impairment was associated with a notable early demise, generating a hazard ratio (HR) of 6.13 (95% confidence interval): 2.07-18.09; p = 0.001. Other variables related to cognitive impairment, such as patients' loss of autonomy were also associated with reduced survival. Such findings of comparatively poor survival when dementia and cancer occur together have been described by others [2].

Another study from Hopkinson and others provided similar conclusions, emphasizing the pervasive nature of such observations within the published literature [3]. These investigators undertook a systematic review to summarize the literature on cancer treatment and dementia. Providing a comprehensive assessment, these investigators focused on hundreds of studies initially, distilling their efforts to focus on the 9 most relevant of these. Again, these investigators reached similar conclusions as those described above: patients with dementia and cancer do poorly. They are diagnosed with a much more advanced stage of cancer than those patients without dementia, receive less cancer therapy, seem to have higher complication rates from cancer therapy, and, again, manifest worse survival.

How exactly does dementia result in such poor outcomes, including poor survival, in the setting of cancer? The answer to this question is not straightforward but might be answered with a twofold set of observations. First, it is not suprising that other investigators have described that risk factors, such as diabetes and heart disease, predispose to cognitive impairment, as is the case even in a non-cancer setting [4]. Even if one were to argue that cognitive impairment is a direct contributor in its own right to early demise, it must be recognized that dementia tends to comigrate with other health issues, such as diabetes and heart disease, which could also contribute to a more limited survival in patients with these dual diagnoses of cancer and dementia. Thus, it might not be exclusively the dementia that accounts for early demise but rather the possiblity that dementia is a signal of other health problems and that it is the confluence of these other health problems in conjunction with cancer and dementia that give rise to these poor outcomes. Second, as perhaps alluded to above, dementia does appear to influence the decision of whether or not to administer cancer therapy; patients who have dementia receive less aggressive cancer therapy and thereby experience poorer cancer outcomes, although it remains unclear if these poor outcomes are a direct result of compromised cancer therapy.

Martin and others illustrated this latter observation in a large prospective, multicenter study of women who were 70 years of age or older and who had been diagnosed with potentially, surgically resectable breast cancer [5]. A total of 3416 women participated in this study, 478 (14%) of whom had a diagnosis of dementia or cognitive impairment. Notably, 85% of women with normal cognition underwent surgery for breast cancer compared to 74%, 61% and 40% of those who had mild, moderate, and severe cognitive impairment, respectively ($p = 0.001$). Similarly, although not statistically significant, the administraiton of postoperative chemotherapy followed this same pattern: 25% of women with no cognitive impairment received postoperative chemotherapy compared to 20%, 22% and 12% of those who had mild, moderate and severe impairment in cognition, respectively ($p = 0.222$). Patients with cognitive impairment manifested a shorter overall survival, or greater risk of death with a notable hazard ratio: HR: 2.10, 95% CI: 1.77-2.50, $p < 0.001$. Of note, however, these investigators described no statistically significant differences in breast cancer-related survival or cancer progression-free survival -- an observation that raises the question of whether the lower rates of cancer therapy among those patients with cognitive impairement were the real drivers of the compromised cancer outcomes or whether it was the other morbidity and related health factors that were in fact the drivers of poor survival. Suffice it to say these interactions are complex and difficult to untangle, especially from a cause and effect standpoint. And taken together, these two studies in patients with breast cancer suggest that it is perhaps both the underlying morbidity associated with cognitive impairment as well as receipt of cancer therapy (or lack thereof) which together lead to worse outcomes in patients with cancer and dementia. Clearly, such data call for a high-priority agenda that makes sure patients with cancer receive the best possible care – including, if appropriate, limited antineoplastic therapy – to ensure that these patients and their families receive the best possible counseling and subsequent treatment (including non-cancer treatment) and that they are positioned to do as well as they can with these dual diagnoses of cancer and dementia.

Along these lines, Caba and others described an absence of guidelines and underscored the importance of having such guidelines [6]. Having conducted a literature search, these investigators identified 55 relevant studies that enabled them to draw the following salient conclusions. Patients with dementia are more likely to forgo curative therapy and, in fact, are also less likely to receive any cancer therapy, such as chemotherapy, radiation, or surgery. As expected, these patients manifest higher mortality rates compared to patients who had a single diagnosis of cancer with no diagnosis of dementia. Importantly, however, these investigators also reported that qualitative data showed that all stakeholders – patients, their caregivers, and their healthcare providers – all, at times, prefer a less aggressive approach to cancer therapy. This last point underscores the importance of ensuring that patients and their families make good decisions concordant with their wishes about cancer therapy and that all involved believe that the best possible decisions have occurred -- hence, the importance of establishing guidelines to help ensure a balanced, patient-centric approach.

This tension between these diagnoses of dementia and cancer and how to manage this tension is the crux of this clinical challenge. On one hand, all stakeholders ostensibly desire to provide the best care possible to a patient, yet, under circumstances where a patient does not understand the rationale for cancer therapy and its side effects because of dementia, the cancer treatment itself might be viewed as unnecessarily painful, harmful, and perhaps even cruel. Furthermore , the wide spectrum of disease – cancer that might be early stage or late stage or dementia that might manifest as only mild cognitive impairment or more severe cognitive dysfunction – point to one of the major conclusions put forth by Caba and others: guidelines on how to manage these patients are absent and yet very much needed.

So what type of guidelines could help patients with both cancer and dementia? Another important study from Hopkinson and others begins to suggest how this absence of guidelines might be remedied and provides a preliminary answer to the question posed above [7]. Although these investigators did not formally issue guidelines, they did generate relevant preliminary data and suggested clinical areas in need of improvements. These investigators conducted a multisite mixed methods study to better understand the issues at large. Focusing on patients with dementia or milder cognitive impairment and a concurrent cancer diagnosis, these investigators undertook observations in 30 different clinics, witnessing 33 encounters between people with memory problems and medical staff members. These investigators also conducted qualitative interviews to better understand the witnessed patient-healthcare provider encounters and circumstances. This rich set of data prompted these investigators to suggest changes that might improve the experiences of patients with dementia and cancer, as these patients interact with their healthcare providers. As summarized below, these imperative actions are intended for healthcare providers and healthcare facilities and consist of the following: 1) increase awareness among healthcare providers of common problems faced by patients with cognitive impairment, as these patients receive cancer treatment; such common problems could vary from medical center to medical center but perhaps might include working to enable a caregiver to remain with the patient at all times while in a foreign environment such as a medical center; 2) encourage patients and caregivers to disclose to healthcare providers that the patient does in fact have problems with memory; the mere disclosure and statement of the issue will serve as a reminder to healthcare providers to slow down and refrain from making assumptions as medical information is conveyed and explained to the patient and his/her caregiver; 3) provide healthcare providers and their staff the tools and training to identify memory problems in patients, even if the speciality of these healthcare providers is not neurology or psychology; 4) keep tools on hand and accessible in the clinic, such as patients' self-management tools for memory problems; the bridging of resources across medical specialties will make cancer-related conversations easier for patients and their caregivers to hear, to potentially understand, and to potentially retain; and 5) identify ways and resources to support the caregiver because often it is the caregiver who shoulders much of the care and responsibility and who, as a result, needs acknowledgement of the same as well as ongoing help in shouldering the care of the patient and maintaining his/her own health and well being. Perhaps the most interesting aspect of these 5 recommendations, which appear to serve as a stand-in for absent guidelines, is that they are by no means draconian in nature -- for example, these recommendations do not dictate whether cancer therapy should be administered or not. Rather, they are more system- and tool-oriented; they are respectful of the possibility that the decision of whether or not to administer cancer therapy varies widely based on the type of cancer, stage of the cancer, the type of treatment being considered, and, of course, the patient's underlying health and specific circumstances. The real guideline-oriented need is to provide tools, resources, awareness, and a receptive mindset to enable healthcare providers to be open to the needs of specific patients with cancer and dementia.

In addition, to the recommendations described above from Hopkinson and others, Ogawa and others described the importance of integrating the geriatric assessment into the care of older patients who have both cancer and dementia [8]: "Elderly cancer patients undergoing treatment need to be assessed for vulnerability with the comprehensive geriatric assessment (CGA)." Others have also alluded to this aspect of heterogeneity in this population of patients with these dual diagnoses [9]. Indeed, the geriatric assessment, a multidomain assessment tool that helps healthcare providers better understand the capabilities and limitations of a specific patient, has received ongoing widespread interest and has been extensively tested and partially validated [10-12]. The complexity of issues related to implementing the geriatric assessment in a busy clinical practice has also been a point of ongoing discussion. For purposes here, however, the main message is that not all patients with dementia and cancer are the same and that an assessment to gain a sense of severity of the dementia, extent of social support, degree of concomitant symptoms, and insight into several other clinical variables are key to deciding how best – if at all -- to proceed with cancer therapy.

Finally, in attempting to capture the published literature on this topic of cancer and compromised clinical outcomes in patients with dementia, two further points need to be made. First, as alluded to above, the literature on this topic is relatively limited, a situation that leaves open a major unfilled gap that can be filled only with further research. Second, not all patients with dementia and cancer are enrolled in clinical trials and not all have their clinical data included in data bases. By virtue of not having received any cancer therapy, many of these patients are never studied or reported on. As a case in point, we reported on patients who were 90+ years of age, had cancer, and never received cancer therapy [13]. Ninety four patients with a median age 93 years are the focus of this report. Notably, dementia occurred in as many as one-third, making one wonder whether a diagnosis of dementia might have had some influence on the decision to forgo cancer therapy altogether. The main point here is that it is daunting to consider that a sizable proportion of patients – in this case, a third – has dementia, do not receive cancer therapy, and go largely unstudied and underreported in the medical literaure. Yet, there is much we can learn from these patients.

Perhaps the time is now to bring together a renewed interest and focus on these patients with cancer and dementia -- not necessarily with the goal of offering cancer therapy to none, some, or all. But rather the goal would be to increase our understanding of how best to support these patients and their caregivers. Perhaps it is important for healthcare providers and healthcare facilities to do all they can to make sure these patients and their caregivers make decisions on cancer therapy that ultimately result in a sense of peace for all involved.

References

1. Libert, Y., et al. (2016). "Vulnerabilities in Older Patients when Cancer Treatment is Initiated: Does a Cognitive Impairment Impact the Two-Year Survival?" PLoS One **11**(8): e0159734.
2. Robb, C., et al. (2010). "Patterns of care and survival in cancer patients with cognitive impairment." Crit Rev Oncol Hematol **74**(3): 218-224.
3. Hopkinson, J. B., et al. (2016). "People with dementia: what is known about their experience of cancer treatment and cancer treatment outcomes? A systematic review." Psychooncology **25**(10): 1137-1146.
4. Mandelblatt, J. S., et al. (2014). "Cognitive impairment in older patients with breast cancer before systemic therapy: is there an interaction between cancer and comorbidity?" J Clin Oncol **32**(18): 1909-1918.
5. Martin, C., et al. (2021). "Treatment choices for older women with primary operable breast cancer and cognitive impairment: Results from a prospective, multicentre cohort study." J Geriatr Oncol **12**(5): 705-713.
6. Caba, Y., et al. (2021). "The Impact of Dementia on Cancer Treatment Decision-Making, Cancer Treatment, and Mortality: A Mixed Studies Review." JNCI Cancer Spectr **5**(3).
7. Hopkinson, J., et al. (2020). "Potential for identification of memory problems in the cancer clinic to enable improved treatment experience and outcomes: Mixed methods case study research." Eur J Oncol Nurs **48**: 101777.
8. Ogawa, A. (2014). "[Cancer treatment for patients with dementia]." Gan To Kagaku Ryoho **41**(9): 1051-1056.
9. McWilliams, L. (2020). "An Overview of Treating People with Comorbid Dementia: Implications for Cancer Care." Clin Oncol (R Coll Radiol) **32**(9): 562-568.
10. Peil E, Williams GR, Rugo H, Woyach JA, Jatoi A, Le-Rademacher JG. Does the cancer geriatric assessment (GA) introduce bias into clinical trials? Observations from 988 prospectively recruited patients. J Geriatr Oncol. 2022 May;13(4):526-529. doi: 10.1016/j.jgo.2021.12.003. Epub 2021 Dec 15. PMID: 34920971.
11. Guerard E, Dodge AB, Le-Rademacher JG, Kemeny MM, Ojelabi M, Sedrak MS, Hopkins J, Shahrokni A, Harlos E, Muss H, Cohen HJ, Lafky J, Sloan J, Jatoi A, Hurria A. Electronic Geriatric Assessment: Is It Feasible in a Multi-Institutional Study That Included a Notable Proportion of Older African American Patients? (Alliance A171603). JCO Clin Cancer Inform. 2021 Apr;5:435-441. doi: 10.1200/CCI.20.00163. PMID: 33852323; PMCID: PMC8240783.

12. Alliance Cancer in the Older Adult Committee:; Adjei A, Buckner JC, Cathcart-Rake E, Chen H, Cohen HJ, Dao D, De Luca JE, Feliciano J, Freedman RA, Goldberg RM, Hopkins J, Hubbard J, Jatoi A, Karuturi M, Kemeny M, Kimmick GG, Klepin HD, Krok-Schoen JL, Lafky JM, Le-Rademacher JG, Li D, Lichtman SM, Maggiore R, Mandelblatt J, Morrison VA, Muss HB, Ojelabi MO, Sedrak MS, Subbiah N, Sun V, Tuttle S, VanderWalde N, Wildes T, Wong ML, Woyach J. Arti Hurria, M.D.: A tribute to her shining legacy in the Alliance for Clinical Trials in Oncology. J Geriatr Oncol. 2020 Mar;11(2):179-183. doi: 10.1016/j.jgo.2019.05.011. Epub 2019 Jun 11. PMID: 31201095; PMCID: PMC7970716.
13. Wieland, J., et al. (2022). "Understanding "Patient refuses" among 90+ year old patients with cancer or presumed cancer." J Geriatr Oncol.

8

Symptoms Burden and Health Needs of Patients with Dementia in a Low-Income Country – Uganda

Elizabeth Namukwaya[1],
Harriet Nankabirwa[2]
and Amos Deogratius Mwaka[3]

Abstract

Dementia is an increasing health challenge in low- and middle-income countries (LMICs), including Uganda. The rise in the incidence and prevalence of dementia is in parallel with other non-communicable diseases, and many of the risk factors of dementia are similar to those of other non-communicable diseases. Previous studies have shown a wide variation in the prevalence of dementia in African countries and within hospital and community settings. This variation has been attributed to the different tools that are used to identify dementia, most of which have not been validated in the African setting. Early diagnosis of dementia is important, as identifying and promptly treating the reversible causes of dementia and addressing the modifiable risk factors may decrease the rate of progression. In addition, early diagnosis gives a person and their family the opportunity to adjust to the illness and plan for their future. However, dementia is under-recognized, underdiagnosed, and undermanaged in most sub-Saharan African (SSA) countries, including Uganda. Challenges that have been

[1] Department of Medicine, School of Medicine, College of Health Sciences, Makerere University, Kampala, Uganda.

[2] Department of Medicine, Mulago National Super-specialized Hospital, Kampala, Uganda.

[3] Department of Medicine, Faculty of Medicine, Gulu University, Gulu, Uganda.

identified in Uganda regarding the diagnosis and management of dementia include lack of knowledge among healthcare workers, patients, and caregivers on the presentation of the condition (and hence it is thought to be a part of normal aging) and lack of essential drugs for management of dementia in health facilities.

Dementia progresses through three main stages: early, middle, and late stage. In these stages, people have mild, moderate, and severe symptoms, respectively. Dementia is a life-limiting condition and there is a twofold mortality risk among people with dementia, compared to age-matched controls. Dementia leads to dependency in the later stages and affects the quality of life of the people living with it and their caregivers. Palliative care is important in addressing the needs of people living with dementia, as well as their caregivers. Palliative care is applicable at all stages of the condition, with different goals at each stage. In people with mild cognitive impairment, the goal of care is prolongation of life and maintenance of functions, while in moderate and severe disease, the goal of palliative care is maximization of comfort and achieving and maintaining an acceptable quality of life. The goal of care when the patient has died focuses on providing bereavement support for the affected family. Palliative care interventions in people with dementia and their caregivers include person-centered care, appropriate and timely communication, shared decision making, collective setting of care goals, and advanced care planning. The palliative care team often ensures continuity of care, prognostication, and timely recognition of dying, thereby avoiding overly aggressive, burdensome, and futile treatments, while providing optimal treatment of symptoms, comfort, psychosocial and spiritual support, societal and ethical issues, family care and involvement, and education of the healthcare team.

Background

Dementia is a clinical syndrome characterized by a progressive decline in cognitive functions, beyond what might be expected from the usual consequences of biological aging, that interferes with the ability to function independently (Duong et al., 2017; WHO, 2022). Dementia affects memory, thinking, comprehension, calculation, learning capacity, language, judgment, and orientation, but does not affect consciousness. The impairment in cognitive function is commonly associated and sometimes preceded by emotional control problems, and changes in mood, behavior and motivation (WHO, 2022). Dementia is currently the seventh leading cause of death among all diseases globally, and it has major physical, social, economic, and psychological impacts on those living with it, their loved ones, and society. Dementia is a result of diseases or injuries that affect the brain. Alzheimer's disease is the commonest subtype of dementia, accounting for 60%–70% of cases of dementia globally. Other subtypes include vascular dementia, dementia with Lewy bodies, and fronto-temporal dementia (WHO, 2022). Globally, risk factors for dementia include age, physical inactivity, obesity, tobacco use, harmful use of alcohol, hypertension, diabetes mellitus, unbalanced diets, social isolation, low educational level, depression in mid-life, history of stroke, HIV infection, chronic traumatic encephalopathy, and nutritional deficiencies (WHO, 2022; Gauthier et al., 2021). The main risk factor for dementia is advanced age; however, dementia is not exclusively found in the elderly, and about 9% of people have young-age onset of dementia (onset before age sixty-five). On the other hand, people over the age of eighty may have more than one subtype and more than one cause to account for their dementia (Guerchet et al., 2017; Duong et al., 2017; Gauthier et al., 2021).

Burden of Dementia in Uganda

Dementia is an increasing health challenge, affecting both males and females in low- and middle-income countries (LMICs), including countries in Sub-Saharan Africa (SSA). In the last twenty years, over half of the global prevalence of dementia has occurred in LMICs (Livingston et al., 2020; Guerchet et al., 2017). The rapid rise in the burden of dementia in LMICs over the recent decades has been attributed to the aging population and the increase in other risk factors for dementia, including hypertension, diabetes mellitus, dyslipidaemia and peripheral artery disease, homocysteine and folate deficiency, low education levels, having HIV infection, malnutrition, and smoking. Strong evidence has not emerged for other risk factors identified in high-income countries (HIC), such as sex, genetics (no association with the APOE ε4 allele, except in a few West-African countries), in utero exposure to noxious agents, early life psychosocial factors, diet, physical activity, and alcohol (Akinyemi et al., 2022). Increasing age was the main risk factor identified in a systematic review of dementia in SSA and in one study in Uganda (Mubangizi et al., 2020; Akinyemi et al., 2022). A meta-analysis of studies on dementia conducted in SSA showed that the prevalence of dementia in both sexes increased from 1.74% for ages sixty to sixty-four to 23.31% in those aged eighty-five and above (Guerchet et al., 2017). Having formal education, exercising regularly, and having a well-ventilated kitchen were associated with lower prevalence of dementia in the same study (Mubangizi et al., 2020).

Studies in Africa have shown a variation in the prevalence of dementia between and within countries, ranging from 2.3% to 20% in the period of 1995 to 2021 (Akinyemi et al., 2022) with the lower prevalence rates being noted in West Africa and Egypt (Mavrodaris et al., 2013). In Uganda, the prevalence of dementia was found to be 6.3% among 127 hospitalized patients in a national referral hospital in Uganda (Nakasujja et al., 2007), 2.2% among 405 patients in another study conducted in 2021 in another referral hospital in Uganda (Kaddumukasa et al., 2022), and 20% among community-dwelling older adults in Western Uganda (Mubangizi et al., 2020). The huge differences in the prevalence of dementia in different African countries and within the same country, and among hospitalized and community-dwelling older people, have been partly explained by the differences in the tools used and in expertise in the assessment and diagnosis of dementia (Akinyemi et al., 2022). In SSA, it is estimated that 2.15 million people were living with dementia in 2015, and it is projected that there will be 3.48 million people with dementia in the same region by 2030, and 7.62 million by 2050 (Guerchet et al., 2017). The largest increases are expected to occur in East Africa, with the disorder being driven by rapid population growth and aging (Prince et al., 2014). The risk factors for dementia are similar to those of other non-communicable diseases (NCDs), and in SSA the rise in dementia prevalence parallels that of NCDs (Guerchet et al., 2017). In Uganda, the prevalence of some of the risk factors for dementia is increasing; for example, the prevalence of hypertension increased from 26.4% in 2014 to 31.5% in 2018 (Guwatudde et al., 2015; Lunyera et al., 2018). Although there has been a 60% decline in the incidence of new HIV infections in Uganda in the last decade (from 94,000 in 2010 to 38,000 in 2020), the number of people living with HIV has increased from 1.2 million to 1.4 million because of the 61% decline in AIDS-related deaths over the last ten years. The decline in HIV-related mortality has been attributed to the increased number of people receiving antiretroviral therapy (Uganda AIDS Commission, 2021).

It is estimated that people with dementia in SSA have a two-fold increased mortality risk compared to those who do not have it, and the risk of mortality is higher in those with advanced disease (Guerchet et al., 2017). Living in urban areas and malnutrition are associated with increased mortality from dementia in SSA (Ojagbemi et al., 2016). However, data on dementia death are sparse, mainly because death in dementia is often not directly attributable to dementia but to comorbid conditions.

Subtypes of dementia and symptoms of dementia

Confirmation of dementia phenotypes is usually on post-mortem, which is rarely done in most of Sub-Saharan Africa. However, current literature shows that Alzheimer's disease and vascular cognitive impairment and dementia are the commonest phenotypes in Africa. Other dementia phenotypes in Africa include fronto-temporal dementia, dementia with Lewy bodies, Parkinson's disease-related dementia, dementia associated with sickle cell disease, and dementia associated with the Creutzfeldt-Jakob and Huntington diseases (Akinyemi et al., 2022). There is currently limited data on the prevalence of the different subtypes of dementia in Uganda, as the available literature does not make such a differentiation. Symptoms of dementia vary with the stage of the disease but also with the underlying causes and comorbidities and cognitive function before becoming ill.

Generally, there are three stages of dementia: early, middle, and late stages. These are also known as mild, moderate, and severe dementia, respectively. People with early stage dementia are often unnoticed, and they are generally independent, occasionally requiring assistance in just a few aspects of life. Symptoms in this stage include forgetfulness, visual perception difficulties and poor orientation, leading to being lost in familiar environments. These people may find it harder to make complex decisions and or engage in planning; they may also have changes in mood and emotion and may be prone to depression (WHO, 2022; Alzheimer's Association, 2022). The middle stage is easier to recognize, and people in this stage need more support in their activities, such as self-care and hygiene. This is usually the longest stage of dementia. In this phase, forgetfulness worsens, especially of recent events, as well as communication difficulties: people may have difficulty in finding the right words and may stop mid-sentence because they forget what they were trying to say. Problems of orientation may become worse, and they may be confused about the time of the day. At this stage, behavior changes begin to manifest, such as wandering, agitation and restlessness, screaming, disturbed sleep patterns, and loss of social disinhibitions (e.g., saying inappropriate things or undressing in public); delusions, paranoia, and visual and/or auditory hallucinations may also develop. People with dementia with Lewy bodies may have visual hallucinations in early stages (Alzheimer's Association, 2022). Using the toilet may start getting harder at this stage.

The late stage of dementia is one of complete dependency of the person living with the illness on others for personal care and for all activities of daily living including eating, bathing, and dressing. In this stage, life expectancy is limited. This is the shortest stage, lasting about one to two years. Symptoms in this stage include worsening memory, with 'time shifting'—patients may think they are at an earlier period of their life and may even ask for people who died—and they may stop recognizing familiar faces, objects, and even their faces in the mirror because they remember their old self. Communication challenges worsen as their speech may be reduced to a few remembered words or none at all, and they will lose languages they learned later in life if they spoke more than one language. Patients become depressed and apathetic, and delusions and hallucinations become more common. They may become more agitated. They also develop physical problems, such as difficulty in walking, and spend more time in the chair or bed. There is an increased incidence of falls, difficulty in eating and swallowing, and incontinence of urine and stool. Reduced mobility predisposes them to venous thrombosis and pulmonary embolism, which can lead to their death (WHO, 2022; Alzheimer's Association, 2022).

Diagnosis of dementia in low- and middle-income settings

Dementia in SSA, like in other LMICs, is an under-recognized challenge because it is considered to be part of old age by both family and health care professionals (Gauthier et al., 2021). Dementia is also often considered a form of mental illness by most communities in SSA. Therefore, it is often stigmatized and diagnosed in advanced stages, which leads to missed opportunities for treating reversible causes of dementia (e.g., vitamin B12 deficiency, hypothyroidism), with consequent unnecessary suffering for the patients and their families, and a high economic burden that could have been avoided. Guidelines on the assessment of people with probable dementia include taking a medical history, performing a physical examination, and conducting appropriate laboratory tests, functional and behavior assessments, cognitive assessment, and brain imaging (Gauthier et al., 2021). The diagnostic criteria for dementia, based on the *Diagnostic and Statistical Manual of Mental Disorders Fifth Edition* (DSM 5; American Psychiatric Association, 2013) include the presence of the following:

a) Modest or significant cognitive decline in one or more cognitive domains based on observed mild or significant decline, expressed by the individual or a reliable informant, or observed by a clinician.
b) Substantial or modest impairment, documented by objective cognitive assessment. Interference with independence in everyday activities; there may be no interference with independence in

everyday activities, although these activities may require more time and effort, accommodation, or compensatory strategies.

c) Not exclusively during delirium.
d) Not better explained by another mental disorder.
e) Identification of one or more etiologic subtypes of dementia (Hugo and Ganguli, 2014)

A study in Uganda showed that healthcare professionals without mental health training diagnosed dementia based on history and physical examinations, while the majority of healthcare professionals with specialized mental health training were more likely to do neuropsychological testing, laboratory workup, and neuroimaging (Kamoga et al., 2019). Therefore, it is likely that many people with early dementia are not diagnosed or are misdiagnosed, and the reversible causes of dementia not treated promptly. The study by Kamoga et al. (2019) also showed that healthcare professionals regarded dementia as part of normal aging and concentrated on treating other coexisting morbidities but did not treat the dementia. It has also been observed (Akinyemi et al., 2022) that culturally sensitive tools for screening of dementia and functional assessment in this population are lacking. Different tools have been used in research in Africa and have led to inconsistent results that may not be comparable. The brief community screening instrument and the international HIV dementia scale that was developed in Uganda have been used in research in the general population as well as among people living with HIV/AIDS, respectively (Mubangizi et al., 2020; Namagga et al., 2019; Nakku et al., 2013). In clinical practice, the mini-mental status exam and the DSM 5 criteria are usually used by healthcare professionals with mental health training and geriatricians (Kamoga et al., 2019; Nakasujja et al., 2007).

Management of patients with dementia

The usefulness of screening and early diagnosis of dementia has been subject to debate, given that to date there are no effective, disease-modifying agents that can reverse the disease or change its natural history (Fox et al., 2013). The challenges identified with early diagnosis include causing anxiety and ethical concerns related to subjects' privacy and confidentiality. An early diagnosis may impact subjects' ability to find employment, insurance premiums, holding a driving license, and financial management—even when they are perfectly capable of carrying out these activities (Rasmussen and Langerman, 2019). However, the benefits of early diagnosis abound and these include allowing time for the one affected and their loved ones and community to adjust. Also, when the person can still engage with others in early dementia, they can get advice and information on the disease and how to plan for the future and also get access to optimal care and treatment that can allow them to live a substantial number of years with a good quality of life. In some cases of dementia, it may be possible to delay progression of dementia by modifying exposure to common risk factors (Rasmussen and Langerman, 2019).

The overall goal of management of dementia is to reduce the impact of the cognitive decline and delay its progression. This is achieved using both pharmacological and non-pharmacological means. Non-pharmacological means include a healthy diet, adequate sleep, support with personal hygiene, ensuring safety at home and outside, effective communication, supporting psychological well-being, exposing subjects to activities that stimulate cognition (e.g., physical exercise), encouraging social interactions with others, and advice on advance care directives and financial planning. The current pharmacological treatments available for Alzheimer's disease offer limited symptomatic benefit for cognitive symptoms; these medications include acetylcholinesterase inhibitors (e.g., donepezil, rivastigmine, and galantamine). The other class of drugs is the NMDA receptor antagonist (e.g., memantine). Given their limited benefit and side effects, it is important to discuss expectations with patient and family when initiating these medications (Arvanitakis et al., 2019). Rivastigmine can be used in Parkinson's disease dementia. There are no approved drugs for fronto-temporal dementia or dementia with Lewy bodies (Arvanitakis et al., 2019).

The capacity to manage dementia was found to be generally lacking in a review of thirty-two health facilities in Uganda, with significant knowledge gaps regarding its management among healthcare workers. In addition, less than half of the facilities had essential medicines in stock to manage dementia and its symptoms, and only about two in ten facilities had guidelines on the management of dementia (Joloba, 2020; Karungi et al., 2019). Most of the care for people living with dementia should take place in the community. However a study conducted in Uganda showed that village health team workers did not recognize dementia as an illness but as part of the aging process, and only referred people for care if they had another illness (Karungi et al., 2019). Multidisciplinary care is very important in dementia in order to meet the complex needs of those living with the disease. The primary doctors are usually geriatricians and sometimes psychiatrists but given the life-limiting nature of the illness and the impact on caregivers the multidisciplinary team should involve palliative care specialists as well as other specialists including speech therapists, social workers, occupational therapists, and others.

Palliative care for patients with dementia

Palliative care aims at relieving severe health-related suffering for both patients and their families when faced with chronic, life-limiting illnesses such as dementia. This suffering is multidimensional and involves physical, psychological, social, and spiritual/existential aspects of the affected person and their families. Relieving the suffering resulting from loss of one's cognitive abilities should be considered an integral part of care for this condition right from diagnosis. The disease trajectory of dementia is not as straightforward as in most cancers, making it difficult to prognosticate. The course of dementia involves an early phase of minimal cognitive impairment, which progresses to a stage of moderate disability, and then an advanced stage of severe disability and dependence. Survival rates vary, so that some people progress to advanced stages while others die earlier due to dementia-related physical problems, associated psychiatric conditions, accidents, and other associated comorbidities. Dementia-specific palliative care approaches have been proposed because of the different trajectories of decline in dementia (Van der Steen et al., 2014). These approaches include appropriate communication skills, being adept at managing comorbid conditions as well as assessing and managing physical, behavioral, and cognitive problems, and supporting the family (Van der Steen et al., 2014).

Goals of palliative care in dementia

The European Association of Palliative Care (EAPC) recommends goals of palliative care that are tailored to the level of cognitive impairment. In patients with mild cognitive impairment, the goal of care is prolongation of life and maintenance of function, while in moderate and severe disease, the goal of palliative care is maximization of comfort and achieving and maintaining an acceptable quality of life. The goal of care when the patient has died focuses on providing bereavement support for the affected family (Van der Steen et al., 2014). The suggested areas for palliative care in patients with dementia include person-centered care, appropriate and timely communications and shared decision making, collective setting of care goals and advanced care planning, continuity of care, prognostication and timely recognition of dying—and therefore avoiding overly aggressive, burdensome, and futile treatments. The palliative care team aim to provide optimal treatment of symptoms, including providing comfort, psychosocial and spiritual support, family care and involvement, education of the healthcare team, and appropriate coping with societal and ethical issues (Van der Steen et al., 2014). Palliative care for dementia in high-income countries includes support of 'meaningful living', support of family, provision of information for people living with dementia (PLWD), family education and training of healthcare workers, and early advanced care planning (Van der Steen et al., 2014). Understanding context-specific palliative care needs of people with dementia and their families is central in providing patient-centered care and in meeting the above aims. In Uganda and most LMICs, palliative care for patients with dementia is under-developed, partly because geriatrics care is yet an upcoming specialty; in previous years, the population was young, and medical and nursing training was therefore more focused on acute medical conditions and conditions that are more prevalent in younger populations. As a result of this epidemiologic transition, dementia is under-recognized by medical professionals, palliative care needs are not explored, and there is a lack of knowledge about care and treatment; therefore, these people are not referred to palliative care. There is also limited research on palliative care for dementia in Uganda.

Palliative care needs of patients with advanced dementia

Appropriate management of patients with dementia requires systematic assessment and determination of individual patients' diverse needs. These needs include the following:

(i) Need for information

There is evidence of inadequate information about dementia among the population in Uganda, which influences health-seeking when symptoms of dementia arise (Awuol et al., 2022). In a study in south-western Uganda, only 53% of patients or their caregivers sought care in a hospital when they first recognized the symptoms of dementia; the rest went to traditional healers and religious sites of worship and healing because they thought the illness needed supernatural treatment. Even those who went to hospitals first did so because they thought the symptoms were a result of another illness and not dementia. Half of those who first went to hospitals eventually ended up at religious places after the third and fourth visits of seeking care, when they noticed no improvement (Kakongi et al., 2020).

Hallucinations were a common reason for attending religious sites, as they caused people to think they were under demonic attacks. Dementia in the community in Uganda is attributed to chronic diseases such as cancer and syphilis, and being on chronic medication, aging, worrying a lot, misuse of alcohol, tobacco and marijuana, and poverty (Owokuhaisa et al., 2020). Sensitization of the community about dementia was reported to be an important need in a study conducted in western Uganda (Owokuhaisa et al., 2020). Studies in other African countries, including in the Democratic Republic of Congo (DRC) and Tanzania, have shown similar findings of attributing dementia to spiritual causes and seeking care from traditional healers, witchcraft, and churches (Hindley et al., 2017; Kehoua et al., 2019). In DRC and South Africa, people living with dementia (PLWD) are stigmatized and viewed as witches (Mkhonto and Hanssen, 2018). This has led to abuse of PLWD (Khonje et al., 2015, Mkhonto and Hanssen, 2018).

(ii) Need for support with medication management

A systematic review of medicine and management issues of people living with dementia revealed that they often forget their medications, and may under- or overdose themselves and therefore need help with medicine management (Lim and Sharmeen, 2018). There is evidence that in Uganda, patients with dementia have challenges with adherence to medicines because of memory challenges that they experience (Kakongi et al., 2020).

(iii) Communication challenges

Communication difficulties are common among patients with dementia and include difficulty in expressing themselves as well as comprehending what is being said to them. This can cause a lot of frustration for the patients, especially if they cannot express their needs. Caregivers of people living with dementia in Uganda reported that their patients found difficulty explaining their symptoms and needs, which impeded proper diagnosis; hence the need to have proper communication skills and tools that help in symptom assessment (Kakongi et al., 2020). A qualitative study among healthcare workers who cared for people with dementia identified the following as facilitators in communicating with people with dementia: having knowledge about dementia so that one has realistic expectations of what may be achieved in communication; having good communication skills, including building relationships and being able to deal with abnormal behavior; employing appropriate verbal and non-verbal communication strategies (e.g., using simple language, speaking slowly, keeping eye contact); and having a conducive environment in which to communicate (Stanyon et al., 2016).

(iv) Need for rehabilitation services

People with dementia develop gait disorders as the illness progresses and may be prone to falls and require gait rehabilitation to improve mobility and coordinate walking (Gupta et al., 2021). Patients with cognitive disorders can also benefit from rehabilitation, including cognitive training (Gupta et al., 2021). In Uganda, patients in advanced stages of dementia had increasing immobility (Ainamani et al., 2020) and depended on others for mobility. They also required mobility devices such as a walking stick, wheel walkers, or wheelchairs as well as rehabilitation services, including physiotherapy. Exercise programs in dementia can prevent dependency later on as dementia progresses (Zucchella et al., 2018). In another study in Central Africa, mobility problems were present in up to 62.2% of people living with dementia (Mbelesso et al., 2016). A study in Tanzania also showed an association between dementia and disability and mobility challenges (Dotchin et al., 2015).

(v) Need for personal care and protection

As cognitive decline progresses, PLWD may not exercise proper judgment about personal care and may not pay attention to personal hygiene; they also have challenges with bladder or bowel continence. Caregivers of people with dementia in Uganda reported that their patients with advanced dementia had urine and fecal incontinence and that they were unable to independently perform personal care, personal hygiene, or go to the toilet. In addition, they were unable to feed themselves or bathe themselves and needed to be supported for these activities (Owokuhaisa et al., 2020; Ainamani et al., 2020). It was also observed that these patients were at risk of home accidents and injuries, such as cutting or burning themselves when preparing food, and needed support in these activities. They were also at increased risk of infections and poisoning, as they had lost judgment and could eat unhygienic food and food unfit for consumption. When they manifest aggressive behavior, they may cause harm to themselves and others (Wang et al., 2014).

Care homes have been suggested for abandoned PLWD, those who live alone with no caregivers, and those who have no homes (Owokuhaisa et al., 2020). Professional caregivers cited a need for protecting PLWD from abuse, which might take place through rape or by physical abuse, especially if their behavior is not acceptable in the home or in the community. Protection from homicide—by families or the community when PLWD behave abnormally— and also from abandoning of patients alone in houses, is necessary too (Owokuhaisa et al., 2020). In other sub-Saharan communities, such as the Central African Republic, the Democratic Republic of Congo, and South Africa, people with dementia were accused of being witches and this led to being stigmatized; some were physically, psychologically, and financially abused, raising the need for protection (Mbelesso et al., 2016; Mkhonto and Hanssen, 2018; Khonje et al., 2015).

(vi) Need for psychological and emotional support

A diagnosis of dementia causes a great deal of anxiety for the diagnosed person and the family, especially if they have previous experience with it, and also because dementia is considered by many to be a mental illness, which is always stigmatized. A diagnosis of dementia may lead to patients reflecting on their lives and achievements, and may lead to worry about their future. Also, people with dementia face a lot of grief as they lose the ability to perform certain functions such as expressing themselves, remembering their families, and activities such as driving (Alzheimer's Society, 2022). Therefore, there is a need for counseling, peer support, and personal therapy.

Emotional, behavioral, and psychological symptoms are common among patients with dementia. Among patients in Uganda, emotional challenges faced by patients with dementia included anger, crying, loneliness, regret, sadness, self-rejection, hopelessness, suicidal ideation, going naked, and wearing torn clothes. Caregivers reported that PLWD need empathic communication and counseling and to be supported by the family and the community through visiting them and loving them and not blaming them for their disease (Ainamani et al., 2020). A systematic review of psychological and behavioral interventions in LMICs, including African countries, showed that cognitive stimulation therapy and a multidisciplinary cognitive rehabilitation program improved behavioral and psychological symptoms in people with dementia (Stoner et al., 2021).

(vii) Need for access to care and medication

Services for dementia diagnosis and treatment, including medicines for dementia, are often lacking at health services in the community (Owokuhaisa et al., 2020). A survey of health centers in one district in Uganda revealed knowledge gaps about dementia among the healthcare workers, lack of medicines used, and also that in most centers, care for dementia was inexistent (Joloba, 2020). These findings are echoed in other LMICs (Prince et al., 2014). In SSA particularly, there are few specialists who care for people with dementia; task shifting to other healthcare professionals has been suggested as a solution to this challenge (Ferri and Jacob, 2017). A basic dementia care package has been suggested for improvement of care in LMICs that propose integrating dementia care in activities of primary care teams, other chronic diseases, and elderly care programs. This integration process need to include diagnosis, provision of information, regular needs assessments, physical health checks, and caregivers' support and training, and care should have a community outreach component (Prince et al., 2009). Training of community/village health teams to identify dementia cases and refer them for treatment has also been suggested as important in improving access for those who are in the communities (Karungi et al., 2019).

(viii) Need for spiritual support

Spiritual care has been identified as a source of strength and a coping aid for patients and their caregivers in chronic diseases. In high-income countries (HICs), spiritual care has allowed people with dementia to express their faith and religious beliefs and helped them experience connectedness to self, God, and other persons. Spiritual care also confirmed people as valuable and helped them experience meaning in life (Ødbehr et al., 2017). In African settings, studies have shown that spiritual care was sought for with the hope of healing the symptoms of dementia and in an attempt to avert spiritual curses and chase demons thought to cause the symptoms of dementia, especially hallucinations (Kakongi et al., 2020; Owokuhaisa et al., 2020; Kehoua et al., 2019).

Caregiver burden and support for family caregivers of people with dementia

Most people with dementia are cared for by their relatives and other community-based caregivers. However, the demands of care increase as dementia advances, putting more strain on the caregivers. Studies in LMICs have demonstrated the multidimensional impact of caregiving on the caregivers, affecting their health, and financial and social wellbeing (Narayan et al., 2015; Fam et al., 2019; Wang et al., 2014, 2015). In a study conducted in western Uganda, caregivers reported impact in the physical, psychological, and socio-economic domains of their lives. Physical symptoms that developed as a result of caregiving included back strain, fatigue, and body aches. The social impact of caregiving included loss of jobs and conflict with other caregivers who wished to kill the patients by poisoning. There are also serious financial challenges that result from high costs of medications, hospital visits, diapers, and paying non-family caregivers. Caregivers also had to live with the psychological impacts of the illness because dementia was stigmatized; this led to the patients and their families being discriminated against and isolated. Caregivers also reported a lot of anxiety about their loved ones getting lost because patients tended to wander off. They also had difficulty in coping with the responsibilities of caregiving, and some caregivers used maladaptive behaviors, such as smoking and excessive alcohol use (Ainamani et al., 2020b, Ainamani et al., 2020a). A relatively high prevalence of depression has been found among caregivers of people with dementia in other parts of the world(Huang, 2022, Alfakhri et al., 2018).

Approaches to the effective support of caregivers include psychosocial and educational interventions (Australia, 2018). Caregivers should be taught about self-care and encouraged to practice it. This includes maintaining good health with a good diet and regular exercise, being involved in social activities, being able to discuss issues with family or friends who understand the impact of caring for someone with dementia, having enough rest and respite, and having realistic goals. Caregivers should also be encouraged to become more knowledgeable about dementia and its impact on the caregiver, construct a consistent schedule for the person with dementia, and recognize that their difficult behavior is a result of the dementia.

Management of common symptoms and concerns in dementia

(i) Delirium

This is a common symptom found in 54% of people with advanced dementia (Sampson et al., 2018). It is a distressing symptom for both the patient and the family (Ainamani et al., 2020). In this state, the patients may be a danger to themselves and others. Delirium may be precipitated by pain, infections, sensory impairment, side effects of medicines, inadequate sleep, metabolic derangements, constipation, stress, and surgery. Delirium may lead to worsening cognition and may put patients at risk of falls, accidents, and premature mortality (Alzheimer's Society, 2022). Timely diagnosis of delirium is important for improving patient outcomes. Diagnosis involves a detailed history and investigation of the possible risk factors in the patient

(Malhi et al., 2021). Non-pharmacological management is the mainstay of treatment and includes family involvement, speaking calmly, reassurance, medication review, soothing environment and music, adequate hydration, rest, and removal of likely causes. Pharmacological management with atypical antipsychotics should only be considered if patients have serious behavioral disturbances. Benzodiazepines should not be used.

(ii) Pain

Pain is a common symptom among PLWD and is often caused by infections, arthritis, and limited mobility, which results in stiffness and pain in the muscles and joints. Pain was present in 11% and 64% of dementia patients in the UK, at rest and during movement, respectively (Sampson et al., 2018). Advanced dementia has a higher prevalence of severe pain (Hendriks et al., 2015). Pain may precipitate agitation, depression, and abnormal behavior if not promptly and adequately treated. There are challenges in pain assessment in this population because of patients' communication difficulties and loss of executive functions and memory. Caregivers in Uganda reported that their patients found it difficult to explain where their pains were (Ainamani et al., 2020). The Pain Assessment in Advanced Dementia tool (PAINAD) is a behavioral tool that is used in this population (Malhi et al., 2021; Eisenmann et al., 2020). Pain management involves use of pharmacological agents such as paracetamol and non-steroidal anti-inflammatory drugs; however, caution should be used as they may have side effects. Non-pharmacological means such as massage and physiotherapy are also useful.

(iii) Feeding problems

Eating and drinking problems are common in advanced dementia and lead to weight loss (Sampson et al., 2018). Therefore, there is need for support with eating and drinking. Eating and drinking problems may result from deteriorating cognitive functions, depression, or poor oral hygiene, leading to mouth ulcers. PLWD also have swallowing problems, which can lead to aspiration pneumonia. Care involves educating caregivers on mouth care, offering preferred foods, and feeding in the upright position to avoid aspiration (Eisenmann et al., 2020). There is no evidence that feeding tubes improve functional status or reduce aspiration; however, they can cause pain and are associated with greater health care use because of tube related complications, they lead to agitation that may require physical or chemical restraints and are associated with recurrent aspiration and development of new pressure sores, therefore they are not recommended (American Geriatrics Society Ethics Committee and clinical Practice and Models of care Committee, 2014) .

(iv) Mouth care

As cognitive decline progresses in moderate and advanced dementia, people may pay less attention to oral hygiene, which predisposes them to periodontal diseases. In addition, they may be on medications that cause dry mouth (e.g., tricyclic antidepressants). Poor oral hygiene and dry mouth predispose to stomatitis and oral ulcers. All these problems will cause difficulty in chewing, swallowing, and pain on eating (Eisenmann et al., 2020). Therefore, it is important for caregivers to support with oral hygiene.

(v) Dyspnea

Dyspnea is common in PLWD close to death, and the causes usually include respiratory infections, comorbidities such as heart failure, functional decline, fatigue and frailty, and side effects of treatments. Treatment involves management of reversible causes, and where possible, the use of non-pharmacological interventions including respiratory exercises, circulating air to the face (fan or fresh air), positioning and breathing techniques, and providing oxygen when oxygen saturation is critically low. Opioids can be used to improve the sensation of breathlessness (Australia, 2018; Eisenmann et al., 2020).

(vi) Constipation, and stool and urine incontinence

Constipation is a common symptom in older people and can be caused by reduced peristalsis (caused by aging), anal disorders, dehydration, electrolyte disorders, comorbid conditions such as hypothyroidism, and medications including diuretics, opioids, antidepressants, and some antihypertensives. The risk is even higher in patients with dementia, who may delay the urge to go to the toilet because of difficulty in remembering where the toilet is or in removing their clothes or due to failure to communicate that they want to use the toilet. Constipation can lead to pain, fecal incontinence, anal fissures, fecal impaction, and bowel obstruction (Alzheimer's Society, 2022). In a study in the United Kingdom, the prevalence of constipation among dementia patients was 13% (Sampson et al., 2018). Therefore, it is important to ensure bowel care to prevent constipation. This should be individualized based on patients' bowel habits.

Management includes non-pharmacological methods such as ensuring adequate intake of fluids and fibers, and encouraging mobility. Laxatives should be used in those with constipation and as prophylaxis for those on opioids (Australia, 2018). In advanced dementia, there may be a disconnect between the neurological signals that raise awareness of a full rectum and the nerve-muscle responses that control defecation, leading to incontinence. Bowel incontinence has been found to be up to four-folds greater in people with dementia compared to a matched sample without dementia, with a prevalence of 30%–50% in dementia care homes. Fecal incontinence affects people's quality of life negatively (Goodman et al., 2017). Bladder incontinence is also common. Incontinence may be caused by a person forgetting to use the toilet, by side effects of medicines (e.g., diuretics), urinary tract infections, constipation, prostate problems, stroke, diabetes mellitus, a disability which prevents the PLWD from reaching the toilet, and wearing clothes which are difficult to remove (Alzheimer's Association, 2022). Strategies to help with incontinence include prompted and scheduled toileting, habit training, establishing a bowel program, pelvic floor exercises if possible, not limiting fluid intake unless there are medical indications, diet adjustments, review of medications that may cause incontinence, support emptying rectum if there is fecal impaction, and use of absorbent products at night for night incontinence (National Institute on Ageing, 2021).

(vi) Pressure injuries and ulcers

Older people are at a high risk of pressure sores, and this risk is even greater among those with advanced dementia because of reduced mobility, poor nutrition, incontinence, frailty, failure to communicate when they want to move, agitation and rubbing skin on bed causing skin injuries, and medications that cause skin drying and drowsiness (National Institute on Ageing, 2021). Prevention of pressure injuries involves actively inspecting the skin when cleaning the patients for signs of early pressure sores, encouraging patients to move about regularly, turning the patients in bed regularly, and teaching caregivers how to move patients safely, keeping patients dry, providing good nutrition, and avoiding tight-fitting clothing (National Institute on Ageing, 2021). If pressure sores develop, an effort should be made to turn patients regularly and use pressure relief devices. Pressure sites are usually painful, and pain medication should be given. Clinicians need to regularly assess for signs of infections and promptly treat the infections if present. Clinicians should refer to guidelines of management of pressure ulcers.

(vii) Multi-morbidity in patients with advanced dementia

Dementia is associated with multi-morbidity in both HICs and LMICs, including Africa (Guerchet et al., 2020). However, a study in Uganda did not find this association, probably because of a small sample size (Mubangizi et al., 2020). Secondly, it is not uncommon for older people in the LMICs to live with undiagnosed chronic illnesses, and this may lead to underestimation of multi-morbidity in these settings. Common multi-morbidities that have been identified in people with dementia include diabetes mellitus, chronic obstructive pulmonary disorders (COPD), chronic heart failure, vascular diseases, and musculoskeletal disorders (Lee et al., 2009; Schubert et al., 2006). There is a complex relationship between these entities: multi-morbidity in early or mid-adulthood is associated with an increased risk for dementia. On the other hand, dementia may predispose to comorbidities, including osteoporosis and fractures, and this may alter the natural history of the comorbid conditions (Hassen et al., 2022). Multi-morbidity is associated with poorer outcomes (poor functional status, accelerated decline in health, poor quality of life, poly-pharmacy and related drug side effects, and frequent hospitalizations (Welsh, 2019; Melis et al., 2013).

(viii) Appropriate use of medicines among patients with advanced dementia

Poly-pharmacy is common among dementia patients in both HICs and LMICs, and several studies have shown the association between the two (Park et al., 2017; Mueller et al., 2018; de Lima et al., 2020). Multiple medications in dementia patients may lead to further cognitive and intellectual decline, falls, and death (Chippa and Roy, 2022; National Institute on Ageing, 2021). In general, anticholinergics and medicines that cause anticholinergic side effects—including antidepressants, antipsychotics, antihistamines, anti-Parkinson agents, and smooth and skeletal muscle relaxants—should be avoided in dementia. People with dementia have reduced acetylcholine, so that anticholinergics make this worse, leading to further cognitive decline. In addition, anticholinergics may also lead to falls.

The following conditions are common among people with dementia, and caution should be employed when treating them because some common medicines used to treat such conditions may be harmful to people with dementia:

a) Delusions, hallucinations, agitation, and aggression

Neuropsychiatric symptoms are common among dementia patients, and clinicians tend to prescribe for them antipsychotic drugs. However, the risk-benefit ratio for the use of antipsychotic medicines in Alzheimer's dementia is high because they lead to accelerated cognitive and functional decline, and potentially cause more morbidities (for example, may accelerate heart diseases), and are also associated with increased mortality and sudden death, while not making much difference in symptom control. It is recommended to conduct a thorough assessment to rule out other causes of these symptoms, and to use non-pharmacological means to manage the symptoms first, before considering medications (Lauretani et al., 2020; Masopust et al., 2018).

Memory medications and antidepressants can be helpful with hallucinations and agitation and are considered first-line medications. However, if the first-line medicines fail, atypical antipsychotics such as quetiapine, olanzapine, and risperidone should be considered. Low doses of antipsychotics may also be used as first-line medications in managing delusions and hallucinations in people with fronto-temporal dementia and dementia with Lewy bodies. However, first-generation antipsychotics such as haloperidol and chlorpromazine should be avoided in those with muscle stiffness because they worsen the condition, and they also worsen thinking, impair movement, and are associated with stroke and death. Non-pharmacological treatments should always be employed, including music therapy and physical therapy, in addition to exploring and managing the causes of the neuropsychiatric symptoms, such as infections (UCSF Institute for Neurosciences, 2022).

b) Anxiety treatment

In the management of anxiety and related disorders, clinicians need to avoid benzodiazepines and anticholinergics because they cause more confusion and increase the risk of falls and sedation; if these medicines have to be used, then clinicians need to use the smallest amount for the shortest amount of time. Safer medicines for anxiety include citalopram, escitalopram, and mirtazapine (Masopust et al., 2018; UCSF Institute for Neurosciences, 2022).

c) Insomnia

Assess and diagnose causes of insomnia, such as pain, anxiety, depression, and diabetes mellitus causing polyuria and sleep disturbance. Avoid benzodiazepines, zolpidem, and drugs containing diphenhydramine. Safer options include melatonin, low-dose mirtazapine, and low-dose trazodone (UCSF Institute for Neurosciences, 2022).

d) Depression

Assess and treat causes of depression and also use non-pharmacological means of care. Selective serotonin reuptake inhibitors (SSRIs) are most commonly used in dementia to improve apathy, mood, and aggressive impulses. However, it is important to note that fluoxetine in particular should be avoided because of the multiple-drug interactions and long half-life. Other antidepressants that should be avoided because of their anticholinergic effects (worsening of cognitive function, vision impairment, dizziness, lead to falls) include amitriptyline, nortriptline, and paroxetine (UCSF Institute for Neurosciences, 2022; Masopust et al., 2018).

e) Pain

Many analgesics used in the elderly with dementia cause adverse effects and some directly affect memory. Opioid analgesics and muscle relaxants can worsen memory and thinking and may lead to constipation, dry mouth, dizziness, drowsiness, and falls. Non-steroidal anti-inflammatory drugs may lead to gastrointestinal bleeding and precipitate or worsen heart failure. Therefore, if the above classes of medicines must be used, they should be used at the lowest effective dose and for a short duration. Paracetamol, non-pharmacological methods of pain control, and topical analgesics should be used more in these patients. Selective Noradrenaline Reuptake Inhibitors (SNRIs) such as duloxetine and venlafaxine may be useful for neuropathic pain in these patients (UCSF Institute for Neurosciences, 2022).

Advance directives and decision-making among patients with advanced dementia

Advance care planning (ACP) is very essential in people with dementia to ensure their wishes are met when they lose their decision-making capacity. The availability of an advance care plan also helps to reduce the stress on caregivers of having to make difficult decisions for patients who may have lost their mental capacity. Advance care plans must be prepared early on in the disease trajectory, when the person is still able to participate in the decision-making process (Malhi et al., 2021). Examples of advance care planning documentation are informal statements of wishes and preferences (e.g., place of care and death), a formal advance decision to refuse treatment, and medical power of attorney. It is important to discuss these issues with patients and families early on. Patients may choose a medical power of attorney who will make health decisions for them and who is aware of their wishes. Early referral for palliative care (PC) helps to achieve this and helps prevent unrequired aggressive futile treatments at end of life. Unfortunately, for many people with dementia, conversations on ACP do not take place with the patients because they are often referred late to palliative care and also because some patients may not be willing to discuss these issues. There is evidence that ACP reduces depression, improves quality of life, reduces hospitalisations, leads to adherence to patients and family wishes at end of life and reduces conflict in decision making (Wendrich-van Dael et al., 2020) and that general practitioners (GPs) can be trained to support ACP (Australia, 2018).

Terminal stage and end-of-life care in patients with advanced dementia

The symptoms and signs that may indicate the terminal stage of dementia include loss of ability to communicate meaningfully, difficulty in swallowing and poor nutritional intake, bowel and bladder incontinence, recurrent episodes of infection, sleeping most of the time, high risk of pressure injury, and inability to change position, sit unsupported, and hold head up and smile (Australia, 2018). The dying phase is the last phase of the terminal stage. The signs of imminent dying include noisy respirations, aspirations due to loss of gag reflex with inability to clear oral and tracheal secretions, abnormal breathing patterns such as apnea episodes, Cheyne-Stokes respirations, agonal breathes, agitation, reduced level of consciousness, peripheral and central cyanosis, and mottling of the skin. The goals of care in this phase are comfort and dignity for the person with dementia, providing a supportive environment for the family and staff, and providing required information and psychological support. It is important to assess for and manage the symptoms that are causing distress. Nursing care is also needed, in particular eye care, mouth care, and prevention of pressure injuries to the skin. Family involvement in care helps to maintain connection with the dying person. At this stage, the route of drug administration may need to change to parenteral routes because patients may not be able to swallow safely or swallow at all. Pain medications should be converted to an equivalent parenteral dose for patients already taking opioids, and for opioid-naïve patients these doses are dependent on the patient's age and comorbidities. In older, frail patients, the starting dose should be smaller than that usually given in other older adults.

People with dementia have a higher risk of mortality than those without it, and previous researches have shown that their survival term ranges between three to ten years from the diagnosis of dementia (Brodaty et al., 2012). In the Democratic Republic of Congo, a prospective study that followed older patients for up to two years showed that the risk of death was two and a half times higher in those with dementia than those without. An advanced clinical stage of dementia at diagnosis was associated with shorter prognosis (Samba et al., 2016). In other studies, other factors associated with survival in patients with dementia include age, sex, co-existing conditions, and type of dementia. A systematic review of prognostic indicators of six-month mortality for people with advanced dementia found that decreased appetite, insufficient food intake, malnutrition, weight loss and anorexia, and comorbidities and reduced function were common prognosticators identified across studies (Brown et al., 2013). The FAST score is used to assess the level of function among patients; for people with a score of 7C (cannot walk or sit without assistance and limited speech) and above, the survival term is estimated at six months or less (Sclan and Reisberg, 1992).

References

Ainamani, h. E., Alele, p. E., Rukundo, g. Z., Maling, s., Wakida, e. K., Obua, c. & Tsai, a. C. 2020. Caring for people with dementia in rural Uganda: qualitative study of caregiving burden experienced by informal and formal caregivers. *Journal of global health reports,* 4 (2020).

Ainamani, Herbert E., Paul E. Alele, Godfrey Z. Rukundo, Samuel Maling, Edith K. Wakida, Celestino Obua, and Alexander C. Tsai. "Caregiving burden and mental health problems among family caregivers of people with dementia in rural Uganda." *Global Mental Health* 7 (2020).

Akinyemi, R. O., Yaria, J., Ojagbemi, A., Guerchet, M., Okubadejo, N., Njamnshi, A. K., Sarfo, F. S., Akpalu, A., Ogbole, G & Ayantayo, t. 2022. Dementia in Africa: Current evidence, knowledge gaps, and future directions. *Alzheimer's & Dementia,* 18, 790-809.

Alfakhri, Abdullelah S., Ahmed W. Alshudukhi, Ali A. Alqahtani, Abdulrahman M. Alhumaid, Omer A. Alhathlol, Abdullah I. Almojali, Muteb A. Alotaibi, and Meshal K. Alaqeel. "Depression among caregivers of patients with dementia." *INQUIRY: The Journal of Health Care Organization, Provision, and Financing* 55 (2018): 0046958017750432.

Alzheimer's Association. 2022. *Incontinence* [Online]. Available: https://www.alz.org/help-support/caregiving/daily-care/incontinence [Accessed 14/11/2022 2022].

Alzheimer'sSociety. 2022. *The psychological and emotional impact of dementia* [Online]. Available: https://www.alzheimers.org.uk/get-support/help-dementia-care/understanding-supporting-person-dementia-psychological-emotional-impact#

American Geriatrics Society Ethics Committee and Clinical Practice and Models of Care Committee. "American Geriatrics Society feeding tubes in advanced dementia position statement." *Journal of the American Geriatrics Society* 62, no. 8 (2014): 1590-1593.

American Psychiatric Association. (2013). Diagnostic and statistical manual of mental disorders (5th ed.). https://doi.org/10.1176/appi.books.9780890425596

Arvanitakis, A., Shah, R. C. & Bennett, D. A. 2019. Diagnosis and management of dementia. *Jama,* 322**,** 1589-1599.

Australia, p. C. 2018. Palliative care and dementia. *Dementia Australia paper*.

Guerchet, M. M., Gbessemehlan, A., Mbelesso, P., Bandzouzi, B. N., YaffE, K., Clement, J. P., Dartigues, J. F., Preux, P. M. & Epidemca 2020. Multimorbidity as a correlate of dementia among older people in Central Africa: The EPIDEMCA study: New insights in determinants of dementia to advance prevention strategies: A view from Latin America and African countries. *Alzheimer's & Dementia,* 16**(**2020**):** e038315.

Awuol, Machuor Daniel Arok, Besigye K. Innocent, and Ayenyo Winfred. "Prevalence, Factors Associated and Knowledge of Dementia in a Sample of Older Ugandans." (2022).

Brodaty, Henry, Katrin Seeher, and Louisa Gibson. "Dementia time to death: a systematic literature review on survival time and years of life lost in people with dementia." *International psychogeriatrics* 24, no. 7 (2012): 1034-1045.

Brown, Meghan A., Elizabeth L. Sampson, Louise Jones, and Anna M. Barron. "Prognostic indicators of 6-month mortality in elderly people with advanced dementia: a systematic review." *Palliative medicine* 27, no. 5 (2013): 389-400.

Chippa V, Roy K. Geriatric Cognitive Decline and Polypharmacy. In: StatPearls. StatPearls Publishing, Treasure Island (FL); 2022. PMID: 34662089.

de Lima, Juliana Dias, Ivan Abdalla Teixeira, Felipe de Oliveira Silva, and Andrea Camaz Deslandes. "The comorbidity conditions and polypharmacy in elderly patients with mental illness in a middle income country: a cross-sectional study⋆." *IBRO reports* 9 (2020): 96-101.

Dotchin, Catherine L., Stella-Maria Paddick, William K. Gray, Aloyce Kisoli, Golda Orega, Anna R. Longdon, Paul Chaote, Felicity Dewhurst, Matthew Dewhurst, and Richard W. Walker. "The association between disability and cognitive impairment in an elderly Tanzanian population." *Journal of epidemiology and global health* 5, no. 1 (2015): 57-64.

Duong, Silvia, Tejal Patel, and Feng Chang. "Dementia: What pharmacists need to know." *Canadian Pharmacists Journal/Revue des Pharmaciens du Canada* 150, no. 2 (2017): 118-129.

Eisenmann, Yvonne, Heidrun Golla, Holger Schmidt, Raymond Voltz, and Klaus Maria Perrar. "Palliative care in advanced dementia." *Frontiers in Psychiatry* 11 (2020): 699.

Fam, Johnson, Rathi Mahendran, and Ee Heok Kua. "Dementia care in low and middle-income countries." *Current opinion in psychiatry* 32, no. 5 (2019): 461-464.

Ferri, Cleusa Pinheiro, and K. S. Jacob. "Dementia in low-income and middle-income countries: different realities mandate tailored solutions." *PLoS medicine* 14, no. 3 (2017): e1002271.

Fox, Chris, Louise Lafortune, Malaz Boustani, and Carol Brayne. "The pros and cons of early diagnosis in dementia." *British Journal of General Practice* 63, no. 612 (2013): e510-e512.

Gauthier, Serge, Pedro Rosa-Neto, J. A. Morais, and Claire Webster. "World Alzheimer Report 2021: Journey through the diagnosis of dementia." *Alzheimer's Disease International* (2021).

Goodman, Claire, Christine Norton, Marina Buswell, Bridget Russell, Danielle Harari, Rowan Harwood, Brenda Roe et al. "Managing Faecal INcontinence in people with advanced dementia resident in Care Homes (FINCH) study: a realist synthesis of the evidence." *Health Technology Assessment (Winchester, England)* 21, no. 42 (2017): 1-219.

Guerchet, Maelenn Mari, Rosie Mayston, Peter Lloyd-Sherlock, Martin James Prince, Isabella Aboderin, Rufus Akinyemi, Stella-Maria Paddick et al. "Dementia in sub-Saharan Africa: challenges and opportunities." (2017).

Gupta, Anupam, Naveen B. Prakash, and Gourav Sannyasi. "Rehabilitation in dementia." *Indian Journal of Psychological Medicine* 43, no. 5_suppl (2021): S37-S47.

Hassen, C. B., Fayosse, A., Landré, B, Raggi, M., Bloomberg, M., Sabia, S. & Singh-manoux, A, Association between age at onset of multimorbidity and incidence of dementia: 30 year follow-up in Whitehall II prospective cohort study. *bmj,* 376 (2022).

Guwatudde, David, Gerald Mutungi, Ronald Wesonga, Richard Kajjura, Hafisa Kasule, James Muwonge, Vincent Ssenono, and Silver K. Bahendeka. "The epidemiology of hypertension in Uganda: findings from the national non-communicable diseases risk factor survey." *PloS one* 10, no. 9 (2015): e0138991.

Hendriks, Simone A., Martin Smalbrugge, Francisca Galindo-Garre, Cees MPM Hertogh, and Jenny T. van der Steen. "From admission to death: prevalence and course of pain, agitation, and shortness of breath, and treatment of these symptoms in nursing home residents with dementia." *Journal of the American Medical Directors Association* 16, no. 6 (2015): 475-481.

Hindley, Guy, John Kissima, Lloyd L. Oates, Stella-Maria Paddick, Aloyce Kisoli, Christine Brandsma, William K. Gray, Richard W. Walker, Declare Mushi, and Catherine L. Dotchin. "The role of traditional and faith healers in the treatment of dementia in Tanzania and the potential for collaboration with allopathic healthcare services." *Age and Ageing* 46, no. 1 (2017): 130-137.

Huang, Si-Sheng. "Depression among caregivers of patients with dementia: Associative factors and management approaches." *World Journal of Psychiatry* 12, no. 1 (2022): 59.

Hugo, Julie, and Mary Ganguli. "Dementia and cognitive impairment: epidemiology, diagnosis, and treatment." *Clinics in geriatric medicine* 30, no. 3 (2014): 421-442.

Joloba, Stephen Samuel. "Capacity of the health facilities to manage Alzheimer's and related dementia diseases in Mukono district: Challenges and recommendations: Improving dementia care within health systems." *Alzheimer's & Dementia* 16 (2020): e038904.

Kaddumukasa, Mark, Felix Bongomin, Levicatus Mugenyi, Micheal Kiyingi, Elly Katabira, and Martha Sajatovic. "Cognitive functioning and prevalence of seizures among older persons in Uganda: A hospital-based, cross-sectional study." *Medicine* 101, no. 41 (2022): e31012.

Lee, P. G., Cigolle, C. & Blaum, C. 2009. The co-occurrence of chronic diseases and geriatric syndromes: The Health and Retirement Study. *Journal of the American Geriatrics Society,* 57, 511-516.

Kakongi, Nathan, Godfrey Zari Rukundo, Bizu Gelaye, Edith K. Wakida, Celestino Obua, and Elialilia S. Okello. "Exploring pathways to Hospital Care for Patients with Alzheimer's disease and related dementias in rural

South Western Uganda." *BMC health services research* 20, no. 1 (2020): 1-12.

Kamoga, Ronald, Godfrey Z. Rukundo, Edith K. Wakida, Gladys Nakidde, Celestino Obua, and Stephanie S. Buss. "Dementia assessment and diagnostic practices of healthcare workers in rural southwestern Uganda: a cross-sectional qualitative study." *BMC Health Services Research* 19, no. 1 (2019): 1-7.

Karungi, Christine, Celestino Obua, Godfrey Zari Rukundo, Samuel Maling, Jessica E. Haberer, and Edith K. Wakida. "Community-based management and care of people with dementia: A training needs assessment among village health teams in Uganda based on WHO guidelines." (2019).

Kehoua, Gilles, Catherine-Marie Dubreuil, Bébène Ndamba-Bandzouzi, Maëlenn Guerchet, Pascal Mbelesso, Jean-François Dartigues, and Pierre-Marie Preux. "People with dementia in sub-Saharan Africa: from support to abuse by caregivers: results of EPIDEMCA-FU program in Congo." *Dementia and geriatric cognitive disorders extra* 9, no. 1 (2019): 163-175.

Khonje, V., C. Milligan, Y. Yako, M. Mabelane, K. E. Borochowitz, and C. A. De Jager. "Knowledge, attitudes and beliefs about dementia in an urban Xhosa-speaking community in South Africa." *Advances in Alzheimer's Disease* 4, no. 02 (2015): 21.

Lauretani, Fulvio, Giuseppe Bellelli, Giovanna Pelà, Simonetta Morganti, Sara Tagliaferri, and Marcello Maggio. "Treatment of delirium in older persons: what we should not do!" *International Journal of Molecular Sciences* 21, no. 7 (2020): 2397.

Lim, Rosemary H., and Taniya Sharmeen. "Medicines management issues in dementia and coping strategies used by people living with dementia and family carers: a systematic review." *International Journal of Geriatric Psychiatry* 33, no. 12 (2018): 1562-1581.

Livingston, Gill, Jonathan Huntley, Andrew Sommerlad, David Ames, Clive Ballard, Sube Banerjee, Carol Brayne et al. "Dementia prevention, intervention, and care: 2020 report of the Lancet Commission." *The Lancet* 396, no. 10248 (2020): 413-446.

Lunyera, Joseph, Bruce Kirenga, John W. Stanifer, Samuel Kasozi, Thys van der Molen, Wenceslaus Katagira, Moses R. Kamya, and Robert Kalyesubula. "Geographic differences in the prevalence of hypertension in Uganda: Results of a national epidemiological study." *PloS one* 13, no. 8 (2018): e0201001.

Malhi, Raja, Jennifer McElveen, and Linsey O'Donnell. "Palliative Care of the Patient with Dementia." *Delaware Journal of Public Health* 7, no. 4 (2021): 92.

Mavrodaris, Angelique, John Powell, and Margaret Thorogood. "Prevalences of dementia and cognitive impairment among older people in sub-Saharan Africa: a systematic review." *Bulletin of the World Health Organization* 91 (2013): 773-783.

Mbelesso, Pascal, Angélique Faure-Delage, Maelenn Mari Guerchet, Bébène Ndamba-Bandzouzi, Alain M. Mouanga, André Tabo, Leslie Cartz-Piver, Pierre-Marie Preux, Jean-Pierre Clément, and Philippe Nubukpo. "Social aspects of dementia in Central Africa (EDAC survey): Les aspects sociaux de la demences en Afrique Centrale (etude EDAC)." *African Journal of Neurological Sciences* 35, no. 1 (2016).

Masopust, Jiří, Dita Protopopová, Martin Vališ, Zbyšek Pavelek, and Blanka Klímová. "Treatment of behavioral and psychological symptoms of dementias with psychopharmaceuticals: a review." *Neuropsychiatric disease and treatment* 14 (2018): 1211.

Melis, Rene JF, Alessandra Marengoni, Debora Rizzuto, Steven Teerenstra, Miia Kivipelto, Sara B. Angleman, and Laura Fratiglioni. "The influence of multimorbidity on clinical progression of dementia in a population-based cohort." *PloS one* 8, no. 12 (2013): e84014.

Mkhonto, Flora, and Ingrid Hanssen. "When people with dementia are perceived as witches. Consequences for patients and nurse education in South Africa." *Journal of clinical nursing* 27, no. 1-2 (2018): e169-e176.

Mubangizi, V., Maling, S., Obua, C. & Tsai, A. C. 2020. Prevalence and correlates of Alzheimer's disease and related dementias in rural Uganda: cross-sectional, population-based study. *BMC geriatrics,* 20**,** 1-7.

Mueller, Christoph, Mariam Molokhia, Gayan Perera, Nicola Veronese, Brendon Stubbs, Hitesh Shetty, David Codling, Jonathan Huntley, and Robert Stewart. "Polypharmacy in people with dementia: associations with adverse health outcomes." *Experimental gerontology* 106 (2018): 240-245.

Namagga, Jane Kasozi, Godfrey Zari Rukundo, and Joachim G. Voss. "Prevalence and risk factors of HIV-associated neurocognitive disorders in rural Southwestern Uganda." *The Journal of the Association of Nurses in AIDS Care: JANAC* 30, no. 5 (2019): 531.

Nakasujja, Noeline, Seggane Musisi, James Walugembe, and Daphne Wallace. "Psychiatric disorders among the elderly on non-psychiatric wards in an African setting." *International psychogeriatrics* 19, no. 4 (2007): 691-704.

Nakku, Juliet, Eugene Kinyanda, and Susan Hoskins. "Prevalence and factors associated with probable HIV dementia in an African population: a cross-sectional study of an HIV/AIDS clinic population." *BMC psychiatry* 13, no. 1 (2013): 1-7.

Narayan, Suzanne M., Mathew Varghese, Kenneth Hepburn, Marsha Lewis, Isabel Paul, and Rozina Bhimani. "Caregiving experiences of family members of persons with dementia in south India." *American Journal of Alzheimer's Disease & Other Dementias®* 30, no. 5 (2015): 508-516.

NationalInstituteOnAgeing. 2021. *The dangers of polypharmacy and the case of deprescribing in older adults* [Online]. Available: https://www.nia.nih.gov/news/dangers-polypharmacy-and-case-deprescribing-older-adults [Accessed 14/11/2022 2022].

Ødbehr, Liv S., Solveig Hauge, Lars J. Danbolt, and Kari Kvigne. "Residents' and caregivers' views on spiritual care and their understanding of spiritual needs in persons with dementia: A meta-synthesis." *Dementia* 16, no. 7 (2017): 911-929.

Ojagbemi, Akin, Toyin Bello, and Oye Gureje. "Cognitive reserve, incident dementia, and associated mortality in the ibadan study of ageing." *Journal of the American Geriatrics Society* 64, no. 3 (2016): 590-595.

Owokuhaisa, Judith, Godfrey Zari Rukundo, Edith Wakida, Celestino Obua, and Stephanie S. Buss. "Community perceptions about dementia in southwestern Uganda." *BMC geriatrics* 20, no. 1 (2020): 1-12.

Park, Hae-Young, Ji-Won Park, Hong Ji Song, Hyun Soon Sohn, and Jin-Won Kwon. "The association between polypharmacy and dementia: a nested case-control study based on a 12-year longitudinal cohort database in South Korea." *PLoS One* 12, no. 1 (2017): e0169463.

Prince, Martin, Emiliano Albanese, Maelenn Guerchet, and Matthew Prina. "World Alzheimer Report 2014: Dementia and risk reduction: An analysis of protective and modifiable risk factors." (2014).

Prince, Martin J., Daisy Acosta, Erico Castro-Costa, Jim Jackson, and K. S. Shaji. "Packages of care for dementia in low-and middle-income countries." *PLoS medicine* 6, no. 11 (2009): e1000176.

Rasmussen, Jill, and Haya Langerman. "Alzheimer's disease–why we need early diagnosis." *Degenerative neurological and neuromuscular disease* 9 (2019): 123.

Samba, Harielle, Maelenn Guerchet, Bebene Ndamba-Bandzouzi, Pascal Mbelesso, Philippe Lacroix, Jean-Francois Dartigues, and Pierre-Marie Preux. "Dementia-associated mortality and its predictors among older adults in sub-Saharan Africa: results from a 2-year follow-up in Congo (the EPIDEMCA-FU study)." *Age and ageing* 45, no. 5 (2016): 681-687.

Sampson, Elizabeth L., Bridget Candy, Sarah Davis, Anna Buylova Gola, Jane Harrington, Michael King, Nuriye Kupeli et al. "Living and dying with advanced dementia: a prospective cohort study of symptoms, service use and care at the end of life." *Palliative medicine* 32, no. 3 (2018): 668-681.

Schubert, C. C., Boustani, M., Callahan, C. M., Perkins, A. J., Carney, C. P., Fox, C., Unverzagt, F., hui, s. & Hendrie, h. C. 2006. Comorbidity profile of dementia patients in primary care: are they sicker? *Journal of the American Geriatrics Society,* 54, 104-109.

Sclan, Steven G., and Barry Reisberg. "Functional assessment staging (FAST) in Alzheimer's disease: reliability, validity, and ordinality." *International psychogeriatrics* 4, no. 3 (1992): 55-69

Stanyon, Miriam Ruth, Amanda Griffiths, Shirley A. Thomas, and Adam Lee Gordon. "The facilitators of communication with people with dementia in a care setting: an interview study with healthcare workers." *Age and ageing* 45, no. 1 (2016): 164-170.

Stoner, Charlotte R., Monisha Lakshminarayanan, Helen Durgante, and Aimee Spector. "Psychosocial interventions for dementia in low-and middle-income countries (LMICs): a systematic review of effectiveness and implementation readiness." *Aging & Mental Health* 25, no. 3 (2021): 408-419.

UCSF Institute For Neurosciences. *medications and dementia* [Online]. Available: https://memory.ucsf.edu/treatments-stays/medications-dementia# [Accessed 15/11/2022 2022].

UGANDA AIDS COMMISSION 2021. Facts on HIV and AIDS in Uganda 2021.

Van der Steen, Jenny T., Lukas Radbruch, Cees MPM Hertogh, Marike E. de Boer, Julian C. Hughes, Philip Larkin, Anneke L. Francke et al. "White paper defining optimal palliative care in older people with dementia: a Delphi study and recommendations from the European Association for Palliative Care." *Palliative medicine* 28, no. 3 (2014): 197-209.

Wang, Jing, Lily Dongxia Xiao, Guo-Ping He, and Anita De Bellis. "Family caregiver challenges in dementia care in a country with undeveloped dementia services." *Journal of advanced nursing* 70, no. 6 (2014): 1369-1380.

Wang, Jing, Lily Dongxia Xiao, Xiaomei Li, Anita De Bellis, and Shahid Ullah. "Caregiver distress and associated factors in dementia care in the community setting in China." *Geriatric Nursing* 36, no. 5 (2015): 348-354.

Wendrich-van Dael, Annelien, Frances Bunn, Jennifer Lynch, Lara Pivodic, Lieve Van den Block, and Claire Goodman. "Advance care planning for people living with dementia: an umbrella review of effectiveness and experiences." *International Journal of Nursing Studies* 107 (2020): 103576.

World HealthOrganisation. 2022. *Dementia* [Online]. Available: https://www.who.int/news-room/fact-sheets/detail/dementia [Accessed 14/11/2022 2022].

Welsh, T. J. Multimorbidity in people living with dementia. *Case reports in women's health,* 23 (2019).

Zucchella, Chiara, Elena Sinforiani, Stefano Tamburin, Angela Federico, Elisa Mantovani, Sara Bernini, Roberto Casale, and Michelangelo Bartolo. "The multidisciplinary approach to Alzheimer's disease and dementia. A narrative review of non-pharmacological treatment." *Frontiers in neurology* 9 (2018): 1058

9

CARING FOR PEOPLE WITH ADVANCED DEMENTIA AND THEIR FAMILY CAREGIVERS IN CHILE

PAMELA TURRILLAS AND MARILÚ BUDINICH

Palliative care needs in patients with dementia

Approximately 1% of the total population in Chile, almost 200,000 people, suffers from dementia. The number may even be higher due to low rates of diagnosis and registration (Fuentes and Albala 2014). Only 26,314 people diagnosed with Alzheimer's disease and other dementias are registered in the public health system, of whom 29% have been classified at an advanced stage of the disease (Ministry of Health of Chile 2022). Dementia represents the leading cause of death in people over 80 (Ministry of Health of Chile 2023). An increased prevalence of cognitive impairment is observed after age 65. Therefore it may be assumed that the comorbidities affecting people with dementia are similar to those affecting this age group, such as hypertension, dyslipidemia, diabetes, and chronic pain, associated with increased morbidity and mortality and healthy life-years lost (Herrera, Fernandez, and Rojas 2019).

Chile is one of the oldest countries in Latin America, with a life expectancy at birth of 80.4 years and 12% of the population over the age of 65 (Global AgeWatch 2015; National Institute of Statistics of Chile 2018a). The increasing prevalence of cognitive impairment has been related to this demographic transition and other social determinants such as low sociocultural level and rurality (González, Massad, and Lavanderos 2009). Data obtained from a national survey revealed that 8.5% of the population aged 60 years or over suffer from some degree of cognitive impairment, affecting over 40% of people over 85. Further, almost 25% of the elderly show some degree of dependence, reaching a severe degree in half of the cases (National Institute of Statistics of Chile 2017). In long-term care facilities, the prevalence of cognitive impairment rises to 78%, associated with severe dependence in 70% of the cases (Massad and Herrera 2019).

The high burden of physical and mental illness faced by people with dementia determines their needs in multiple dimensions. These needs are also influenced by social, cultural, and economic aspects, confirming that the complexity of caring for those people goes beyond a biomedical perspective (Budinich et al 2019). Care needs are related to psychological-behavioral symptoms, communication disorders, sleep disorders, gait disorders, immobility, incontinence, multimorbidity and frequent medical intercurrences such as pneumonia and urinary tract infections (Eisenmann et al 2020), making noteworthy the need to train family members and health care staff in long-term care management (Walsh et al 2021).

The underdiagnosis of people with dementia reflects the "invisibilisation" problem. They often receive care from health teams that are undertrained to address their needs and the needs of their family caregivers. In addition, the psychological and behavioural symptoms of people with dementia are sometimes confused with episodes of refusal of treatment or events of mistreatment of health personnel. Suspicion of dementia generally occurs during interventions by general practitioners or specialists with insufficient knowledge of referral algorithms, and national care plans offered to attend to this population (Ministry of Social Development of Chile 2017).

Due to governmental guarantees, primary health care serves most of the elderly in a referral-counter-referral system coordinated at the secondary and tertiary specialized levels. In this regard, 17,937 people were admitted to the dementia program in the public health service and 475 in the private health service in 2022. Low-level access to the private health system results from the high cost of care, which explains why only a minority of older people can access it (Superintendence of Health 2022).

The absence of curative treatments for dementia has led international organizations to recommend initiating palliative care in the early stages following diagnosis to prevent and alleviate suffering through the early identification of needs, multidimensional assessment, and appropriate management in the physical, psychosocial and/or spiritual dimensions (Alliance, Worldwide Palliative Care, and World Health Organization 2014).

Although there are no Chilean studies on palliative care in patients with dementia, international publications mention issues relevant to health staff and families, such as the relevance of hospitalizations, establishment of care guidelines, transitions of care, prescription and de-prescription of medications, prevention and management of acute events such as pneumonia or urinary tract infections, assessment and management of dysphagia, feeding techniques, prevention and management of psychosocial symptoms, prevention and control of psychological and behavioral symptoms, prevention and management of discomfort, decision-making and updating the family, diagnostic and therapeutic proportionality, and symptomatic management of end-of-life care (Budinich et al 2019).

Within these issues, the perspective of therapeutic proportionality and advance care directives are commonly discussed in hospital settings and intensive care units concerning unit admissions and decisions about tube feeding, cardiopulmonary resuscitation, and the use of invasive or noninvasive mechanical ventilation (Slachevsky, Abusleme, and Arenas 2016).

The costs of caring: family and social impact of dementia

The physical and mental deterioration associated with dementia implies that gradually yet progressively, the person with dementia will reach a situation of dependence to perform instrumental and basic activities of daily living, decreasing participation in decision-making and community life, creating inequity gaps (Gajardo and Abusleme 2016).

The disease burden associated with disability and dependency considerably impacts the patient's family, related to caregiver overload and the high economic costs associated with caregiving for both the families and the state (Wimo et al 2010).

A 2011 study showed that the cost of caring for people with dementia in Chile reaches 1,463 dollars per month, of which 20% correspond to direct medical expenses, 5% to direct social expenses (institutionalization and remuneration of caregivers), and 75% to indirect expenses, existing a direct correlation between condition severity and higher economic expenditure. By contrast, differences exist in the type of expenditure according to the socioeconomic level of the household; that is, a higher income level is related to higher direct expenditure and a lower income level with higher indirect expenditure (Hojman et al 2017).

In Chile, care and support for people with dementia are predominantly provided by the family, and secondly, in long-term care facilities (Massad and Herrera 2019). In the first case, the support networks are usually made up of family members, friends, or community members, who usually do not receive stipends for care (González, Massad, and Lavanderos 2009).

A survey of Chilean informal caregivers revealed that 98.9% are relatives of the person with dementia, mostly women in their role as wives or daughters. Only one of every five cases received paid caregiver support. The prevalence of caregiver overload is high, severe in more than 60% of the cases, and is associated with mental pathology in almost half of the caregivers. This overload correlates to emotional stress, family dysfunction, and the severity of neuropsychiatric symptoms and functional impairment of the person with dementia (Slachevsky and Budinich 2013). It has also been noted that formal caregivers working in long-term care facilities have a high workload and suffer emotional exhaustion, which may influence the quality of care received by the elderly (Massad and Herrera 2019).

Most caregivers spend much of their day supporting basic daily living activities and supervising people with dementia. As described by Chilean informal caregivers, more than 50% of them have provided care for more than five years, implying a reduction of hours in paid work and, in some cases, the total cessation of paid work to assume the role of caregiver fully (Slachevsky et al 2013).

Female-headed households represent almost 50% of households in Chile, which leads to tension by coexisting with the female predominance in long-term care. This gender role in care maintains gender inequalities in access to paid work; consequently, care for these patients generates or perpetuates poverty in many homes where long-term care is provided (National Institute of Statistics Chile 2015). Furthermore, new forms of families with smaller sizes, composed of 3.1 members per household, impact the willingness and availability of their members to assume a caregiving role, thus reducing the capacity to generate an adequate care network (National Institute of Statistics Chile 2018b).

The family structure changes and long-term care's impact on families are concerning because 50% of households experiencing multidimensional poverty have one or more older adults living in it.[21] This implies that people with dementia are more exposed to neglect, loneliness, poverty, leading to the progression of chronic diseases, mental illness and disability which is associated with higher health resource use and mortality (Martínez-Sanguinetti et al 2019). In the case of people with dementia living in rural areas, there is also a greater risk of isolation and barriers to accessing to health services, thus deepening the problem (González, Massad, and Lavanderos 2009).

A national dementia strategy

Public Policies: National Framework

In the early 2000s, the National Service for the Elderly in Chile convened a roundtable to discuss the implications of population aging on health, economic, social, cultural, and political issues, sparking a series of milestones and governmental socio-health initiatives (Gajardo and Abusleme 2016). In 2006, the Ministry of Health began implementing the home care program for people with severe dependency, mainly serving older adults with cognitive impairment and their caregivers. The program provides comprehensive physical, emotional and social home care, promotes rehabilitation and autonomy, and improves the quality of life. Program implementation has been gradual, reaching 6% of the target population in 2017 (Budget Directorate 2017). In addition, family caregivers can access a stipend of approximately 40 dollars per month (Ministry of Social Development and Family 2023).

After several years of work, a strategy for a national dementia plan was created in 2015, aiming to identify and strengthen existing systems or services that address the needs of people with dementia. The strategy is to enhance and implement actions to reduce disability and improve psychosocial well-being and environmental conditions for patients and their families (Ministry of Health of Chile 2017).

In this vein, the government declared dementia a condition requiring guarantees of timeliness, quality of care, and financing by the public and private health systems in 2019, while considering diagnostic and management benefits, regardless of the disease's severity. Implementation of this measure was interrupted by the COVID-19 pandemic, so it is expected that in the coming years, data will be available to evaluate the scope of this program, which involves family training, accompaniment, and case management (Official Gazette of the Republic of Chile 2019).

Another Health strategy, still in the pilot stage, consists of comprehensive care focused on people with multimorbidity. This strategy considers dementia a double risk that requires care coordination. Its principles are promotion and prevention, personal responsibility and autonomy, continuity of care, and efficient interventions adapted to needs. The strategy incorporates case management, population stratification, and person-centered medicine (Vargas et al 2021).

Motivated by milestones on the rights of persons with disabilities and their care, the National System of Support and Care of the Ministry of Social Development was created in 2016 in order to shift the responsibility for care from households—specifically women as primary caregivers—to one of co-responsibility between households, the community and the state (Budget Directorate 2021). This system created a local support and care network program to provide home services for moderately and/or severely dependent elderly adults experiencing socioeconomic vulnerability. Support for the person and their family caregiver consists of visits by care assistants, the existence of local coordinators, and technical and professional guidance and support for the assistants.[27] Thus far, coverage reaches 17% of the country's municipalities (National Service for the Elderly 2017).

National strategies have also been established to improve the care provided in long-term care facilities. These strategies utilize regulatory frameworks of the National Service for the Elderly and the Ministry of Health regarding care, rehabilitation, accompaniment, and social interaction for people with advanced chronic diseases and dependency. Although progress has been made, monitoring the implementation of the right policies and procedures and hiring adequately trained personnel is still needed (Massad and Herrera 2019).

Dementia-friendly community initiatives are still scarce, and the level of development and integration of these initiatives in the country is unknown. There are, however, isolated initiatives to strengthen the community network for the care of people, such as community monitors, respite care, and volunteering (Slachevsky, Abusleme, and Arenas 2016).

To reduce the economic burden of patients at the end-of-life, Law 21.309 was implemented in 2021 by the Ministry of Labor and Social Security. This law establishes a new pension system and benefit people with advanced chronic illness and life expectancy of less than 12 months. The beneficiary has the right to receive a temporary income for twelve months, which supports expenses freely determined by the person (Ministry of Labor and Social Security, 2021).

The palliative care model for people with advanced dementia and their family was integrated into the Chilean health system after repeated international urging (World Health Assembly Resolution, 2014). The development of the Palliative Care Program emerged in the 1990s to provide care for oncological patients and was codified in 2005 as a health guarantee. In 2021, the rights of people suffering from terminal illnesses were enshrined in Law 21.375, granting universal access to palliative care, including those diagnosed with advanced dementia (Ministry of Health of Chile, 2022). Enforcement of this law poses a great challenge for the Chilean social and health care system, which must respond with a restructuring of the health system to ensure the adequate implementation and provision of palliative care services at all levels of care. This transition requires adequate funding for human resources training and the purchase of essential medicines and supplies to meet the objectives of health improvement outcomes for individuals and their families (Gómez-Batiste et al 2017).

Existence of guidelines and standards of end-of-life care for advanced dementia patients

The national clinical practice guideline on dementia includes two specific recommendations on the management of advanced dementia: de-prescription of dementia-specific drugs and favouring feeding by mouth. Further, the technical guideline for the implementation of explicit health guarantees for people with dementia mentions various activities aimed at the advanced stage in different sections (Ministry of Health of Chile, 2021). Also, the technical guidelines for implementing universal palliative care contain recommendations for end-of-life management of physical and psychological symptoms, spiritual care, and socio-familial aspects, including education and psychological support for the caregiver. Recommendations also include management of the last days' situation, feeding, hydration, medication pathways, and palliative sedation (Ministry of Health of Chile, 2022).

Advance care planning and end-of-life decision making

Various Chilean studies in palliative, intensive, and medical care show professional acknowledgment of the importance of people being able to plan end-of-life care based on their wishes and preferences, although the degree of specific knowledge and legislation regarding advance directives varies among disciplines (Dittborn 2018; Valdebenito 2015).

In this vein, Law 21.331 was enacted in 2021, regulating the recognition and protection of the rights of people in mental health care, addressing the use of advance directives as an instrument to safeguard the wishes and preferences of each person concerning personal areas including the body itself, the disease, and the manner of death (Marshall and Gómez, 2022). Further, the regulations of Law 21.375, enacted in 2022, specify those persons and institutions involved in the advance care planning document and defines its contents (Comptroller's Office, 2022). Both laws are in the nascent stages of implementation, and a period of evaluation of the impact of this tool in healthcare practice is required.

Challenges ahead

The coming years will be crucial for consolidating palliative care and long-term care in Chile to improve the quality of life of people with advanced dementia and their families. Acknowledging the needs of people with dementia and their families is central to a comprehensive understanding of how services should provide care to this population. The training of professionals should respond to these needs with a person-centered focus and respect for patients' wishes and preferences in management. This model will allow for a better approach to and execution of care that considers best practices at all levels and fair use of existing resources, thus avoiding ineffective practices and mismanagement in care transitions.

With the entry into force of the Universal Palliative Care Law, several training initiatives have originated in the Ministry of Health, universities, and scientific societies. In this sense, the gap in palliative care education for health professionals should be reduced. However, better governmental guidelines are needed to promote curricular changes in undergraduate and postgraduate in health careers courses, and increase coverage by training professionals already caring for this population.

Several government strategies are still in the implementation stage, during which the COVID-19 pandemic has decelerated. Consequently, there needs to be more data on the access, coverage, and benefits individuals and their families receive. Likewise, plans depend on an inter-ministerial network of systems and sub-systems that require coordination at both the central and regional levels by case managers to enable the expected system integration.

Generating more binding decisions and actions with a gender-based approach is necessary to provide practical solutions for headed-female households caring for people with advanced dementia. In this regard, there should be support mechanisms, such as an adequate caregiver stipend, that accords with the families' out-of-pocket expenses and caregivers lack of access to paid jobs. This will help avoid, as far as possible, the risk of multidimensional poverty in these households. Additionally, the home care assistance and local network system implementation should be extended and strengthen training and psychosocial support for family caregivers with better instruction on network navigation to find solutions to their own problems, together with a community network that supports care. These interventions may extend the functionality and autonomy of the person with dementia, avoiding crises and inadequate transitions between hospital, outpatient, and home care.

References

Alliance, Worldwide Palliative Care, and World Health Organization. "Global Atlas of Palliative Care at the End of Life." *London: Worldwide Palliative Care Alliance* (2014).

Budinich, M, JM Aravena, J Gajardo, and P Fuentes. "Dementias: A Biopsychosocial View." Self-publishing, 2019.

Budget Directorate. "Executive Summary of the Evaluation of the Governmental Program for Home Care for Persons with Severe Dependency." Government of Chile, 2017. Accessed January 2, 2023. https://www.dipres.gob.cl/597/articles-163132_r_ejecutivo_institucional.pdf.

Budget Directorate. "Social Programs Report, Local Care and Support Network - SNAC." Ministry of Social Development and Family of Chile, 2021. Accessed January 2, 2023. https://www.dipres.gob.cl/597/articles-212577_doc_pdf1.pdf.

Comptroller's Office. "Regulations Regarding Palliative Care and the Rights of Persons Suffering from Terminal or Serious Illness. "Government of Chile, April 21, 2022. Accessed January 2, 2023. https://www.contraloria.cl/documents/451102/3103767/Reing.+Dto+41-22+Salud.pdf/5128d75c-9790-d2d1-75b7-81533cd9bb

Dittborn Bellalta, Mariana. "Knowledge and Attitudes of Palliative Care Professionals on Advance Directives in the Metropolitan Region, Chile." *Colombian Bioethics Journal* (2018): 36-49.

Eisenmann, Yvonne, Heidrun Golla, Holger Schmidt, Raymond Voltz, and Klaus Maria Perrar. "Palliative Care in Advanced Dementia." *Frontiers in Psychiatry* 11 (2020): 699.

Fuentes, Patricio, and Cecilia Albala. "An Update on Aging and Dementia in Chile." *Dementia & Neuropsychologia* 8 (2014): 317-22.

Gajardo, Jean, and María Teresa Abusleme. "Nacional Plan of Dementias: Global Background and Summary of the Chilean Strategy." *Clinica Las Condes Medical Journal* 27, no. 3 (2016): 286-96.

Global AgeWatch. "Global AgeWatch Index 2015: Insight Report, Summary and Methodology | Reports | Global AgeWatch Index 2015," 2015. Accessed January 2, 2023. http://www.globalagewatch.org/reports/global-agewatch-index-2015-insight-report-summary-and-methodology/.

Gómez-Batiste, Xavier, Scott A Murray, Keri Thomas, Carles Blay, Kirsty Boyd, Sebastien Moine, Maxime Gignon, *et al.* "Comprehensive and Integrated Palliative Care for People with Advanced Chronic Conditions: An Update from Several European Initiatives and Recommendations for Policy." *Journal of Pain and Symptom Management* 53, no. 3 (2017): 509-17.

Herrera, M, M Fernández, and M Rojas. "Chile and its Elders: Results of the 5th national survey on quality of life during old age 2019 UC-Caja Los Andes." Santiago: Pontificia Universidad Católica de Chile AND Caja Los Andes (2020).

Hojman, Daniel A, Fabian Duarte, Jaime Ruiz-Tagle, Marilu Budnich, Carolina Delgado, and Andrea Slachevsky. "The Cost of Dementia in an Unequal Country: The Case of Chile." *PLoS One* 12, no. 3 (2017): e0172204.

González, F, C Massad, and F Lavanderos. "National survey on dependency of the elderly. SENAMA Government of Chile, 10-12." 2009.

Marshall, Pablo, and Hernán Gómez Yuri. "Advance Directives in Mental Health and the Problem of Revocation." *Bioethics Act* 28, no. 2 (2022): 205-14.

Martínez-Sanguinetti, María Adela, Ana María Leiva, Fanny Petermann-Rocha, Claudia Troncoso-Pantoja, Marcelo Villagrán, Fabián Lanuza-Rilling, Gabriela Nazar, *et al.* "Factors Associated with Cognitive Impairment in Older Persons in Chile." *Chile Medical Journal* 147, no. 8 (2019): 1013-23.

Massad, Cristián, and Herrera, Felipe. "Living Conditions of The Elderly Inside Senama's Long-Stay Facilities For Older Adults" (2019).

Ministry of Health of Chile. "National Dementia Plan 2017." Government of Chile, 2017. Accessed January 2, 2023. https://www.minsal.cl/wp-content/uploads/2017/11/PLAN-DE-DEMENCIA.pdf.

Ministry of Health of Chile. "Basic Health Indicators Chile." Department of Health Statistics and Information (DEIS) Reports, 2019. Accessed January 2, 2023. https://informesdeis.minsal.cl/SASVisualAnalytics/?reportUri=%2Freports%2Freports%2Fe9928c9c-d555-40dc-b9e6-14497037c21a§ionIndex=0&sso_guest=true&sas-welcome=false.

Ministry of Health of Chile. "Technical Guidance Universal Palliative Care." Division of Disease Prevention and Control, 2022. Accessed January 2, "Executive Summary Clinical Practice Guideline Dementia Type Alzheimer's Disease." Division of Disease Prevention and Control, 2021. Accessed January 2, 2023. https://diprece.minsal.cl/wp-content/uploads/2021/12/Resumen-Ejecutivo-GPC-Demencia-tipo-Alzheimer2021-12-09-V2.pdf.2023. https://diprece.minsal.cl/cuidados-paliativos-universales/.

Ministry of Health of Chile. "Mental Health Reports." Department of Statistics and Health Information Reports, December 22, 2022. Accessed January 2, 2023. https://informesdeis.minsal.cl/SASVisualAnalytics/?reportUri=%2Freports%2Freports%2Fad0c03ad-ee7a-4da4-bcc7-73d6e12920cf§ionIndex=0&sso_guest=true&reportViewOnly=true&sas-welcome=false.

Ministry of Labor and Social Security. "Technical Standards for Terminal Patient Certification, According to Law 21.309." Superintendency of Pensions, 2021. Accessed January 2, 2023. https://www.spensiones.cl/portal/institucional/594/articles-14608_recurso_1.pdf.

Ministry of Social Development of Chile. "Social Programs Monitoring Report (Closing as of June 30, 2017). Home Care for Persons with Severe Dependency". Social Programs, 2017. Accessed January 2, 2023. https://programassociales.ministeriodesarrollosocial.gob.cl/pdf/2017/PRG2017_5_100059207.pdf.

Ministry of Social Development and Family. “Payment Program (Stipend) for caregivers of people with disabilities.” Chileatiende, February 14, 2023. Accessed February 20, 2023. https://www.chileatiende.gob.cl/fichas/49627-programa-de-pago-de-cuidadores-de-personas-con-discapacidad-estipendio.

National Institute of Statistics Chile. "WOMEN IN CHILE AND THE LABOR MARKET. Female Labor Participation and Wage Gaps." Government of Chile, January 2015. Accessed January 2, 2023. https://www.ine.gob.cl/docs/default-source/ocupacion-y-desocupacion/publicaciones-y-anuarios/publicaciones/mujeres-en-chile-y-mercado-del-trabajo---participaci%C3%B3n-laboral-femenina-y-brechas-salarialesa.pdf?sfvrsn=ade344d4_3.

National Institute of Statistics of Chile. "Estimates and Projections of The Population of Chile 1992-2050 Total Country," 2018a. Accessed January 2, 2023. https://www.ine.gob.cl/docs/default-source/proyecciones-de-poblacion/publicaciones-y-anuarios/base-2017/ine_estimaciones-y-proyecciones-de-poblaci%C3%B3n-1992-2050_base-2017_s%C3%ADntesis.pdf?sfvrsn=c623983e_6.

National Institute of Statistics Chile. "2017 CENSUS RESULTS SUMMARY." Census 2017, June 2018b. Accessed January 2, 2023. http://www.censo2017.cl/descargas/home/sintesis-de-resultados-censo2017.pdf.

National Service for the Elderly. "Technical Orientation Guide. Home Care Program," 2017. Accessed January 2, 2023. http://www.senama.gob.cl/storage/docs/Guia_de_Orientaciones_Tecnicas_PCD_VERSION_RESOLUCION_09_08_2017_-_copia.pdf.

Official Gazette of the Republic of Chile, No. 42.449. September 7th, 2019. Accessed January 2, 2023. https://auge.minsal.cl/website/doc/decreto.pdf

Slachevsky Ch, Andrea, Mª Abusleme, and Ángela Arenas Massa. "Palliative Care in Persons with Severe Dementia: Reflections and Challenges." *Chile Medical Journal* 144, no. 1 (2016): 94-101.

Slachevsky, Andrea, Marilu Budinich, Claudia Miranda-Castillo, Javier Núñez-Huasaf, Jaime R Silva, Carlos Muñoz-Neira, Sergio Gloger, *et al.* "The Cuideme Study: Determinants of Burden in Chilean Primary Caregivers of Patients with Dementia." *Journal of Alzheimer's Disease* 35, no. 2 (2013): 297-306.

Superintendence of Health. Quarterly statistics of accumulated GES cases, 2005- 2022. Accumulated GES cases September 2022. Accessed January 2, 2023. http://www.supersalud.gob.cl/difusion/665/w3-propertyvalue-1962.html#acordeonDocumentos

Valdebenito Aguilar, Guillermo Humberto. "Advance Directives in Clinical Decision Making at the End Of Life: Knowledge and Attitudes Towards Advance Directives In Medical And ICU Professionals And In Patients

With End-Stage Renal Failure On Hemodialysis Therapy, From The 4th Region Of The Country" (2015).

Vargas, Irma, Ximena Barros, María José Fernández, and Macarena Mayol. "Redesign in Approach to People with Chronic Multimorbidity: From Fragmentation to Integral Care Centered on People". *Clinica Las Condes Medical Journal* 32, no. 4 (2021): 400-13.

Walsh, Sharon C, Edel Murphy, Declan Devane, Elizabeth L Sampson, Sheelah Connolly, Patricia Carney, and Eamon O'Shea. "Palliative Care Interventions in Advanced Dementia." *Cochrane Database of Systematic Reviews*, no. 9 (2021).

Wimo, Anders, Linus Jönsson, John Bond, Martin Prince, Bengt Winblad, and Alzheimer Disease International. "The Worldwide Economic Impact of Dementia 2010." *Alzheimer's & Dementia* 9, no. 1 (2013): 1-11. e3.

World Health Assembly Resolution. "Strengthening of Palliative Care as a Component of Comprehensive Care Throughout the Life Course: Resolution WHA67. 19." *Geneva: World Health Organization* (2014).

10

COMMUNITY AS CARERS – NEED TO STRENGTHEN THE INFORMAL CARER SYSTEM IN DEMENTIA

DR SURESH KUMAR[1]

Abstract

Dementia is a progressive neurological disease that affects millions worldwide and significantly impacts physical, psycho-social, and spiritual well-being. Preventable risk factors have been identified, but gaps in access to care and resources hinder effective management and support, particularly in low- and middle-income countries. Caregiving responsibilities often fall to families, burdening healthcare systems, as institutions like hospitals and care homes have limitations in cost, personalised care, and round-the-clock support. Home care programs are an alternative but have resource and support limitations. Community-based care delivery models are emerging as an effective way to provide care to individuals with dementia, focusing on meeting their physical, emotional, and social needs. Four primary home care delivery models have been identified: case management, integrated care, consumer-directed care, and restorative care. Layperson caregivers are vital for individuals with dementia, and capacity building for them is crucial to ensure they have the skills, knowledge, and resources to provide high-quality care.

Advanced care planning (ACP) is associated with decreased hospitalizations, increased concordance between care received and prior wishes, and increased completion of advance care planning documents.

[1] Director, WHO Collaborating Centre for Community Participation in Palliative Care and Long Term Care, Institute of Palliative Medicine, 673008, Calicut, Kerala, India

Dementia friendliness is a significant shift that supports the well-being of individuals with dementia within the community. Networking is a crucial aspect of improving dementia care as it enables healthcare professionals, caregivers, and people with dementia to exchange information, share best practices, and access resources to enhance the quality of care.

Collaboration among different organizations and stakeholders involved in dementia care through networking can lead to more coordinated and effective care. The informal care system plays a crucial role in low and middle-income countries, but stigma and a sense of helplessness can hinder its effectiveness. Coordination and capacity building between informal and formal care systems can overcome these barriers.

The formal care delivery system comprises primary, secondary, and tertiary healthcare systems, each with specific roles and responsibilities. Infrastructural arrangements and care facilities can be better organized at all three levels, avoiding duplication of services and need-based capacity building of professionals. Decentralized dementia care services engaging informal and formal care systems are cost-effective and sustainable but require informed decisions, solid policies, access to essential drugs, and availability of care devices from state and national governments.

Overall, a comprehensive approach that addresses the diverse needs of patients and their families is essential for effective dementia care delivery. Effective care systems need to be built on four pillars: government policies and resources, integration with mainstream healthcare, involvement of the formal social support system, and community participation.

Background

Dementia is a progressive neurological disease affecting millions worldwide (World Health Organization [WHO] 2021). According to WHO, around 50 million people currently live with dementia, and this number is expected to triple by 2050 (WHO 2021). Dementia is a leading cause of disability and dependency among older adults and significantly impacts their quality of life and their families.

Dementia is a complex disease affecting cognitive functions and individuals' physical, psycho-social, and spiritual well-being. Common symptoms include memory loss, difficulty with communication, mood swings, and behavioural changes. The symptoms of dementia can vary from person to person, and the disease progresses at different rates in different individuals.

Various risk factors for dementia have been identified. Preventable among them include lower education level, hypertension, smoking, hearing loss, obesity, depression, physical inactivity, diabetes, limited social interaction, excessive alcohol consumption, traumatic brain injury, and air pollution. The Lancet Commission suggests that it may be possible to prevent or delay approximately 40% of dementia cases worldwide if these 12 modifiable risk factors are addressed. (Livingston et al. 2020)

There is currently no cure for dementia, and the available treatment options are limited (Alzheimer's Association 2022). The management of dementia focuses on controlling the symptoms, providing support and care to the individual, and improving their quality of life. Current management options include pharmacotherapy and non-pharmacological interventions. Pharmacotherapy includes drugs that target the cognitive symptoms of dementia, such as cholinesterase inhibitors and memantine. Non-pharmacological interventions include cognitive stimulation therapy, music therapy, reminiscence therapy etc. Care is the most important component of dementia management, and it is crucial to ensure that individuals with dementia receive high-quality care that meets their physical, emotional, and social needs.

Gaps in Dementia Care

While there has been some progress in the field of dementia care, there are still significant gaps in access to care, particularly in low- and middle-income countries (LMICs). (WHO 2017). There are often limited resources and infrastructure to support dementia care, resulting in a lack of diagnosis and treatment options. Additionally, there may be a cultural stigma surrounding dementia, which can lead to social isolation and a lack of community support for those living with the condition. Furthermore, there may be a lack of trained healthcare professionals who can provide specialised care for individuals with dementia, as well as limited access to medications and other supportive therapies. This can result in a lower quality of life for those living with dementia and their caregivers and an increased burden on healthcare systems and families. (Prince et al. 2015)

Identifying dementia in low- and middle-income countries (LMICs) is also difficult because of inadequate screening tools, limited awareness and understanding, and social stigma. In LMICs, families are primarily responsible for caring for people with dementia, and there is a shortage of dementia services in the community (Fam et al. 2019, 461-464). Difficulties include inadequate facilities for formal long-term care, disparities in health due to social and economic factors, gender-based imbalances, and the recent COVID-19. It is vital to identify the specific needs of caregivers, implement evidence-based interventions at the local level, counter gender biases, and enhance community support. Innovative, evidence-based solutions and the strengthening of public policies are necessary to overcome the disparities in dementia caregiving (Ibáñez et al. 2021).

Institution-based care

Institutions, such as hospitals and care homes, play a significant role in providing care to individuals with dementia (Brodaty and Donkin 2009). However, there are limitations to institutional care, including the high cost, lack of personalized care, and inability to provide care round the clock. Home care programs are an alternative to institutional care, but they too have limitations, such as lack of support and resources for caregivers and the inability to provide specialized care to individuals with complex needs. The decline in the availability of care homes has had a significant impact on individuals with dementia, who constitute the largest group of care home residents and will continue to drive demand. According to a study, more than half of all UK dementia patients are currently residing in care homes, and projections indicate that by 2043, over twice as many care home places as presently available will be needed to maintain the current balance between institutional and community-based care services for dementia. The study warns that an availability crisis is looming and recommends investing in affordable in-home care and enhancing staff ratios and training in long-term care facilities. (Macdonald and Cooper 2007, 16)

Moving from hospitals to care homes or community settings is frequently needed. This transition can be challenging and often difficult for patients and their families. The move can be physically demanding and emotionally overwhelming for patients because they are often confused, frail, elderly, or have complex health needs. To help ease this transition, it is essential to make appropriate preparations and ensure that communication and care are of high quality. it is crucial to ensure that care is provided in a compassionate and person-centred manner, considering the individual's unique needs, preferences, and goals. It is essential to involve family members in the process, as they can provide valuable insights into the patient's needs, preferences, and history. Family members can also play an essential role in providing emotional support and helping to facilitate the transition to the new setting. (Richardson et al. 2019)

Community-Based Care

Community care delivery systems have emerged as an effective way to provide care to individuals with dementia (Batsch and Mittelman 2012). Community-based care delivery models involve a range of healthcare professionals, caregivers, and community organizations working together to provide high-quality care to individuals with dementia. These models are based on the principles of person-centered care, which focus on meeting the individual's physical, emotional, spiritual and social needs and promoting their well-being.

The growing number of individuals with dementia and the need to transfer their care from institutionalised settings to home care due to economic and workforce pressures have resulted in the development of home care models of care. Four primary home care delivery models for community-dwelling people with dementia have been identified: case management, integrated care, consumer-directed care, and restorative care. There has been limited research on these models, and no direct comparison has been made between them. Consequently, more research is necessary to develop evidence-based policies and service delivery for people with dementia, including assessing the impact of these models on outcomes and identifying optimal delivery methods to enhance outcomes (Low and Fletcher 2015, 1595).

Home-Based Dementia Care (HBDC) is a promising paradigm shift to improve care for those living with dementia. A consensus panel formed recently to develop recommendations for HBDC identified the advantages and challenges of shifting to HBDC and developed five core recommendations. The recommendations include considering HBDC as the nexus of new dementia models, implementing new payment models, preparing a diverse workforce, testing and integrating new technologies, and targeted dissemination efforts (Samus et al., 2018).

Lay Person Care Givers

Layperson caregivers are vital for individuals with dementia (Covinsky et al. 2021). Caregiving can be a rewarding experience, but it is very often challenging and stressful. Caregivers often face physical, emotional, and financial burdens, which can affect their well-being and that of individuals with dementia. While interventions targeting caregivers have shown promise in reducing caregiver burden and improving patient outcomes, there needs to be more standardisation in the definition, goals, and outcome measurement tools for caregiver participation in dementia care. Not many studies focusing on this area have come out. A recent scoping review showed that caregivers in African countries lack formal education and support systems, spending an average of 13 hours per day in caregiving (Adedeji et al., 2022). Chiao, Wu, and Hsiao (2015, 340), in their systematic review focussing on possible factors contributing to the caregiver burden for informal caregivers of people with dementia living in the community, found that behavioural problems or psychological symptoms of the person with dementia were the primary factors associated with caregiver burden, while caregiver socio-demographic factors and psychological factors were also significant contributors. The paper suggests that healthcare professionals should deliver appropriate assistance to relieve the caregiver burden and improve the quality of care for people with dementia. Capacity building for layperson caregivers through professional assistance is crucial to ensure they have the skills, knowledge, and resources to provide high-quality care to individuals with dementia.

Multicomponent community programs, caregiver education, respite programs, and care management can delay long-term care admission to institutions. Such community support and services can also help reduce the distress experienced by caregivers. It has been recommended that all community-based healthcare providers should be aware of available local support and services for people with dementia (Warrick, Prorok, and Seitz 2018).

Advanced care planning (ACP) is discussing and documenting a person's wishes and preferences for future medical care if they cannot make their own decisions. This process typically involves conversations between the person, their family members, and their healthcare providers. Advanced care planning aims to ensure that the person's healthcare wishes are respected and that they receive care that aligns with their values and preferences, even if they cannot communicate those wishes at the time (Piers et al. 2018).

Advanced Care Planning (ACP) was associated with decreased hospitalisations, increased concordance between care received and prior wishes, and increased completion of advance care planning documents.

Views of ACP for people with dementia clustered around six themes, with diminishing decision-making capacity over time being a key overarching feature (Wendrich-van Dael et al. 2020). The process needs to be initiated early in the course of the disease.

It has also been pointed out that targeting individuals at high risk for dementia can help detect it early. It is advisable to detect dementia early when it is in the mild cognitive impairment or early dementia stages, but not when no symptoms are present. Detecting dementia early has its advantages such as getting early access to treatments and support networks, but there are also disadvantages such as causing psychological harm and false positive diagnoses. Although there are various screening tests available, they are not accurate enough to avoid false positives. Early detection might postpone institutionalization, but it could place a significant strain on social and human resources. To effectively implement early detection, it is necessary to improve diagnostic capabilities, care and support systems, and community involvement. A community-based integrated care system is recommended to meet each community's specific health needs, health status, and values (Maki and Yamaguchi 2014).

The importance of "dementia friendliness" in improving the quality of life for the growing number of people with dementia is widely accepted. This concept, similar to the idea of age-friendliness, represents a significant shift from solely addressing the physical and health needs of dementia patients to a more comprehensive approach that supports their well-being within the community. The concept of dementia friendliness is applicable in various settings, including hospitals, nursing homes, and neighbourhoods, with dementia-friendly communities (DFC) being the most prevalent (Alzheimer's Disease International 2016).

Dementia Friendly Initiatives (DFIs) that strive to enhance the dignity, empowerment, engagement, and independence of individuals with dementia and their caregivers throughout dementia can be the foundational components of a DFC. Examples include instances such as supermarkets in the area with staff members that have received training to deliver considerate services to those with dementia and Alzheimer's Cafes where individuals can gain knowledge about the condition. These measures can be implemented at either a small or large level. (Hebert and Scales 2019, 1858)

Integration with Palliative Care

Palliative care focuses on improving the quality of life for individuals with serious or life-limiting illnesses, such as dementia. Palliative care teams are composed of healthcare professionals and community volunteers who work together to manage patients' and their families' physical, emotional, social and spiritual needs. Patients with dementia and their family members can benefit greatly from palliative care interventions. These interventions can include managing symptoms such as pain, anxiety, and depression and providing emotional and spiritual support. Palliative care teams can also help with decision-making, advance care planning, and ensure patients receive appropriate end-of-life care. Additionally, palliative care teams can educate and support family members, helping them understand the disease and providing them with resources and guidance on caring for their loved ones. This can be particularly important as the disease progresses and the caregiving responsibilities become more demanding (World Health Organization 2014).

A recent scoping review concluded that although the integration of dementia and palliative care services holds potential, further high-quality research is required to recognize the essential elements of palliative care for individuals who are living with dementia. This is critical for empowering individuals with dementia to take part in their own care, live at home for as long as possible, and pass away when appropriate. Research on end-of-life care for people with dementia has yet to develop interventions that address the particular challenges that dying with dementia poses. (O'Connor et al. 2022) A systematic review conducted recently identified four main areas where palliative care consultations demonstrated benefits or potential benefits if implemented. These areas include discussions about care goals and end-of-life, symptom management, emergency room visits, and prescribing behaviour. However, the current literature supporting or opposing these findings is limited, and more extensive randomized controlled trials with longer follow-up periods are necessary to confirm the patterns highlighted in the review. Furthermore, qualitative research is required to optimize referrals to palliative care, implement palliative care suggestions, and enhance targeted education on palliative care (Senderovich and Retnasothie 2020)

Networking

Networking is an essential factor that can contribute to improving dementia care. When healthcare professionals, caregivers, and people with dementia network, they can exchange information, share best practices, and access resources that can enhance the quality of care. Networking can also promote collaboration among different organizations and stakeholders involved in dementia care, leading to more coordinated and effective care. One of the benefits of networking is that it can help to connect local support groups with national organizations. These connections can facilitate the sharing of resources and information, ultimately leading to better support for people with dementia and their caregivers. Furthermore, networking can help to build relationships between healthcare professionals and community-based organizations, such as churches and senior centres. This collaboration can lead to more integrated care, with healthcare professionals and community-based organizations working together to provide comprehensive support to people with dementia and their families. (Gaugler and Kane 2019)

Community Participation

Dementia care is a complex and multifaceted issue that requires a comprehensive approach to address the diverse needs of patients and their families. The needs of patients with dementia are not limited to physical care but also include psychosocial, spiritual, and legal aspects. Caregivers also undergo stress and strain-related issues. These needs can be met through informal and formal care systems, including family and community networks, primary, secondary, and tertiary healthcare systems, and specialist dementia care services.

One of the key challenges in providing effective dementia care is the lack of resources (World Health Organization 2017). Dementia care systems cannot be effective if they are developed as an add-on to the health care system. The care system, instead, needs to be built on four pillars to be effective and sustainable: government policies and earmarked resources, integration with mainstream healthcare, involvement of the formal social support system, and participation of the community. The support system should be set up through a range of action areas, including developing policies and committed funding, improving service coverage and capacity building, engaging the community as partners in care, ensuring reliable access to essential medicines and assistive devices, and additional emphasis on services for children.

In low and middle-income countries, the informal care system plays a crucial role in meeting the needs of patients with dementia (Alzheimer's Disease International, 2013). The informal system consists of family members, friends, and neighbourhood members of the patient, as well as civil society organisations, religious institutions, and other informal community networks. However, barriers such as stigma and a sense of helplessness in the face of a chronic, severe condition such as dementia can hinder the effectiveness of the informal system. To overcome these barriers, it is essential to develop a supportive environment that enables the coordination between the informal and formal systems and enhances their dementia care skills and knowledge.

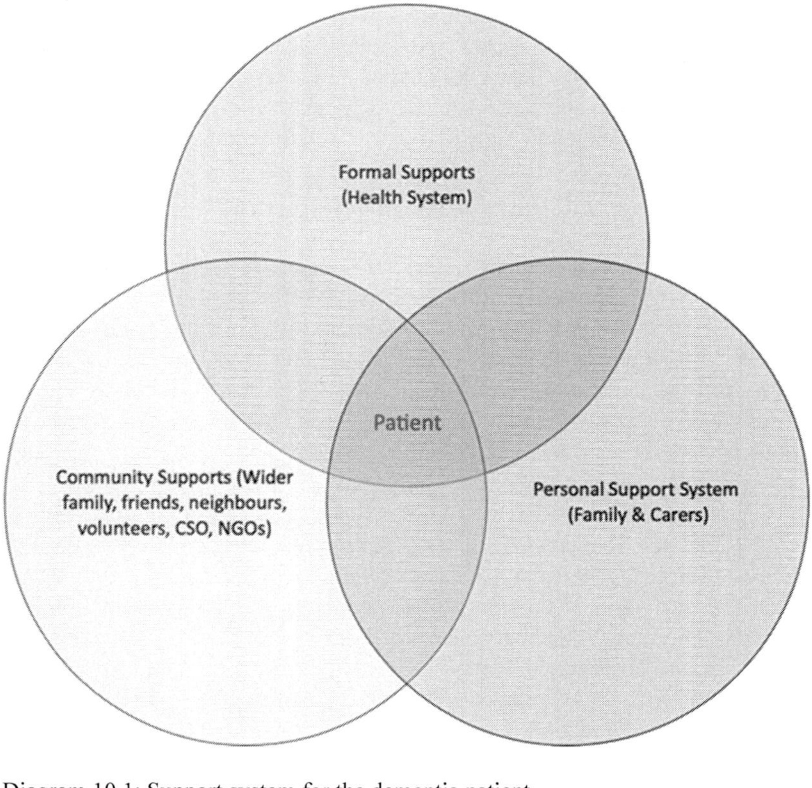

Diagram 10.1: Support system for the dementia patient

The formal care delivery system comprises primary, secondary, and tertiary healthcare systems operated by public, private, and third sectors. The primary healthcare workforce includes general practitioners, community nurses, and healthcare and support workers. The secondary and tertiary systems in dementia care constitute specialist dementia care services, mostly institution-based and led by a multi-professional team of physicians, nurses, psychologists, and social workers. They provide inpatient and outpatient services besides attending to symptom management and handling complex clinical procedures. Education and training programs for healthcare professionals in dementia care are also run mainly by secondary and tertiary sectors.

To ensure effective dementia care delivery, it is crucial to define the roles and responsibilities of primary, secondary, and tertiary levels concerning dementia care. (Jha and Tavan 2019). This can help avoid duplication of services and need-based capacity building of professionals working in each sector. Infrastructural arrangements and care facilities can be better organised at all three levels fruitfully, based on the specific roles of these systems.

Caring environments can enable a supportive stance in all aspects of the community that interface with the care process (World Health Organization 2012). Decentralised dementia care services engaging informal and formal care systems will be successful in achieving scale, efficiency, and sustainability (Prince et al. 2015). Cost-effectiveness and accountability are reportedly better in the case of such services in health compared to other models. State and national governments should ensure a caring environment through informed decisions, solid and efficient policies, access to essential drugs, and availability of care devices to mark the will and interest of governments in achieving quality care for patients suffering from long-term and life-threatening illnesses.

In conclusion, providing effective dementia care requires a comprehensive approach that addresses the diverse needs of patients and their families. This can be achieved through informal and formal care systems, which government policies, resources, and funding should support. Coordination between the informal and formal systems and capacity building and training can help ensure a robust dementia care delivery model that is accessible, sustainable, and cost-effective.

A proposed approach for encouraging community involvement in caring for people with dementia

Step 1: Provide training and orientation for healthcare professionals (HCPs) to educate caregivers and family members on providing home-based care. This will empower HCPs to facilitate community and family participation in continued care for the patient through structured educational activities. The training and orientation program should focus on developing the skills and knowledge of healthcare professionals in providing home-based care for dementia patients. The program should cover dementia diagnosis, symptom management, communication strategies, and the importance of engaging family and community members in the care process. The program should also include interactive sessions where caregivers and family members can share their experiences and ask questions.

Step 2: Conduct a community assessment to identify the current need and the status of the community's willingness and ability to participate in Dementia Care activities and to identify barriers to community involvement. This can be done through various means, including interviews, surveys, and meetings with community organisations and leaders. The assessment should be comprehensive and involve various stakeholders, including dementia patients, caregivers, healthcare professionals, and community leaders. The assessment should identify the current level of awareness and knowledge of dementia care in the community and the specific challenges people face in accessing care. The assessment should also identify the resources available in the community, such as support groups and care facilities, and any gaps in service provision.

Step 3: Identify stakeholders and potential volunteers during the assessment activity, such as beneficiaries, local government representatives, village leaders, religious leaders, healthcare officials, youth club leaders, teachers, journalists, and local businesspeople. Volunteers are essential for the success of the Dementia Care program. They can provide support, advocacy, and resources to the program. Identifying and engaging with stakeholders early in the process can help build relationships and create a sense of ownership for the program within the community.

Step 4: Conduct sensitisation programs for stakeholders and potential volunteers, such as short presentations on Dementia Care, awareness programs in collaboration with public events and media, and awareness programs in schools and universities. Sensitisation programs are essential for creating awareness about dementia care and the importance of community involvement. The programs should be tailored to different stakeholders and delivered culturally appropriately. The programs can be delivered through various channels, including community meetings, media campaigns, and educational institutions.

Step 5: Develop a training module for stakeholders and potential layperson carers, with regular training programs, certification of courses, and reward programs. Training programs for stakeholders and layperson carers should include dementia care, communication, symptom management and self-care. The training should be structured, with regular sessions and opportunities for participants to practice their skills. Certification and reward programs can help motivate participants and recognise their achievements.

Step 6: Implement the project by developing program policies, protocols, and procedures, soliciting involvement from community leaders, meeting with policymakers to support policy implementation concerning Dementia Care, and contacting businesses and NGOs for financial support. Start with a few Dementia Friendly initiatives, review, modify, replicate and later expand these into a wider Dementia Friendly Community in the locality. Implementing the program should involve developing policies and procedures to guide service provision and ensure consistency and quality of care. The program should also involve engaging policymakers to advocate for policy changes supporting dementia care. Financial support from businesses and NGOs can help sustain the program long-term. The program should be started with a few dementia-friendly initiatives and then gradually expanded as resources and support become available.

Step 7: Sustain the project by involving the maximum possible stakeholders in the planning, establishing a good rapport with communities and stakeholders, providing information about Dementia Care, and maintaining collaboration with hospitals, care homes and other institutions in the region. Involving multiple stakeholders ensures everyone knows the project's goals, objectives, and progress. It also helps to generate support and enthusiasm for the project. Collaboration with hospitals, care homes, and other regional institutions is critical to sustaining a dementia care project. Resources, expertise, and best practices can be shared by working together. Collaboration also helps build relationships and networks to support the project over time. Maintaining open communication channels with these institutions is vital to ensure that the project meets their needs and priorities.

Step 8: Establish a monitoring and evaluation system with culturally appropriate and validated measurement tools to measure outcomes monthly and quarterly. Sample outcome indicators may include patient/family reports, training, process, and social indicators. Monitoring and evaluation are critical to measuring the program's impact and identifying improvement areas. A monitoring and evaluation system should track progress against program goals and objectives. The system should use culturally appropriate and validated measurement tools to ensure that the data collected is accurate and meaningful. The outcome indicators used to measure the program's impact should be based on the goals and objectives of the program. For example, the indicators may include patient and family reports on the quality of care, the number of caregivers trained, the number of community members engaged in the program, and social indicators such as changes in attitudes towards dementia care. The collected data should be analysed and reported to stakeholders to ensure transparency and accountability.

References

Adedeji, I. A., Ogunniyi, A., Henderson, D. C., & Sam-Agudu, N. A. (2022). Experiences and practices of caregiving for older persons living with dementia in African countries: A qualitative scoping review. Dementia: The International Journal of Social Research and Practice, 21(3), 995-1011. https://doi.org/10.1177/14713012211065398

Alzheimer's Disease International. (2016). Dementia friendly communities: Key principles. Alzheimer's Disease International. https://www.alzint.org/u/dfc-principles.pdf

Alzheimer's Association. (2021). 2021 Alzheimer's disease facts and figures. Alzheimer's & Dementia, 17(3), 327-406.

Alzheimer's Disease International. (2013). World Alzheimer Report 2013: Journey of caring, an analysis of long-term care for dementia. Alzheimer's Disease International. https://www.alzint.org/u/WorldAlzheimerReport2013.pdf

Blomqvist, K., & Hallberg, I. R. (2005). "To be acknowledged as myself": Experiences of persons with Alzheimer's disease living in group dwellings. International Psychogeriatrics, 17(2), 255-270.

Brodaty, H., & Arasaratnam, C. (2012). Meta-analysis of nonpharmacological interventions for neuropsychiatric symptoms of dementia. The American Journal of Psychiatry, 169(9), 946-953.

Chan, W. C., Ngai, E. K., Kwok, T. C., & Wong, S. Y. (2011). A systematic review of the effects of social support on caregivers of people with dementia. Journal of Social Work in End-of-Life & Palliative Care, 7(3), 158-175.

Chiao, C. Y., Wu, H. S., & Hsiao, C. Y. (2015). Caregiver burden for informal caregivers of patients with dementia: A systematic review. International Nursing Review, 62(3), 340-350. https://doi.org/10.1111/inr.12194

Cohen-Mansfield, J., Golander, H., Arheim, G., & Garfinkel, P. M. (2000). A nursing aide training program for improving dementia care in nursing homes: A randomized controlled trial. The Journals of Gerontology: Series A, 55(10), M634-M640.

Fam, J., Mahendran, R., & Kua, E. H. (2019). Dementia care in low and middle-income countries. Current Opinion in Psychiatry, 32(5), 461-464. https://doi.org/10.1097/YCO.0000000000000523

Gaugler, J. E., Kane, R. L., Kane, R. A., & Newcomer, R. (2007). Early community-based service utilization and its effects on institutionalization in dementia caregiving. The Gerontologist, 47(6), 785-794. https://doi.org/10.1093/geront/47.6.785

Gitlin, L. N., Hodgson, N., Jutkowitz, E., & Pizzi, L. T. (2010). The cost-effectiveness of a nonpharmacologic intervention for individuals with dementia and family caregivers: The tailored activity program. The American Journal of Geriatric Psychiatry, 18(6), 510-519

Hebert, C. A., & Scales, K. (2019). Dementia friendly initiatives: A state of the science review. Dementia, 18(5), 1858-1895.

Ibáñez, A., Pina-Escudero, S. D., Possin, K. L., Quiroz, Y. T., Peres, F. A., Slachevsky, A., Sosa, A. L., Brucki, S. M. D., & Miller, B. L.(2021). Multi-Partner Consortium to Expand Dementia Research in Latin America. "Dementia caregiving across Latin America and the Caribbean and brain health diplomacy." Lancet Healthy Longev, 2(4), e222-e231. doi: 10.1016/s2666-7568(21)00031-3.

Jha, A., & Tavan, H. (2019). Dementia care in Southeast Asia: current challenges and future directions. Current Opinion in Psychiatry, 32(5), 467-472. doi: 10.1097/YCO.0000000000000532

Lee, E., Rhee, H., & Kim, Y. (2016). Factors affecting quality of life of family caregivers of community-dwelling elderly with dementia. Journal of Clinical Nursing, 25(1-2), 44-53.

Livingston, G., Huntley, J., Sommerlad, A., Ames, D., Ballard, C., Banerjee, S., Brayne, C., et al. (2020). Dementia prevention, intervention, and care: 2020 report of the Lancet Commission. Lancet, 396(10248), 413-446. doi: 10.1016/S0140-6736(20)30367-6

Low, L. F., & Fletcher, J. (2015). Models of home care services for persons with dementia: a narrative review. International Psychogeriatrics, 27(10), 1593-1600. doi: 10.1017/S1041610215000137

Macdonald, A., & Cooper, B. (2007). Long-term care and dementia services: An impending crisis. Age and Ageing, 36(1), 16-22. doi: 10.1093/ageing/afl126

Maki, Y., & Yamaguchi, H. (2014). Early detection of dementia in the community under a community-based integrated care system. Geriatrics & Gerontology International, 14(Suppl 2), 2-10. doi: 10.1111/ggi.12259.

O'Connor, N., Fox, S., Kernohan, W. G., Drennan, J., Guerin, S., Murphy, A., & Timmons, S. (2022). A scoping review of the evidence for community-based dementia palliative care services and their related service activities. BMC Palliative Care, 21(1), 32. doi: 10.1186/s12904-022-00922-7.

Piers, R., Albers, G., Gilissen, J., De Lepeleire, J., Steyaert, J., Van Mechelen, W., Steeman, E., Dillen, L., Vanden Berghe, P., & Van den Block, L. (2018). Advance care planning in dementia: recommendations for healthcare professionals. BMC Palliative Care, 17(1), 88. doi: 10.1186/s12904-018-0332-2.

Prince, M., Wimo, A., Guerchet, M., Ali, G., Wu, Y. T., & Prina, M. (2015). World Alzheimer Report 2015: The Global Impact of Dementia. Retrieved from https://www.alz.co.uk/research/WorldAlzheimerReport2015.pdf

Richardson, A., Blenkinsopp, A., Downs, M., & Lord, K. (2019). Stakeholder perspectives of care for people living with dementia moving from hospital to care facilities in the community: A systematic review. BMC Geriatrics, 19(1), 202. doi: 10.1186/s12877-019-1220-1. PMID: 31366373

Samus, Q. M., Black, B. S., Bovenkamp, D., Buckley, M., Callahan, C., Davis, K., Gitlin, L. N., Hodgson, N., Johnston, D., Kales, H. C., Karel, M., Kenney, J. J., Ling, S. M., Panchal, M., Reuland, M., Willink, A., & Lyketsos, C. G. (2018). Home is where the future is: The BrightFocus Foundation consensus panel on dementia care. Alzheimer's & Dementia, 14(1), 104-114. doi: 10.1016/j.jalz.2017.10.006

Senderovich, H., & Retnasothie, S. (2020). A systematic review of the integration of palliative care in dementia management. Palliative & Supportive Care, 18(4), 495-506. doi: 10.1017/S1478951519000968.

Søgaard, R., & Sørensen, J. (2014). Cost-effectiveness of community-based dementia care. International Journal of Geriatric Psychiatry, 29(5), 465-472.

Steinberg, M., Shao, H. W., Zandi, P., et al. (2008). Point and 5-year period prevalence of neuropsychiatric symptoms in dementia: The Cache County Study. International Journal of Geriatric Psychiatry, 23(2), 170-177.

Warrick, N., Prorok, J. C., & Seitz, D. (2018). Care of community-dwelling older adults with dementia and their caregivers. Canadian Medical Association Journal, 190(26), E794-E799. doi: 10.1503/cmaj.170920.

Wendrich-van Dael, A., Bunn, F., Lynch, J., Pivodic, L., Van den Block, L., & Goodman, C. (2020). Advance care planning for people living with dementia: An umbrella review of effectiveness and experiences. International Journal of Nursing Studies, 107, 103576. doi: 10.1016/j.ijnurstu.2020.103576. PMID: 32380259.

World Health Organization. (2012). Dementia: A Public Health Priority. Retrieved from https://www.who.int/mental_health/publications/dementia_report_2012/en/

World Health Organization. (2014). Palliative Care for Older People: Better Practices. Geneva, Switzerland: World Health Organization.

World Health Organization. (2017). Global action plan on the public health response to dementia 2017-2025. Retrieved from https://www.who.int/publications/i/item/global-action-plan-on-the-public-health-response-to-dementia-2017---2025

11

COMMUNITY-BASED PALLIATIVE CARE MODEL FOR THE IRANIAN PATIENTS WITH ALZHEIMER'S DISEASE

MARYAM RASSOULI[1], HADIS ASHRAFIZADEH[2], AND AZAM ESHAGHIAN DORCHEH[3]

Abstract

With the growth of elderly population in the world, debilitating diseases are increasing significantly. Aging has a significant effect on both cognitive and metacognitive processes and increases the likelihood of cognitive failures. The lack of timely diagnosis of these disorders and symptoms will cause irreversible diseases and, concurrently, numerous hospitalizations in medical centers. One of the degenerative diseases that develop in old age is Alzheimer's disease. The diversity and the multiplicity of social, family, and personal problems and outcomes caused by Alzheimer's complicates the care provision for these patients and their caregivers, and since there is no definitive treatment, patients need palliative care. This chapter introduces Alzheimer's status in Iran and the necessity of addressing the needs of the patients and their families in the form of palliative care. Then the status of palliative care in Iran, the necessity of its integration into Primary Health

[1] PhD in Nursing, Professor, Cancer Research Center; School of Nursing & Midwifery, Shahid Beheshti University of Medical Sciences, Vali-e Asr Street, Niyayesh Cross, Tehran, Iran.

[2] PhD in Nursing, Assistant Professor, School of Nursing, Student Research Committee, Dezful University of Medical Sciences, Dezful, Iran. Azadegan Street, Azadegan Square, Dezful, Iran

[3] PhD in Nursing, Kashani Hospital, Isfahan University of Medical Sciences, Isfahan, Iran. Ayatollah Kashani Main Street, Ayatollah Kashani Hospital, Esfahan, Iran.

Care (PHC) and the need for developing a palliative care service package for patients with Alzheimer's will be investigated. In the next step, the components and the dimensions of the developed package including the different settings of service provision, care givers, funding, the physical and psychological dimensions, and the ethical-legal, cultural-social, and spiritual-religious aspects of it will be discussed in detail, as well as the end-of-life care.

Keywords: Community-Based, Palliative Care, Alzheimer's disease, End-of-Life care, Service Package, Iran.

Introduction

Alzheimer's disease, as the most common form of untreatable dementia, accounts for 60-70% of people with dementia (World Health Organization 2019). Every three seconds, one person in the world is affected. Almost 50 million people worldwide live with Alzheimer's disease, around 60% of whom live in low- or middle-income countries. In addition, 10 million new cases are diagnosed every year. The estimated ratio of the people over 60 with Alzheimer's to the general population at a given time is 5 to 8% (World Health Organization 2019, Assocciation Alzheimers in Iran 2018). The prevalence of this disease has been reported to be 3.6% in the Middle East and 2.3% in Iran (Adlimoghaddam, Roy, and Albensi 2018, Navipour et al. 2019). It is estimated that there are 750,000 elderly people living with Alzheimer's disease in Iran, and every 11.5 minutes, one more person is affected by it (Assocciation Alzheimers in Iran 2018, Salehi 2011). According to the latest World Health Organization data published in 2020, deaths due to Alzheimer's and dementia in Iran reached a total of 11046 cases, accounting for 3.32% of all deaths. The age adjusted death rate in Iran is 18.63 per 100,000 people, ranking 74th globally (Wold Health Ranking 2022). Moreover, more than half of these patients are not aware of their disease, resulting in a slow treatment process and an unfavorable outcome due to delayed diagnosis (Iran Dementia & Alzheimer's Association 2019).

According to the report of the World Health Organization (WHO) and the Alzheimer's Disease International, the costs related to the support and the treatment of the people with dementia are more than one percent of the Gross Domestic Product (GPD), i.e. 604 billion dollars in 2010, and 818 billion dollars in 2015 (Wimo et al. 2011). This estimate includes the costs of health and social services as well as the loss of the affected people and their caregivers' incomes (Wimo et al. 2013). The results of recent research in Iran show that the direct costs of a patient in the early stages of the disease at minimum is about 625 $ per year, reaching 1125 $ in the advanced stages. The indirect costs of the disease, such as caregivers' quitting their jobs, family's mental health, as well as family breakup, are not included in these statistics (Iran Dementia & Alzheimer's Association 2016).

There is no known cure for dementia and its variants and, in elderly societies, people are increasingly dying of dementia or the complications that often occur as part of it (Mitchell et al. 2009, Weuve et al. 2014). Dementia can be considered as a chronic-progressive and at the same time terminal disease, which leads to the complicated needs of the patient and the family. In terms of the burden of the disease, dementia is in some ways like cancer (Mitchell et al. 2009, Van der Steen et al. 2014). However, unlike the trajectory of cancer palliative care, people with advanced stage dementia may live for several years, and some never reach a detectable end stage (Gill et al. 2010, Goodman et al. 2015, Hendriks SA 2016). The World Atlas of Palliative Care has placed diseases such as dementia, which may not have a predictable prognosis, in the category *trajectories to death*. As a result, care providers may be unable to determine or accept a 6-month prognosis or curative treatment for a terminal illness. Therefore, trying to provide end-of-life Alzheimer's patients with palliative care as quickly as possible may be a way to reduce additional costs (World Health Organization 2020b).

Dementia caregivers experience high levels of disease burden for reasons such as patients' loss of judgment, their inability to communicate effectively, as well as personality and behavioral changes (Feast et al. 2016, Vaingankar et al. 2016). Cognitive deterioration associated with dementia, which leads to patients' not being aware of the disease, also complicates their participation in care-related decision making (van der Steen et al. 2017). Therefore, family members' participation is particularly important. Family members are both caregivers and surrogate decision makers, who need additional support and information to anticipate future events and understand the terminal nature of the disease (Caron, Griffith, and Arcand 2005, Robinson et al. 2014, Van der Steen et al. 2014). In addition, dementia caregivers are expected to take more responsibilities as the patients' condition deteriorates, leading to an increased burden experienced by caregivers (Hsiao 2015).

Studies have shown that compared to the caregivers of other chronic diseases that require long-term care, according to the caregivers of the people with dementia, caregiving activities are very stressful and higher levels of disease burden in various financial, emotional, physical, and psychological dimensions are reported (Kasper et al. 2015, Iran Dementia & Alzheimer's Association 2019). Along with the anticipated grief, they are involved in the aspects of care that are not experienced by other dying patients. Caregivers have understood the positive and negative dimensions of care provision for Alzheimer's patients and, of course, they are mostly impacted by the negative aspects (Boogaard et al. 2017).

In an Iranian study, the negative experiences of the family caregivers of Alzheimer's patients are categorized in 8 main themes including *caregiving pressure*, *caregiving captivity*, *disruption in family relationships*, *occupational disorders*, *fear of stigma*, *maintaining patient's dignity*, *temporal confusion,* and *caregiver's reactive emotions* (Shafei et al. 2017), where the positive experiences are categorized in 3 themes including *Caregiver's personal growth* (feeling of maturity, highlighted positive personality traits and spiritual growth), *satisfaction with care* (self-satisfaction, self-awareness of the patient's condition, self-awareness of the patient's appreciation, and the joy of being with the patient), and *caregiving achievements* (social appreciation by others and the feeling of mastering one's role) (Farhadi et al. 2018).

Furthermore, in another study, the experiences of family caregivers of Alzheimer's patients are classified in 2 categories. The first category is *burnout and exhaustion* with the 6 sub-categories *mental regression*, *physical burnout*, *role disorder*, *entrusting a family member with care*, *ignoring the patient,* and *economic burden of disease,* and the second one is *growth and transcendence* with 3 subclasses including *resilience and endurance*, *spiritual growth,* and *inner satisfaction with care* (Ashrafizadeh et al. 2021a).

Although caregivers are aware of the importance of their own health in care provision, they sometimes ignore their physical and mental health. In addition to these issues, the economic burden of the disease also causes a great challenge for caregivers. Moreover, the fear of stigma leads some families to feel ashamed of the presence of these patients in their family and try to hide them due to other's inappropriate judgments (Shafei et al. 2017). The diversity and the multiplicity of the problems and the personal, family, and social outcomes caused by Alzheimer's make care provision for these patients and their caregivers complicated. The dynamics of Alzheimer's care focus on multiple factors including the patient, the family, the organization providing care, and the community. In fact, it can be said that caring for these patients goes far beyond the medical and nursing instructions which focus on physical needs and is considered a psychological and social phenomenon (Boyd 2001, Chu and Chi 2008, Machnicki et al. 2009, Mendez-Luck, Kennedy, and Wallace 2009). Considering the complicated nature and the needs of this disease, people with dementia and their families can and should benefit from palliative care (World Health Organization 2020b, van der Steen et al. 2014).

The Status of Palliative Care in Iran

Palliative care, as one of the dimensions of human rights, is an important part of health services, which aims to improve the quality of life in incurable patients and their families through prevention, screening, early diagnosis, the relief of pain and suffering, as well as the assessment and the treatment of physical, psychological, spiritual, and social problems (World Health Organization 2020a). This care was first used for patients with cancer and HIV/AIDS, and later dementia, Alzheimer's and other cognitive disorders were added to the groups in need of palliative care (Batiste and Connor 2017, World Health Organization 2020b). In a report, World Health Organization states that among adult diseases, the ones that cause the most serious pain and suffering and require palliative care include cancer, HIV/AIDS, strokes, Alzheimer's and other types of dementia, and lung diseases (World Health Organization 2020b).

Providing palliative care in the form of simple and accessible services leads to better symptom control, clinical pain management, reduced patient and family anxiety, reduced unnecessary diagnostic and therapeutic actions, a better perception of the patients' needs in the final stages of life, reduced treatment costs, increased patient and family satisfaction, and the improved quality of provided care (Centeno et al. 2016, Gaertner et al. 2015, Shin et al. 2016). Unmet needs are the needs that are either not addressed or inappropriately addressed (Sandman and Hofmann 2019), including many palliative needs of Alzheimer's patients (World Health Organization 2020a). The results of a study showed that in 75% of the patients with dementia who received palliative care, the pain was clinically severe, and 93% of them required morphine treatment; in most of these cases pain control was achieved (Romem et al. 2015).

The World Atlas of Palliative Care has classified the countries of the world according to the level of palliative care development, where Iran is placed in level 3a (isolated palliative care provision) in the EMRO region. The countries in this category are characterized by the development of palliative care activities which is still small in scope and not well supported. Funding is mostly dependent on charities. Limited access to morphine is a major problem and the services provided are insignificant compared to the population. In addition, limited services are mostly provided at home and hospice care is not developed (World Health Organization 2020b).

In Iran, care services for incurable patients, especially those in end-of-life stages, are provided by family members. Although hospitals accept and deliver services to these patients, palliative care is still unknown and limited services are provided (Rassouli and Sajjadi 2014). Most of the patients are deprived of this type of care and it has no place in the Iranian health system (Rassouli and Sajjadi 2016). The patients with incurable diseases who need palliative care are confused about receiving these services and unable to reduce the pain and the suffering caused by their diseases; in most cases, they are not provided with proper and timely services (Asadi-Lari, Madjd, and Akbari 2008). In addition, the health staff's traditional perspective on managing the treatment of incurable diseases, the lack of clear laws in support of health staff to stop unnecessary treatments or ignore the patient or the family's unreasonable expectations, and socio-cultural differences will prevent the improvement of palliative care in the Iranian society. Deficiencies in the process of payment and insurance coverage for these patients is another problem in the delivery of community-based palliative care (Heydari et al. 2016, Mobasher et al. 2013). Moreover, the absence of a healthcare follow-up system in the country after the patient' discharge has caused this care approach to be focused on by Iranian health policymakers in the past years, and the development of palliative care service packages is considered as a perceived need (Silbermann 2014).

In line with WHO's announcement regarding nations' responsibility to prepare plans to deal with Alzheimer's, certain plans have been prepared and commenced in Iran, including the development of the National Document on Dementia, conducting diagnostic-screening tests, creating a comprehensive law for protecting the disabled people, and establishing the field of geriatric medicine in universities. Moreover, Iran Dementia & Alzheimer's Association is known as the first educational, treatment, care, and rehabilitation NGO for the affected people, the offices of which are active in 11 province capitals in cooperation with the Civil Servants Pension

Organization. In addition, research has been conducted on palliative care for Alzheimer's patients in Iran. In one study, the most important unmet palliative care needs of Alzheimer's patients are categorized in 7 dimensions, including *care structures and processes*, *physical aspects of care*, *psychological aspects of care*, *cultural aspects of care*, *social aspects of care*, *ethical-legal aspects of care* and *care provision for end-of-life patients* (Ashrafizadeh et al. 2021b).

Nevertheless, in some countries of the region, such as Oman and Jordan, which are culturally and religiously similar to Iran, the situation is better, and these countries are placed in the category “3b” (generalized palliative care provision) of the World Atlas. The countries in this category are characterized by the development of palliative care activities in multiple locations with increasing local support. These countries have numerous financial resources, convenient access to morphine, palliative care service providing centers and hospices with a wide range of healthcare service providers, as well as certain educational innovations offered by these centers (World Health Organization 2020b).

Oman Alzheimer’s Society was established in 2013 and is a member of Alzheimer's disease International (ADI) since 2018. Oman Alzheimer’s Society recently launched a dementia-friendly program; the services provided by this society include educational events, support, the preparation of educational pamphlets (datasheets, reading materials), as well as educational seminars, webinars, and workshops (international federation of Alzheimer and dementia 2020). In Jordan, Al-Malath Foundation, a voluntary NGO established in 1993, has a nursing home with a team of volunteer nurses who provide social, spiritual, mental and nursing care for the Alzheimer's patients at the end of life stages (Stjernswärd et al. 2007, Zeinah, Al-Kindi, and Hassan 2013). In Jordan, instead of developing a separate plan for Alzheimer's, the disease is integrated as a priority into the existing national/subsidiary regulations or programs that address the related issues such as mental health, aging, disability, or non-communicable diseases (NCD) (World Health Organization 2018).

A codified system of palliative care in every society tries to address the needs of a wide range of patients in healthcare settings such as clinics and home-based care, inpatient and outpatient centers, through creating various processes and structures according to the status quo of the health system. In addition, there are different structures for providing these types of care which vary depending on the structure of the health system in every country.

Developing an organized care plan in accordance with the society, including palliative care programs for patients with Alzheimer's, is a perceived need for the Iranian health system (Rassouli and Sajjadi 2014), which will be explained as follows.

The Necessity of Integrating Palliative Care into Primary Health Care (PHC)

According to the first global monitoring reports on Universal Health Coverage (UHC), at least 400 million people do not have access to one or more essential health services (White 2015). This is mainly due to public health systems' focus on expensive, vertical, disease-specific prevention and treatment programs, insufficient funding for PHC (including community-based palliative care), and the lack of integration between vertical programs and PHC (White 2015). Disease treatment and palliative care should be integrated at all they levels of health care systems. The goal of providing patient-centered palliative care is to formulate and implement care plans in accordance with the goals and preferences of the patient and the caregiver. Integrating PC into PHC improves the quality of life among end-of-life patients (Ray, Najmi, and Sadasivam 2019). Waiting until the final stage of a disease to apply for palliative care results in patients' missing out on improvements in their QoL in the course of treatment (Alshammary et al. 2015).

Mechanisms to ensure the smooth and continuous transition of care between different levels of health care systems, e.g. between hospital care and home care, should be established for all patients, including chronic end-of-life patients such as Alzheimer's (Baillieu et al. 2019). According to the classification of services and the referral system (Mojen et al. 2018), the only community-oriented programs in the structure of PHC in Iran include therapeutic, diagnostic, and preventive health care provision for non-communicable diseases such as vaccination, mental health plan, and IRAPEN program for preventing and controlling 4 non-communicable diseases, i.e. diabetes, hypertension, cancer, and chronic respiratory disease (Heydari et al. 2017). Therefore, the majority of people, especially those living in less privileged areas, do not receive other types of care, especially palliative care (Wang, Kindzierski, and Kaul 2015). Despite the policy of the Ministry of Health for improving the quality of care, reducing the costs of services in community-based care (Hays et al. 2006) and improving the PHC program in Iran, there is still no codified plan to provide patients and their families with palliative care (Asadi-Lari, Madjd, and Akbari 2008).

Due to the growth of elderly population in Iran, increased non-communicable diseases and raised health care costs, fragmented health care systems can no longer effectively address the increased demand for care, and the integration of PC into PHC is an undeniable necessity as mentioned in the WHO statement, required to be carried out by all countries. Obviously, this requires a consensus between policy makers and health care service providers, and the necessary infrastructure should be created with the cooperation of charitable organizations, NGOs, and volunteers (Barasteh et al. 2021, Heydari et al. 2017).

In explaining the policies and drafting the national plans, the realization of a comprehensive health approach and increasing the quality of life are of great importance. Increasing the cost-effectiveness of healthcare and reducing the burden of health costs are among the issues that have been emphasized in the law of the 5th development plan and the health system transformation plan of Iran (Rassouli and Sajjadi 2014). How health care is delivered is an important issue in all countries, and health workers make efforts to provide the highest quality care using the available resources (Nabiloo 2002).

One way to provide quality care is to provide cost-effective service packages. The package of basic health services is a set of basic and prioritized services, for the development of which the economic, social, cultural, and political status of the target community are taken into consideration. Besides, a prioritization process is used to select the related interventions in order to accomplish specific social and technical goals. Iran has just taken the first steps towards developing a service package, and the project for the development of healthcare service packages of health care centers was designed in 2012, in accordance with the comprehensive and universal health network of Iran as a part of the health system transformation plan (Iranian Ministry of Health & Medical Education. 2014b).

In this project, all the communicated and pilot programs of the health sector will be reviewed with the aim of integrating the society's priority needs and maintaining the success of the health system. After reviewing the design of the appropriate model, the draft plan will be submitted to the technical and the executive committees for finalization. The implementation of this package requires the development of infrastructure for service delivery. Therefore, if the services are designed based on the principles of the classification system, the referral system, service packages, guidelines, and a fair financial system, and if the prerequisites are addressed for empowering people regarding self-care, investing in the prevention sector, establishing intersectoral coordination and cooperation, as well as developing healthcare-supporting policies, the package for supporting the elderly with chronic diseases such as Alzheimer's can be implemented (Iranian Ministry of Health & Medical Education. 2014a).

According to the statistics of Alzheimer's and the studies conducted in Iran on the care needs of the patients and their families on the one hand and the need for symptom management and disease treatment on the other hand, the palliative care service package for the elderly with Alzheimer's in the Iranian primary healthcare system has been designed in the form of two service categories:

1- Essential services are related to the structure and the procedures of care provision, the physical dimension of care, the psychological dimension of care, as well as the religious, spiritual, and existential dimension of care.
2- Augmented services include care provision for the patients at end-of-life stages, the ethical and legal aspect of care, the social aspect of care, and the cultural aspect of care.

Obviously, each of the above-mentioned packages has dimensions and components that will be discussed separately as follows:

A) Providing palliative care settings for Alzheimer's patients

Community-Based Care

One of the strategies for managing and providing services to the patients with non-communicable diseases and Alzheimer's is intersectoral cooperation (hospitals and community health centers) and detailed community-based planning. WHO has also presented a community-based care strategy (Javadi M 2011, Xu et al. 2016). This strategy aims to control health care costs and improve the quality of care, and results in reducing the patients' length of hospital stay, moving towards community-based care and using non-hospital resources, as well as providing appropriate and quality home care (Gonçalves-Bradley et al. 2016). Changing policy priorities, using community-based approaches to solve healthcare issues, demographic changes, and the increased need for long-term care, changes in the family structure from extended to nuclear, greater participation of women in the society as a workforce, changes in the people's attitudes and expectations of medical and care services, and the increased demand for private services in the society have persuaded health policymakers to address these needs and to replace community-based care and the traditional approach to hospital care with regard to chronic diseases (Genet et al. 2011, Nikbakht-Nasrabadi and Shabany-Hamedan 2016).

Community-based care has a special place as a result of reduced costs, increased patient satisfaction, minimized need for hospitalization, delivering comprehensive services, controlling chronic diseases, adherence to the treatment, increased quality of life, increasing patients' knowledge of their disease, self-management, as well as the community's participation in care provision (Heydari et al. 2016), and it seems that some community-based approaches such as home care are higher priorities (Ashrafizadeh et al. 2021b).

Home Care

One of the desirable settings of care in the countries with limited resources is home care with the presence of a health care team consisting of a nurse, a volunteer, and a physician under the supervision of hospitals or home care centers. Most of the service centers in the Middle East are based on service provision at home (Rassouli et al. 2021). Today, providing care at home as a model of community-based care is one of the important and necessary needs in developing communities such as Iran and plays an important role in delivering healthcare services through benefiting from the help and the capacity of families, the community, and NGOs (Barati A et al. 2010). Furthermore, services are provided in the form of home care in the health system of many advanced countries, too (Genet et al. 2011).

World Health Organization suggests that home-based palliative care should be provided to patients as a part of PHC, so that all patients can access it in the shortest time possible and benefit from its advantages, regardless of the costs (Genet et al. 2011, Rassouli et al. 2021). This type of care is known to be a favorable care approach in the 21st century and is divided into two groups of specialized and general care. The main goal of this approach is to provide appropriate, quality and cost-effective care to maintain people's ability and independence throughout life. However, its nature may be different from primary health care, secondary level care, and even rehabilitation (Ferrell, Coyle, and Paice 2014, World Health Organization 2018). This type of care, which is considered as one of the community-based care models and one of its key forms, is important in the management of limited resources and is carried out with the aim of reducing patients' length of hospital stay and treatment costs (Barati A et al. 2010).

Nevertheless, in Iran, the services provided to patients are mostly hospital-based, and community-based services are very rare. It seems that one of the goals of establishing palliative care centers, home care, or nursing homes is to create conditions enabling patients to spend the end-of-life stages in a place similar to home with access to care facilities. In the past few decades, the establishment of these centers has grown significantly, and the results show that this increase is associated with a better symptom management in patients and their increased satisfaction (Lysaght and Ersek 2013). Palliative care clinics are the most proper setting for providing care in the hospital, so Iranian health policy makers have come the conclusion that the challenge will be solved by developing a connection between the first and the second levels of care in the form of launching hospital-based palliative care clinics (Rassouli et al. 2021).

Improving home care strategies for the people with cognitive disorders such as Alzheimer's is an urgent need. Home care interventions for these patients include home visits 4-6 times a week for symptom management, medical consultation, checking the complication of medicines, reducing polypharmacy interactions, as well as spiritual and mental support. Home care improves behavioral problems in dementia and Alzheimer's patients, and reduces anxiety and behavioral disorders in them. In addition, the dignity of elderly patients will be maintained as much as possible (Miranda et al. 2019).

In the development of a service package for Alzheimer's patients in Iran, the policymakers focused on providing home-based and community-oriented services in order to cover a wide range of services, and to empower the elderly to live as independent individuals in the community (Shaarbafchi Zadeh et al. 2020).

The care program in Iran's nursing home is not carried out in a comprehensive manner and based on standards, neither does it include all the care needs of the elderly (Parsa et al. 2017). In addition, the current service package of the Welfare Organization's home care program does not even provide individual care at the level of basic healthcare (Safdari et al. 2014).

The Iranian society has a high ethnic diversity and numerous subcultures, and these cultural differences influence people's health beliefs and behaviors in such a way that choosing the places for care delivery, spending end-of-life stages, and death is rooted in their culture (Mogadasian et al. 2014, Saccomano and Abbatiello 2014). On the other hand, dominant religious beliefs in Iran value the provision of care for the sick and the elderly at their own homes, and advise all family members to participate in providing care to the elderly and the disabled. It seems that most people are inclined to receive care primarily at home and then at hospitals and inpatient centers (Heidari, Hosseinkhani, and Norouzadeh 2018). Therefore, home care is consistent with the Iranian culture and can highlight the need to establish this care model.

Hospital care

Due to the poor structure of service provision at the community level, Alzheimer's patients receive most services in the hospital, and mostly visit doctors' offices and different hospital departments. Perhaps one of the most important issues in the current health system is how to establish a connection between the primary level services, i.e. community-based services, and the secondary level services, i.e. hospital services (Rassouli and Sajjadi 2014).

Hospice

One of the settings which had been considered to be important in the service package developed for Alzheimer's patients in Iran by the expert panel was the provision of hospice care as one of the care processes and structures (Ashrafizadeh et al. 2021a, b). The purpose of establishing hospice for Alzheimer's patients in advanced end-of-life stages is to create conditions so that patients can spend the end-of-life stages in a place similar to home with access to care equipment. Moreover, in the past few decades, the establishment of these places has grown significantly, and the results show that this increase is related to better symptom management and increased patient satisfaction (Lysaght and Ersek 2013). However, the lack of awareness of the possibility of care provision for Alzheimer's patients in hospices as well as the lack of familiarity with hospice patient care criteria are the reasons why these patients receive end-of-life care in hospices less frequently. On the other hand, the lack of access to these services can be one of the main obstacles to providing care at end-of-life stages for patients with cognitive disorders. The prerequisite to these cares is the integrity of social and health services and ensuring the continuity of care. The compilation of guidelines, the tools and the standards, planning, and informing people regarding these services help spread these services (Mataqi and Aslanpour 2020).

The results of several Iranian studies have focused on launching and creating the centers that are dedicated to providing care in the end-of-life stages and providing hospice services. However, according to experts, the possibility of establishing these centers is lower comparing to other settings (Ansari et al. 2018, Beiranvand, Rassouli, Hazrati, Molavynejad, Hojjat, Tuvesson, et al. 2022, Beiranvand, Rassouli, Hazrati, Molavynejad, Hojjat, and Zarea 2022). In the meantime, it seems that the establishment of hospice centers and providing comprehensive care in them is a perceived need in the Iranian health system. The existence of hospice centers is essential at least for emergency situations and support, providing temporary care, and also for the patients with special family conditions, and is affected by factors such as changes in the Iranian family structure from traditional and extended families to one-child and nuclear families, or the obstacles to providing home and hospital care (Zarea et al. 2020).

Critically ill patients in the end-of-life stages are generally admitted to intensive care units and much money is spent on their treatment (Ziloochi et al. 2012, JSA 2015, Feizi E EM 2009). In addition, providing care for these patients in the intensive care units of hospitals creates many challenges for nurses and the other members of the medical team, such as the lack of sufficient knowledge and experience in providing end-of-life care, the feeling of providing futile care, mental pressures, and moral issues. Considering that the palliative care system is a nascent care approach in Iran, the establishment of these centers requires conducting more research and fulfilling the necessary prerequisites and facilities for its implementation (Ansari et al. 2018, Borhani, Hosseini, and Abbaszadeh 2014, Valiee, Negarandeh, and Dehghan Nayeri 2012).

Nursing Home

Long-term care includes a variety of services designed to address individuals' health or care needs over a short or long period of time. These services help people who are unable to do their daily activities on their own and need continued care after hospital discharge or care in special environments (Rassouli et al. 2021). This type of care is provided in different places by different caregivers, both formal and informal ones, depending on the individual's needs. Nursing home is defined as a center for providing long-term health care services for the elderly with chronic diseases and disability, especially the ones who need help to carry out their daily life activities. However, there is a lot of concern about the quality of care in nursing homes related to issues such as dignity, abuse, nutrition, and medical care (Bergland and Kirkevold 2006, Shah et al. 2010). Despite the improvements in care provision for the elderly, some challenges emerge in long-term care, as nursing homes are inappropriate and inadequate to address their needs (Batista et al. 2014). Care provision for Alzheimer's patients includes ordinary treatments based on personal experiences without professional attention to other aspects of care (Yektatalab et al. 2012). Sporadic healthcare, inappropriate structure for care provision, and experience-based care are the main forms of nursing home care.

B) Care Providers

In the palliative care package provided for Iranian Alzheimer's patients, the role of volunteers, health liaisons, and family caregivers is very important.

The family members and the friends who regularly visit the patient will play the most important role in providing care for him/her, who are referred to as *informal caregivers*. Furthermore, volunteers and social workers can provide community health center nurses with a report on the status of the patient and the family (World Health Organization 2019). Mainly in the Iranian culture and society, extended families with a traditional structure are inclined to providing care for their patients at home, especially at end-of-life stages (Aseyedali, Sadeghi Mahalli, and Norouzi Tabrizi 2019).

Receiving care at home and being in the familiar environment of home alongside the family members are among the factors that impact patients' quality of life, especially at end-of-life stages (Alborzi et al. 2018, Estebsari and Taghdisi 2015). In Islamic society and the Iranian constitution, the family is considered as a social foundation; using this potential in healthcare helps facilitate the provision of services in the patient's own home with minimized referral to medical centers. In such a situation, the duty of care provision rests on the first-degree family members such as spouse, children, and siblings. Usually, male family members are responsible for the financial, practical, and logistical aspects of care, and females feed, give hope, nurse their patients, and provide care for them. Usually, one of the elder family members, preferably the patient's eldest son, is considered as the head or the leader of the support team (Abedi 2013, Nikbakht-Nasrabadi and Shabany-Hamedan 2016, Rassouli and Sajjadi 2014).

Volunteers and charity donors are effective in the palliative care system of many countries around the world, and the provision of many services, especially hospice services, depends on their participation. These people either have passed formal training courses and are employed in various job positions, or work as informal manpower in various fields, including social support. Palliative care volunteers significantly help terminally-ill patients and their families (Burbeck et al. 2014). The patients who were visited by volunteers were even reported to have a longer survival period than those who did not receive these visits (Candy et al. 2015).

In Iran, most volunteers work in charitable institutions and in the field of community services, especially in the field of psychological and financial support (MKLPT 2018). Using volunteers for providing hospice services is not a priority in Iran compared to other countries (Zarea et al. 2020).

In the service package for Alzheimer's palliative care in Iran, holding ongoing basic and advanced training workshops for all members of the palliative care team is considered important, with the aim of improving and empowering human resources. Standard care in all aspects of the palliative care system requires the use of clinical guidelines and instructions at the national level and the extensive training of service providers. Educating human resources in the palliative care system through dedicating academic degrees and holding training courses, retraining new manpower, and the related disciplines and public volunteers general training are among the processes required to provide services in this system. Moreover, it is required to change the medical education system and the related systems and propose this approach based on new needs and conditions as well as social changes (Ansari et al. 2018).

In 2014, the World Health Assembly explained that addressing the needs of patients and their families in the palliative care system is dependent on the education and the training in the professions relevant to this approach in the health care system. One of the priorities of palliative care for service provider organizations is hiring more employees, and expert staff trained in the field of care services. Providing supportive and palliative care requires specific knowledge, skills, and organization (Connor and Gwyther 2018).

Having information regarding the disease and health care is necessary for family caregivers. How the disease develops, its symptoms, as well as the treatment and the behavior management of Alzheimer's patients are also part of the necessary information that stall the disease and improve the quality of life in patients and their families (Salehi et al. 2017). On the other hand, official caregivers should have the knowledge of the diseases and care provision for these patients and should be able to provide appropriate care. In the nursing undergraduate curriculum, adult/geriatric nursing courses 1-3 investigate health deviations, system by system. In these courses, students learn about Alzheimer's and other cognitive and neurodegenerative disorders. In the geriatric nursing graduate program, students learn about various disorders, including cognitive disorders, how to support the elderly, and the related social and family issues.

Furthermore, geriatric medicine is a specialty clinical discipline which was launched in Iran about 10 years ago and deals with all the medical, psychological, and social issues of the elderly, aiming to help with rehabilitation or maintaining functioning skills or to achieve a good quality of life in the people over 60. Experts in this field evaluate the physical, mental, functional, and social problems of the elderly in order to prevent, diagnose, and treat diseases, besides rehabilitating the elderly. In Iran, caregivers' (i.e. nurses and doctors) level of awareness and attitude towards palliative care delivery has been reported as moderate. Therefore, with the aim of improving this level of awareness, as well as the scientific skills and abilities for addressing the needs of the community, training courses at different levels should be offered in the form of clinical and in-service courses (Ashrafizadeh et al. 2022, Khanali-Mojen et al. 2022).

C) Funding Different Levels of Service Delivery

Providing financial resources to establish a coherent system of palliative care is one of the biggest concerns of most governments regardless of the level of income. In the development of these services, it is necessary to determine the per capita and the costs of medical services at the actual price, develop a coherent communication between the private and public sectors for providing medical services, and explain specific regulations for monitoring how private sector works, design and execute a comprehensive information system, and organize charitable organizations. Diversity in palliative care services exists not only in the type and the content of the services provided, but also in funding methods. Different funding mechanisms may cause differences in the type and the content of services, as well as the number of patients who receive services in the course of disease. In each country, funding models change over time, providing opportunities for palliative care managers to shape future funding mechanisms for palliative care. Privatization in the health system can have positive outcomes. Higher budget and investments in the private sector, and managers' flexibility and freedom in better using the available finances makes them able to carry out more activities with higher diversity in order to attract patients and their families, increase their satisfaction, and provide higher quality services (Nekoeimoghadam, Amiresmaili, and Izadi 2020).

One of the goals of privatization is to improve the access to and the quality of services. Private sector's participation and moving towards decentralization are the most important elements in reforming the health system of each country. In this case, the government should focus on supervisory regulations, the quality of services, and supporting service delivery in the private sector. In other words, the government should manage and monitor the quality of service provision, but should not provide services (Baba and Hain 2012). In Iran, few insurance organizations have covered home-care nursing services. Nursing Office's plan regarding the insurance coverage of costly diseases such as stroke, congestive cardiac failure, cancer, chronic obstructive pulmonary diseases (COPD), and neonatal jaundice, as well as ICU hospitalization is currently awaiting insurance pilot for estimating the costs and assessing cost-effectiveness.

Some NGOs and charity centers, such as Ala Charity Foundation, provide free of charge home care services for the adults with cancer; The Mahak Society to Support Children with Cancer offers services to children with cancer. Some home care centers are also active in the private sector, which provide general services that may include end-of-life care (mostly physical care), but these services are not free of charge. Although there are many charitable organizations in the country which only provide general services to cancer patients, each of them delivers services in only one field; they do not provide comprehensive services, especially end-of-life care, for Alzheimer's patients (Ansari et al. 2018, Mojen 2017).

D) Physical and Psychological Aspects of Care

Since Alzheimer's disease is a complicated disease with behavioral and psychological symptoms (BPSD) including a wide range of physical, emotional, psychological, and behavioral symptoms, which causes great pain and suffering in patients and caregivers, the only solution is adopting comprehensive and holistic approaches (Tible et al. 2017, Zucchella et al. 2018). BPSD management requires a both patient-centered and caregiver-centered method, and interventions are necessary in order to comfort patients and reduce the care burden (Tible et al. 2017). Developing patient-centered care services, focusing on the patient instead of the disease, will only be possible through a better perception of the patient's issues and symptoms, and prioritizing them (Curnow et al. 2019). Care provision for the patients with BPSD includes psychosocial therapies for both the patient and the family. BPSD may respond to environmental and psychological interventions; however, for more severe symptoms, pharmacological treatment is often required (Hersch and Falzgraf 2007). In regard with dementia, the first step in implementing a multidisciplinary and comprehensive plan is a combination of different approaches such as care delivery and pharmacological treatment, epidemiology and genetics, social environment and behavioral issues, as well as biomarkers and health behaviors (Rodriguez Then et al. 2020).

Some programs have been developed and launched in Iran regarding Alzheimer's management. But there is no comprehensive and holistic approach for managing these patients. In addition, the lack of treatment-care centers and the absence of a home care system to provide care for Alzheimer's patients are the main obstacles to achieving comprehensive Alzheimer's management in Iran, where management of BPSD symptoms is mostly done through drug interventions. Expert advice and guidelines mostly focus on non-pharmacological interventions as the first-line approach. Although there is poor evidence in favor of most non-pharmacological strategies, their effectiveness is confirmed through long-term clinical experience. BPSD pharmacological treatment is frequently offered, but is often accompanied by serious complications (Deuschl and Maier 2016, Savaskan et al. 2014). Since Alzheimer's patients are especially vulnerable to the adverse effects of medicines, it is recommended to use non-pharmacological interventions in the first step and then follow pharmacological interventions to better manage the physical and psychological symptoms in these patients (Ashrafizadeh et al. 2021b).

E) Ethical and Legal Aspects of Care

Since Alzheimer's has a progressive nature and the patient's abilities significantly decrease in each phase, it is required to follow some ethical and legal considerations in each phase of the disease. In general, the ethical considerations related to Alzheimer's patients can be expressed in *initial*, *middle*, and *final phases*, and in the 3 sections *care*, *treatment*, and *research* in the form of the principles of ethics consisting of *independence*, *care*, *participation*, *self-fulfillment*, and *dignity* (KhanAhmadi M 2015). One of the important ethical challenges is complicated surrogate decision-making, which is created due to the patient's lack of decision-making competence (DMC) and can be followed by many ethical dilemmas for formal and informal caregivers. Decision-making appears to be impaired in the early phases of Alzheimer's, and even more impaired in later phases. This decline in the decision-making ability seriously impacts the quality of life in the patient and the relatives, for they are often asked to make important decisions, especially regarding health care, finances, or the place of residence (Gaubert and Chainay 2021).

Today, contrary to the rich Iranian culture that recommends respect for the elderly, the ethical and legal principles concerning the elderly are not given much attention. According to the service package developed for these patients, it is necessary to create a framework for solving ethical and legal issues in a way that makes it possible for the patients with Alzheimer's to make their own decisions and choose surrogate decision makers to make decisions regarding the patient's behavior, which includes major decisions around care, treatment, and finances, as well as daily decisions.

Furthermore, this package places special emphasis on misbehavior in Alzheimer's patients. Maltreatment is defined as intentional harm, irrational confinement, intimidation, or punishment, which can lead to physical harm, pain, psychological suffering, or deprivation (Pitman and Metzger 2018, Services. 2019). Maltreatment can come from a variety of sources, including family members, informal and formal caregivers, acquaintances, or other patients during hospitalization (Yon et al. 2019).

Assessment by physicians and nurses, who play an important role in controlling maltreatment, may identify other symptoms that may contribute to the offending behavior, such as inadequate pain treatment, delirium, constipation, or infection, all of which are common among the patients with cognitive impairment and difficult to evaluate (Rosen et al. 2016). Early diagnosis and creating a suitable solution will provide a vital opportunity for both the caregiver and the care recipient. Through training caregivers towards increasing correct coping strategies and improving and correcting ineffective coping behaviors, individuals' abilities to deal with the situations in which they may misbehave (such as dealing with the patients' aggressive behaviors) can be increased (Pourmollamirza et al. 2020).

F) Sociocultural Aspects of Care

Culture is considered a determining factor in health care due to its influence on lifestyle, beliefs and values, individuals' perception of the quality of life and palliative care, interactions with the health care system, as well as decision-making during the illness and the end-of-life stages. Therefore, besides the facilities and the resources available in the health system of each country in the design of the structure of special service provision, the selection of patients is also of particular importance (Park et al. 2016). Early discussion of disease prognosis and end-of-life care options leads to faster acceptance of palliative care in these stages. The desire to tell or know the truth about one's illness or death is considered a value in the western culture, and patients are entitled to be informed about their illness so that they can make decisions around end-of-life care. However, in some communities, talking about diagnosis, prognosis, and death is a taboo, because it leads to losing hope and causes concerns about reduced adherence to treatment (Senel and Silbermann 2017).

In the Iranian culture, it is common to hide the truth of illness and death from the patient, and in these cases, the truth has often kept hidden from the patient at the request of the family. The reason behind it is the belief that telling the truth to the patient leads to losing hope and increases the suffering and the discomfort of the patient. However, patients are willing to know about the condition of the disease, as well as its diagnosis and prognosis (Motlagh et al. 2014, Senel and Silbermann 2017). In addition, the Iranian society has ethnic diversity and numerous subcultures that affect their health beliefs and behaviors (Zamani et al. 2011). Without doubt, cultural differences have had a major impact on the acceptance and the use of hospice and palliative care services, and these differences should be taken into account in the design and the development of these services in any society (Aseyedali, Sadeghi Mahalli, and Norouzi Tabrizi 2019).

One of the important items mentioned in the service package compiled in line with cultural and social aspects is social destigmatization. Being diagnosed with Alzheimer's disease, like mental illnesses, carries significant stigma, due to cultural beliefs about etiology and antisocial behaviors that can result from cognitive impairment (Ashrafizadeh et al. 2021a, b). Caregivers' experiences indicate the fear of being ridiculed by the society and the relatives; their attempts to hide the patient reflect this issue. People in collectivist cultures, like the Iranian culture, pay a lot of attention to relationships with others and care about how they manage their communications with them. When a person cannot establish effective relationships with caregivers and other people, their presence as a member of society will be questioned; as a result, these patients need acceptance from the family, the society, and the medical system (Yektatalab et al. 2013).

Reducing stigma in patients, culture-building, especially through mass media, education, protesting current inequalities, and communicating with the people who have Alzheimer's have great impacts on people's belief systems, and manifesting mental disease and Alzheimer's to people will have a significant impact on how the disease is perceived (Edney 2012, Mukadam and Livingston 2012). Therefore, the necessity of cultural interventions, including education through mass media, to promote and improve the society's attitude towards Alzheimer's patients and their families is felt.

In addition, Alzheimer's patients in Iran receive less social support compared to the similar patients in developed countries (Prince 2004). The studies show that patients with mild to moderate Alzheimer's disease receive the lowest amount of social support, mainly facing the lack of support and reduced self-confidence (Górska, Forsyth, and Maciver 2018, Yang et al. 2020). Besides, providing a model to empower vulnerable Iranian caregivers of the elderly along with the patients has been emphasized in the studies that point to the necessity of emotional, psychological, and informational support for caregivers; it states that empowering caregivers is important in facing the problems of caring for the elderly and managing family care (Mohammadi 2008). Despite the need for social support, there is no support program for Alzheimer's patients in Iran, such as financial, psychological, and social support programs from the governmental organizations, peer groups, family, and society, which may be due to the lack of guidelines, policy making, and planning in this field (Ashrafizadeh et al. 2021a, b). It is recommended to provide a supportive approach for Alzheimer's patients and their family caregivers that combines recreational activities, psychotherapy for the patients, psychotherapy and support groups for caregivers, social activities for the patients and their caregivers, and holding regular meetings in medical centers, the need for which is now felt more than ever.

G) Religious and Spiritual Aspects of Care

According to the service package developed in Iran, providing spiritual care for Alzheimer's patients is one of the ignored basic needs. In Iran, the religious beliefs of the patients with dementia have received less attention compared to other patients, and less spiritual care has been provided for the patients with cognitive disorders (Daaleman et al. 2008, Sampson et al. 2006). The lack of spiritual care provision for Alzheimer's patients at the end-of-life stages creates specific challenges. On the other hand, establishing verbal communication is impossible due to cognitive impairment or comorbidities in Alzheimer's, which makes it difficult to provide this type of care for these patients (van der Steen et al. 2014). Conceptually, needs assessment is a part of spiritual care at the end-of-life stages (Cobb, Dowrick, and Lloyd-Williams 2012, Vachon, Fillion, and Achille 2009).

After the needs assessment, spiritual and religious interventions can be useful in coping with the disease and improving the patient's well-being (Bonelli and Koenig 2013, Ennis and Kazer 2013). Receiving or not receiving spiritual care at the end-of-life stages in the patients with dementia is not precisely known (Daaleman et al. 2008). The religious environments with specific circumstance, such as Iran, where spirituality and religion are interlinked, also create barriers to providing care, as a result of which the spiritual needs of patients may be ignored for various reasons (Farahani et al. 2019). The most important obstacle to providing spiritual care in Iran is the lack of time and the fear of patients discomfort, which prevents their spiritual needs' from being revealed (Farahani et al. 2019). Spiritual care is a part of palliative care (World Health Organization 2002), which should be provided in accordance with the patient and the family's beliefs (van der Steen et al. 2014).

Therefore, one's spiritual history should be taken into consideration and the sensitivities of the patient, and the family should be respected. Given that one of the goals of palliative care is focusing on spiritual approaches, the challenges in this field should be identified. It is possible to address the current issues and spread spiritual care through the organizational and managerial support of health service providers, supplying sufficient workforce, revising the strategies implemented in care environments regarding the allocation of healthcare providers' services, designing and implementing theoretical and practical training courses in the form of in-service training programs.

H) Providing Care for the Patients at End-of-Life Stages

Caring for end-of-life stage patients is a big challenge presented in a challenging environment. The care provided for the patients in this department is mostly in the form of support, which is provided in a comprehensive and humanistic manner focusing on the patient's body and mind. Nevertheless, this issue has not received much attention in Iran's health system and medical centers. The goal of end-of-life care is providing a good and peaceful death, maintaining balance in the patient's daily life, and comforting the family following a long illness (Iranmanesh et al. 2010). End-of-life care is one of the key components of care for the elderly, including Alzheimer's patients. However, evidence shows that people over 85 have less access to specialty end-of-life care (Hunt, Shlomo, and Addington-Hall 2014). A comparison of the cancer and the Alzheimer's patients receiving end-of-life care indicates that analgesics have less frequently been used to control pain and manage end-of-life symptoms in Alzheimer's patients (Sampson et al. 2006).

In Islamic societies like Iran, religious beliefs play an important role in people's attitude about End-of-Life Care (EoLC). These believes affect their decision making around the conditions regarding EoLC, such as futile care and Do-Not-Resuscitate (DNR) order (Rassouli et al. 2021).

According to the definition of futile care, life-saving interventions and treatments have no potential positive effect on the patient's quality of life, and cannot end the patient's dependence on medical care (Meltzer and Huckabay 2004). Therefore, individuals' having different perceptions of the definition of futility and futile care has created many challenges between the treatment team and the patients' families regarding decision making around continuing or quitting this type of interventions (DJ 2011). These data suggest that even when prolonging the patient's life remains as a goal, antimicrobials may be administrated orally, if necessary, avoiding more invasive intravenous treatments or hospitalization.

In addition, in these patients, there are fewer DNR and DNH (Do-Not-Hospitalize) orders, and the probability of receiving palliative care is lower, too (Mitchell, Kiely, and Hamel 2004). The religious background of individuals, including medical staff, has created numerous ethical, legal, and religious challenges (Peimani, Zahedi, and Larijani 2012), many of which are rooted in misunderstandings of resuscitation, ignorance of the evidence related to this intervention, patients' suffering, prolonged death process, as well as direct and indirect costs (Shamsi Goshki E 2014). Some experts believe that if requested by the patient and in case the doctor's clinical judgment indicates that resuscitation will not help the patient, ethical principles such as autonomy, beneficence, and non-maleficence will be taken into consideration, which can solve some of these challenges (Shamsi Goshki E 2014). In this case, since according to Islam, death is considered as a stage of human spiritual life, delaying or prolonging the process of death is not justifiable (Peimani, Zahedi, and Larijani 2012). In many cases, due to its illegality, DNR is performed without informing the patient and the family, and messages will be exchanged verbally without being recorded (Rassouli et al. 2021).

Moreover, the most important rights of a dying person include being cared for as a living person until death, staying hopeful, and being cared for by those who can give him/her hope, not being deceived, being supported by the family to accept death, dying peacefully while maintaining his/her human dignity and respect and not being judged by others, participating in decision making around his/her own care, not dying alone, being relieved of pain, his/her questions being answered correctly, as well as having his/her body purified and respected after death. Besides, there are religious instructions regarding managing this period of the patient's life and his/her relatives in all cultures, especially in the religion of Islam (Bahramnezhad et al. 2018).

Considering the human values in the Iranian society regarding the issue of life and death, the importance of religion, as well as the people and the society's believing that their loved ones should be cared for in the best possible way in the end-of-life stages, it seems that providing these services will be welcomed. In addition to these issues, families' problems and concerns regarding the care provision for their patients in the end-of- life stages, including the lack of knowledge and time shortage, makes the need for these centers even stronger. However, on the other hand, the cultural and religious beliefs and issues of patients and families in the traditional Iranian society may lead to the rejection of this type of services in hospice centers (Azami-Aghdash et al. 2015). Therefore, offering practical solutions for the management of these conditions is necessary and requires the development of national DNR guidelines in accordance with the ethical principles as well as scientific, cultural, local, and religious principles, which has led to start hospital ethics committees for making decisions in emergency situations.

Conclusion

Palliative care is necessary for the elderly with chronic and life-threatening diseases in order to shorten the length of hospital stay and reduce hospital complications and the use of limited hospital resources. This type of care should be provided through empowering the family in care, under the supervision of the treatment team and a multidisciplinary and interdisciplinary experienced care team at all the levels of care. Therefore, teaching palliative care at all the levels and the areas of care, as well as applying it, is important. Based on the service package designed for Alzheimer's patients in the Iranian society, all the needs of Alzheimer's patients should be considered together and comprehensively. The lack of justice in having access to health care services for Alzheimer's patients is one of the important challenges.

Therefore, it is suggested that policy makers pay more attention to the integration of palliative care for Alzheimer's patients in the primary health care system and explaining its position. In addition, it is very important to develop the infrastructure in the health system, which requires paying attention to many factors in the field of policy making. Based on this package, the patients and their families should be provided with services by an interdisciplinary and multidisciplinary expert team. Therefore, it is necessary to implement public awareness programs, provide and train expert manpower, codify clinical guidelines and implement them at the related levels, use the capacity of all the levels of the primary health care system, and encourage the private sector and non-governmental organizations. The palliative care service package for the elderly with Alzheimer's in the primary health care system can be used as a model appropriate to the conditions of the health system and the society in Iran.

Acknowledgements

The authors hereby express their gratitude to Professor Michael Silbermann, who eliminated all geographical boundaries through his amazing efforts and patience. He helped the countries in the region mobilize and take action towards a single goal, which is nothing but the provision of palliative care to cancer patients, regardless of their culture, language and religion. The authors also thank Professor Mohammad Esmaeil Akbari for his guidance and knowledgeable support of the establishment of palliative care in Iran.

References

Abedi, Mojdeh. 2013. "Palliative Care within the Iranian Context: re-defining palliative care, deploying spirituality as a support measure and need for cultural sensitivity." In *Spirituality: New Reflections on Theory, Praxis and Pedagogy*, 249-258. Brill.

Adlimoghaddam, A., B. Roy, and B. C. Albensi. 2018. "Future Trends and the Economic Burden of Dementia in Manitoba: Comparison with the Rest of Canada and the World." *Neuroepidemiology* 51 (1-2):71-81. doi: 10.1159/000490414.

Alborzi, Jila, Fahimeh Sabeti, Shahram Baraz, Mojtaba Miladinia, Vahid Saidkhani, and Asaad Sharhani. 2018. "Investigating of moral distress and attitude to euthanasia in the intensive care unit nurses." *International Journal of Pediatrics* 6 (11):8475-8482.

Alshammary, Sami Ayed, Abdullah Alsuhail, Balaji P Duraisamy, Saad Hamad Alabdullateef, and Savithiri Ratnapalan. 2015. "Interval between first palliative care consultation and death among patients in a comprehensive cancer center in Saudi Arabia." *J Health Spec* 3 (2):61.

Ansari, Mojgan, Maryam Rassouli, Mohamad Esmaiel Akbari, Abbas Abbaszadeh, and Ali Akbari Sari. 2018. "Educational needs on palliative care for cancer patients in Iran: A SWOT analysis." *International journal of community based nursing and midwifery* 6 (2):111.

Asadi-Lari, Mohsen, Z Madjd, and ME Akbari. 2008. "The need for palliative care services in Iran; an introductory commentary." *International Journal of Cancer Management* 1 (1).

Aseyedali, Masoume, Nasim Sadeghi Mahalli, and Kian Norouzi Tabrizi. 2019. "A review on adult daycare centers in the world." *Iranian Journal of Aging* 13 (4):518-528.

Ashrafizadeh, Hadis, Mahin Gheibizadeh, Maryam Rassouli, Fatemeh Hajibabaee, and Shahnaz Rostami. 2021a. "Explain the Experience of Family Caregivers Regarding Care of Alzheimer's Patients: A Qualitative Study." *Frontiers in Psychology* 12. doi: 10.3389/fpsyg.2021.699959.

Ashrafizadeh, Hadis, Mahin Gheibizadeh, Maryam Rassouli, Fatemeh Hajibabaee, and Shahnaz Rostami. 2021b. "Explaining Caregivers' Perceptions of Palliative Care Unmet Needs in Iranian Alzheimer's Patients: A Qualitative Study." *Frontiers in Psychology* 12. doi: 10.3389/fpsyg.2021.707913.

Ashrafizadeh, Hadis, Leila Khanali Mojen, Salman Barasteh, Mohammad Esmaeil Akbari, Samira Beiranvand, Azam Shirinabadi Farahani, Azam Eshaghian Dorcheh, Maryam Karami, Fatemeh Khademi, and Tahereh

Alsadat Khoubbin Khoshnazar. 2022. "Factors Related to Nurses and Physicians' Knowledge and Attitudes Towards Palliative Care." *International Journal of Cancer Management* 15 (2).

Assocciation Alzheimers in Iran. 2018. "Dementia: a health priority ".

Azami-Aghdash, Saber, Morteza Ghojazadeh, Mir Hossein Aghaei, Mohammad Naghavi-Behzad, and Zoleikha Asgarlo. 2015. "Perspective of patients, patients' families, and healthcare providers towards designing and delivering hospice care services in a middle income country." *Indian Journal of Palliative Care* 21 (3):341.

Baba, Megumi, and Richard Hain. 2012. "Paediatric Palliative Care in the United Kingdom." In *Pediatric palliative care: Global perspectives*, 269-298. Springer.

Bahramnezhad, F, P Askari, M Shiri, and N Sanaie. 2018. "Concept of palliative care of the end of life from the perspective of the Quran and Hadith." *Qurʾān va ṭib (Quran and Medicine)* 3 (4):193-198.

Baillieu, Robert, Michael Kidd, Robert Phillips, Martin Roland, Michael Mueller, David Morgan, Bruce Landon, Jennifer DeVoe, Viviana Martinez-Bianchi, and Hong Wang. 2019. "The Primary Care Spend Model: a systems approach to measuring investment in primary care." *BMJ Global Health* 4 (4):e001601.

Barasteh, Salman, Akram Parandeh, Maryam Rassouli, Rouhallah Zaboli, Amir Vahedian-Azimi, and Morteza Khaghanizadeh. 2021. "Integration of palliative care into the primary health care of iran: a document analysis." *Middle East Journal of Cancer* 12 (2):292-300.

Barati A, Janati A, Tourani S, Khalesi N, and Gholizadeh M. 2010. "Iranian Professional's Perception about Advantages of Developing Home Health Care System in Iran." *Hakim Health Systems Research Journal* 13 (2):71-79.

Batista, MRF, F Batista, KM Meneses, LF Pompeu, RRS Silva, and CMM Sousa. 2014. "Elders perception of their lives in long-term care facilities." *J Nurs UFPE line* 8 (7):1988-96.

Batiste, Xavier Gómez, and Stephen R Connor. 2017. *Building integrated palliative care programs and services*: Càtedra de Cures Pal· liatives.

Beiranvand, S., M. Rassouli, M. Hazrati, S. Molavynejad, S. Hojjat, and K. Zarea. 2022. "Developing a Model for the Establishment of the Hospice Care Delivery System for Iranian Adult Patients With Cancer." *Front Psychol* 13:807621. doi: 10.3389/fpsyg.2022.807621.

Beiranvand, Samira, Maryam Rassouli, Maryam Hazrati, Shahram Molavynejad, Suzanne Hojjat, Hanna Tuvesson, and Kourosh Zarea. 2022. "Hospice care delivery system requirements." *International Journal of Palliative Nursing* 28 (12):562-574.

doi: 10.12968/ijpn.2022.28.12.562.

Bergland, Ådel, and Marit Kirkevold. 2006. "Thriving in nursing homes in Norway: contributing aspects described by residents." *International journal of nursing studies* 43 (6):681-691.

Bonelli, Raphael M., and Harold G. Koenig. 2013. "Mental Disorders, Religion and Spirituality 1990 to 2010: A Systematic Evidence-Based Review." *Journal of Religion and Health* 52 (2):657-673. doi: 10.1007/s10943-013-9691-4.

Boogaard, JA, JT van der Steen, AH de Boer, CMPM Hertogh, and MI Broese van Groenou. 2017. "Informal end-of-life care for community dwelling older people with or without dementia: caregiver burden and positive experiences." Abstract accepted for presentation at the 15th Worl Congress of the European Association for Palliative Care (EAPC): Madrid.

Borhani, F, SH Hosseini, and A Abbaszadeh. 2014. "Commitment to care: a qualitative study of intensive care nurses' perspectives of end-of-life care in an I slamic context." *International Nursing Review* 61 (1):140-147.

Boyd, Mary Ann. 2001. "Behavioral disturbances associated with dementia: Nursing implications." *Journal of the American Psychiatric Nurses Association* 7 (6):S14-S22.

Burbeck, Rachel, Bridget Candy, Joe Low, and Rebecca Rees. 2014. "Understanding the role of the volunteer in specialist palliative care: a systematic review and thematic synthesis of qualitative studies." *BMC palliative care* 13 (1):1-12.

Candy, Bridget, Rachel France, Joe Low, and Liz Sampson. 2015. "Does involving volunteers in the provision of palliative care make a difference to patient and family wellbeing? A systematic review of quantitative and qualitative evidence." *International journal of nursing studies* 52 (3):756-768.

Caron, Chantal D, Jennifer Griffith, and Marcel Arcand. 2005. "Decision making at the end of life in dementia: how family caregivers perceive their interactions with health care providers in long-term-care settings." *Journal of Applied Gerontology* 24 (3):231-247.

Centeno, Carlos, Thomas Lynch, Eduardo Garralda, José Miguel Carrasco, Francisco Guillen-Grima, and David Clark. 2016. "Coverage and development of specialist palliative care services across the World Health Organization European Region (2005–2012): Results from a European Association for Palliative Care Task Force survey of 53 Countries." *Palliative Medicine* 30 (4):351-362.

Chu, Leung-Wing, and Iris Chi. 2008. "Nursing homes in China." *Journal of the American Medical Directors Association* 9 (4):237-243.

Cobb, Mark, Christopher Dowrick, and Mari Lloyd-Williams. 2012. "Understanding spirituality: a synoptic view." *BMJ Supportive & Palliative Care* 2 (4):339-343. doi: 10.1136/bmjspcare-2012-000225.

Connor, Stephen R, and Elizabeth Gwyther. 2018. "The worldwide hospice palliative care alliance." *Journal of pain and symptom management* 55 (2):S112-S116.

Curnow, Eleanor, Robert Rush, Donald Maciver, Sylwia Górska, and Kirsty Forsyth. 2019. "Exploring the needs of people with dementia living at home reported by people with dementia and informal caregivers: a systematic review and Meta-analysis." *Aging & mental health*:1-11.

Daaleman, Timothy P, Christianna S Williams, V Lee Hamilton, and Sheryl Zimmerman. 2008. "Spiritual care at the end of life in long-term care." *Medical care*:85-91.

Deuschl, G, and W Maier. 2016. S3-Leitlinie Demenzen. Deutsche Gesellschaft für Neurologie, Hrsg Leitlinien für Diagnostik und Therapie in der Neurologie.

DJ, Wilkinson. 2011. "Savulescu J. Knowing when to stop: futility in the intensive care unit." *Current opinion in anaesthesiology* 24 (2):160-165.

Edney, DR. . 2012. "Mass media and mental illness: Lit. Rev. ."

Ennis, Everol M., Jr., and Meredith Wallace Kazer. 2013. "The Role of Spiritual Nursing Interventions on Improved Outcomes in Older Adults With Dementia." *Holistic Nursing Practice* 27 (2).

Estebsari, Fatemeh, and Mohammad Hossain Taghdisi. 2015. "A Qualitati e Study on Affe ting Fa tors on Quality of Life in End-Stage Patients."

Farahani, Azam S., Maryam Rassouli, Nayereh Salmani, Leila K. Mojen, Moosa Sajjadi, Mehdi Heidarzadeh, Zeynab Masoudifar, and Fateme Khademi. 2019. "Evaluation of Health-Care Providers' Perception of Spiritual Care and the Obstacles to Its Implementation." *Asia-Pacific Journal of Oncology Nursing* 6 (2):122-129. doi: https://doi.org/10.4103/apjon.apjon_69_18.

Farhadi, Akram, Maryam Noroozian, Farahnaz Mohammadi, Mahshid Foroughan, Maryam Rassouli, Liela Sadeghmoghadam, and Shima Nazari. 2018. "Positive Experiences of Caregiving in Family Caregivers of Older Adults with Dementia: a Content Analysis Study." *Iranian South Medical Journal* 21 (4):319-334.

Feast, Alexandra, Esme Moniz-Cook, Charlotte Stoner, Georgina Charlesworth, and Martin Orrell. 2016. "A systematic review of the relationship between behavioral and psychological symptoms (BPSD) and caregiver well-being." *International psychogeriatrics* 28 (11):1761-1774.

Feizi E EM, Ansari M. 2009. "Mortality rate and effective factors of patients in intensive care unit." *Journal of Ardabil University of Medical Sciences* 8 (4):420-423.

Ferrell, Betty R, Nessa Coyle, and Judith Paice. 2014. *Oxford textbook of palliative nursing*: Oxford University Press.

Gaertner, Jan, Waldemar Siemens, Gerd Antes, Joerg J Meerpohl, Carola Xander, Guido Schwarzer, Stephanie Stock, and Gerhild Becker. 2015. "Specialist palliative care services for adults with advanced, incurable illness in hospital, hospice, or community settings—protocol for a systematic review." *Systematic Reviews* 4 (1):1-9.

Gaubert, Fanny, and Hanna Chainay. 2021. "Decision-making competence in patients with Alzheimer's disease: A review of the literature." *Neuropsychology Review* 31 (2):267-287. doi: 10.1007/s11065-020-09472-2.

Genet, Nadine, Wienke GW Boerma, Dionne S Kringos, Ans Bouman, Anneke L Francke, Cecilia Fagerström, Maria Gabriella Melchiorre, Cosetta Greco, and Walter Devillé. 2011. "Home care in Europe: a systematic literature review." *BMC health services research* 11 (1):1-14.

Gill, Thomas M, Evelyne A Gahbauer, Ling Han, and Heather G Allore. 2010. "Trajectories of disability in the last year of life." *New England Journal of Medicine* 362 (13):1173-1180.

Gonçalves-Bradley, Daniela C, Natasha A Lannin, Lindy M Clemson, Ian D Cameron, and Sasha Shepperd. 2016. "Discharge planning from hospital." *Cochrane database of systematic reviews* (1).

Goodman, Claire, Katherine Froggatt, Sarah Amador, Elspeth Mathie, and Andrea Mayrhofer. 2015. "End of life care interventions for people with dementia in care homes: addressing uncertainty within a framework for service delivery and evaluation." *BMC palliative care* 14 (1):1-9.

Górska, Sylwia, Kirsty Forsyth, and Donald Maciver. 2018. "Living with dementia: a meta-synthesis of qualitative research on the lived experience." *The Gerontologist* 58 (3):e180-e196.

Hays, Ross M, Jeanette Valentine, Gerri Haynes, J Russel Geyer, Nanci Villareale, Beth Mckinstry, James W Varni, and Shervin S Churchill. 2006. "The Seattle Pediatric Palliative Care Project: effects on family satisfaction and health-related quality of life." *Journal of palliative medicine* 9 (3):716-728.

Heidari, Mohammad Reza, Seyedeh Navabeh Hosseinkhani, and Reza Norouzadeh. 2018. "Elderly's Attitude toward End-Of-Life Concerns." *JOURNAL OF NURSING EDUCATION (JNE),[online]* 7 (2):35-44.

Hendriks SA, Smalbrugge M, van Gageldonk-Lafeber AB, Galindo-Garre F, Schipper M, Hertogh CMPM, et al. 2016. "Pneumonia, intake problems, and survival among nursing home residents with variable stages of dementia in the Netherlands: Results from a prospective observational study. ." *Alzheimer Dis Assoc Disord Epub ahead of print.*

Hersch, Elizabeth C., and Sharon Falzgraf. 2007. "Management of the behavioral and psychological symptoms of dementia." *Clinical interventions in aging* 2 (4):611-621. doi: 10.2147/cia.s1698.

Heydari, Heshmatolah, Hooman Shahsavari, Abdolrahim Hazini, and Alireza Nikbakht Nasrabadi. 2016. "Exploring the barriers of home care services in Iran: A qualitative study." *Scientifica* 2016.

Heydari, Mohammad Reza, Ahmad Kalateh Sadati, Kamran Bagheri Lankarani, Mohamma Hadi Imanieh, Homataj Baghi, and Mohammad Javad Lolia. 2017. "The evaluation of urban community health centers in relation to family physician and primary health care in southern Iran." *Iranian journal of public health* 46 (12):1726.

Hsiao, CY. 2015. "Caregiver burden for informal caregivers of patients with dementia: A systematic review." *International nursing review.*

Hunt, Katherine J, Natalie Shlomo, and Julia Addington-Hall. 2014. "End-of-life care and preferences for place of death among the oldest old: Results of a population-based survey using VOICES–Short Form." *Journal of palliative medicine* 17 (2):176-182. international federation of Alzheimer and dementia. 2020. "Oman Alzheimer's Society."

Iranian Ministry of Health & Medical Education. 2014a. "ajmoheh dasturolamalhaye barnameh tahavole nezameh salamat ". Iran., Ministry Health of. 2014b. "barnameh tahavol nezame salamat dar hozeh pezeshki."

Iran Dementia & Alzheimer's Association. 2019. "The upward trend of Iran's aging and outbreaks of Alzheimer's and Parkinson's."

Iran Dementia & Alzheimer's Association. 2016. Draft Comprehensive National Action Plan for Dementia In the Islamic Republic of Iran. In *1*. Iran Ministry of Health Medical Education.

Iranmanesh, Sedigheh, Karin Axelsson, Terttu Häggström, and Stefan Sävenstedt. 2010. "Caring for dying people: Attitudes among Iranian and Swedish nursing students." *Indian journal of palliative care* 16 (3):147.

Javadi M, Maroofi M, Yaghoobi M. 2011. "Hospital's new role in chronic disease management: WHO, strategies and the patient self-management." *Proceedings of the 1st National Conference On Community Oriented Care In ChronicDisease* (Dec 23-25 Isfahan).

JSA, Imani E. 2015. "Evaluation of terminal life cost for patients admitted in teaching hospitals affiliated with Kerman university of medical sciences in 2014." *Journal of Health Based Research* 1 (2):133-143.

Kasper, Judith D, Vicki A Freedman, Brenda C Spillman, and Jennifer L Wolff. 2015. "The disproportionate impact of dementia on family and unpaid caregiving to older adults." *Health Affairs* 34 (10):1642-1649.

KhanAhmadi M, Farhood D, Malmir M. 2015. "Ethical Consideration of Aging: Especially Patients with Alzheimer Disease." *Ethics in science and Technology* 10 (1):0-0.

Khanali-Mojen, Leila, Mohammad Esmail Akbari, Hadis Ashrafizadeh, Salman Barasteh, Samira Beiranvand, Azam Eshaghian-Dorcheh, Maryam Karami, Fatemeh Khademi, Eric L Krakauer, and Azam Shirinabadi Farahani. 2022. "Caregivers' Knowledge of and Attitude towards Palliative Care in Iran." *Asian Pacific Journal of Cancer Prevention* 23 (11):3743-3751.

Lysaght, Susan, and Mary Ersek. 2013. "Settings of care within hospice: new options and questions about dying "at home"." *Journal of hospice and palliative nursing: JHPN: the official journal of the Hospice and Palliative Nurses Association* 15 (3):171.

Machnicki, Gerardo, Ricardo F Allegri, Carol Dillon, Cecilia M Serrano, and Fernando E Taragano. 2009. "Cognitive, functional and behavioral factors associated with the burden of caring for geriatric patients with cognitive impairment or depression: evidence from a South American sample." *International Journal of Geriatric Psychiatry: A journal of the psychiatry of late life and allied sciences* 24 (4):382-389.

Mataqi, Mona, and Zoe Aslanpour. 2020. "Factors influencing palliative care in advanced dementia: a systematic review." *BMJ Supportive & Palliative Care* 10 (2):145-156.

Meltzer, Lilia Susana, and Loucine Missak Huckabay. 2004. "Critical care nurses' perceptions of futile care and its effect on burnout." *American journal of critical care* 13 (3):202-208.

Mendez-Luck, Carolyn A, David P Kennedy, and Steven P Wallace. 2009. "Guardians of health: The dimensions of elder caregiving among women in a Mexico City neighborhood." *Social Science & Medicine* 68 (2):228-234.

Miranda, Rose, Frances Bunn, Jennifer Lynch, Lieve Van den Block, and Claire Goodman. 2019. "Palliative care for people with dementia living at home: a systematic review of interventions." *Palliative medicine* 33 (7):726-742.

Mitchell, S. L., D. K. Kiely, and M. B. Hamel. 2004. "Dying with advanced dementia in the nursing home." *Arch Intern Med* 164 (3):321-6. doi: 10.1001/archinte.164.3.321.

Mitchell, Susan L, Joan M Teno, Dan K Kiely, Michele L Shaffer, Richard N Jones, Holly G Prigerson, Ladislav Volicer, Jane L Givens, and Mary Beth Hamel. 2009. "The clinical course of advanced dementia." *New England Journal of Medicine* 361 (16):1529-1538.

MKLPT. 2018. "Designing palliative care system for pediatrics with cancer in Iran." Phd, Shahidbehashti University of Medical Sciences; 2018.

Mobasher, Mina, Nouzar Nakhaee, Mamak Tahmasebi, Farzaneh Zahedi, and Bagher Larijani. 2013. "Ethical issues in the end of life care for cancer patients in Iran." *Iranian journal of public health* 42 (2):188.

Mogadasian, Sima, Farahnaz Abdollahzadeh, Azad Rahmani, Caleb Ferguson, Fermisk Pakanzad, Vahid Pakpour, and Hamid Heidarzadeh. 2014. "The attitude of Iranian nurses about do not resuscitate orders." *Indian journal of palliative care* 20 (1):21.

Mohammadi, F. 2008. "Family caregiving process on Iranian frail elderly." PhD dissertation, Nursing & Midwifery faculty of Iran Medical Sciences University.

Mojen, Leila Khanali. 2017. "Palliative care in Iran: The past, the present and the future." *Supportive & Palliative Care in Cancer* 1 (1).

Mojen, Leila Khanali, Maryam Rassouli, Peyman Eshghi, Kazem Zendedel, Ali Akbari Sari, Majideh Heravi Karimooi, Mamak Tahmasebi, and Azam Shirin Abadi Farahani. 2018. "Pediatric palliative care in Iran: Applying regionalization of health care systems." *Asian Pacific journal of cancer prevention: APJCP* 19 (5):1303.

Motlagh, Ali, Neda Yaraei, Ahmad R Mafi, Farnaz Hosseini Kamal, Mehdi Yaseri, Simin Hemati, Hojatollah Shahbazian, Abdol-Azim Sedighi, Reza Khodabakhshi, and Ali Taghizadeh. 2014. "Attitude of cancer patients toward diagnosis disclosure and their preference for clinical decision-making: a national survey." *Archives of Iranian medicine* 17 (4):0-0.

Mukadam, Naaheed, and Gill Livingston. 2012. "Reducing the stigma associated with dementia: approaches and goals." *Aging Health* 8 (4):377-386.

Nabiloo, B. 2002. "olguhaye bartare sazmani" *mahnameh tadbir* 11 (11):58-61.

Navipour, Elham, Mahbobeh Neamatshahi, Zahra Barabadi, Mohammad Neamatshahi, and Aghilallah Keykhosravi. 2019. "Epidemiology and risk factors of Alzheimer's disease in Iran: a systematic review." *Iranian Journal of Public Health* 48 (12):2133.

Nekoeimoghadam, Mahmood, Mohammad Reza Amiresmaili, and Azar Izadi. 2020. "The Competitive Analysis of the Private Hospital Industry Using Porter's Competitive Diamond Model: A Case Study in Kerman 2014." *Journal of Qualitative Research in Health Sciences* 5 (1):29-45.

Nikbakht-Nasrabadi, Alireza, and Maryam Shabany-Hamedan. 2016. "Providing healthcare services at home-a necessity in Iran: a narrative review article." *Iranian Journal of Public Health* 45 (7):867.

Park, Nan Sook, Yuri Jang, Jung Eun Ko, and David A Chiriboga. 2016. "Factors affecting willingness to use hospice in racially/ethnically diverse older men and women." *American Journal of Hospice and Palliative Medicine®* 33 (8):770-776.

Parsa, Parisa, Forouzan Rezapur-Shahkolai, Maliheh Araghchian, Maryam Afshari, and Alireza Moradi. 2017. "Medical procedure problems from the viewpoint of elderly referrals to healthcare centers of Hamadan: A qualitative study." *Iranian Journal of Ageing* 12 (2):146-155.

Peimani, Maryam, Farzaneh Zahedi, and Bagher Larijani. 2012. "Do-not-resuscitate order across societies and the necessity of a national ethical guideline." *Medical Ethics and History of Medicine* 5 (5):19-35. doi: http://ijme.tums.ac.ir/article-1-99-en.html.

Pitman, Jeffrey A, and Katherine E Metzger. 2018. "Nursing home abuse and neglect and the Nursing Home Reform Act: an overview." *NAELA J.* 14:137.

Pourmollamirza, Afsaneh, Farshad Sharifi, Farnaz Etesam, and Elham Navab. 2020. "Abuse of people with Alzheimer's disease by family caregivers: A Review." *Iranian Journal of Nursing Research* 15 (2):96-108.

Prince, Martin. 2004. "Care arrangements for people with dementia in developing countries." *International journal of geriatric psychiatry*.

Rassouli, Maryam, Leila Khanali Mojen, Azam Shirinabadi Farahani, and Samira Beiranvand. 2021. "The Role of the Nurse in the Community in Running the Palliative Care Interdisciplinary Team: The Iranian Experience." In *Palliative Care for Chronic Cancer Patients in the Community: Global Approaches and Future Applications*, edited by Michael Silbermann, 317-338. Cham: Springer International Publishing.

Rassouli, Maryam, and Moosa Sajjadi. 2014. "Palliative care in the Islamic Republic of Iran."

Rassouli, Maryam, and Moosa Sajjadi. 2016. "Palliative care in Iran: Moving toward the development of palliative care for cancer." *American Journal of Hospice and Palliative Medicine®* 33 (3):240-244.

Ray, Avik, Ahmad Najmi, and Balakrishnan Sadasivam. 2019. "Integrating palliative care with primary care: A synergistic mix." *Journal of Family Medicine and Primary Care* 8 (9).

Robinson, Andrew, Claire Eccleston, Michael Annear, Kate-Ellen Elliott, Sharon Andrews, Christine Stirling, Michael Ashby, Catherine Donohue, Susan Banks, and Christine Toye. 2014. "Who knows, who cares? Dementia knowledge among nurses, care workers, and family members of people living with dementia." *Journal of Palliative Care* 30 (3):158-165.

Rodriguez Then, Francisca S., Jonathan Jackson, Caitlin Ware, Rebekah Churchyard, Bernard Hanseeuw, Alzheimer's International Interdisciplinary Young Investigators, and Dementia. 2020. "Interdisciplinary and Transdisciplinary Perspectives: On the Road to a Holistic Approach to Dementia Prevention and Care." *Journal of Alzheimer's disease reports* 4 (1):39-48. doi: 10.3233/ADR-180070.

Romem, Anat, Sarah E Tom, Michelle Beauchene, Lynn Babington, Steven M Scharf, and Ayal Romem. 2015. "Pain management at the end of life: A comparative study of cancer, dementia, and chronic obstructive pulmonary disease patients." *Palliative medicine* 29 (5):464-469.

Rosen, Tony, Mark S Lachs, Jeanne Teresi, Joseph Eimicke, Kimberly Van Haitsma, and Karl Pillemer. 2016. "Staff-reported strategies for prevention and management of resident-to-resident elder mistreatment in long-term care facilities." *Journal of elder abuse & neglect* 28 (1):1-13.

Saccomano, Scott J, and Geraldine A Abbatiello. 2014. "Cultural Considerations at the end of life." *The Nurse Practitioner* 39 (2):24-31.

Safdari, Reza, Mahtab Alizadeh, Maryam Mohamadiazar, Farshad Sharifi, and Hossein Fakhrzadeh. 2014. "Comparative study of home care program in Iran with other developed countries." *Iranian Journal of Diabetes and Metabolism* 13 (6):439-446.

Salehi, M. 2011. "alzheimer's disease increase in Iran, The age of Amnesia increase in Iran.".

Salehi, NEJAD SIMIN, Mohammad Azami, Fatemeh Motamedi, BEHNAZ SEDIGHI, and ARMITA SHAHESMAILI. 2017. "The effect of web-based information intervention in caregiving burden in caregivers of patients with dementia."

Sampson, Elizabeth L, Vivienne Gould, Dan Lee, and Martin R Blanchard. 2006. "Differences in care received by patients with and without dementia who died during acute hospital admission: a retrospective case note study." *Age and ageing* 35 (2):187-189.

Sandman, Lars, and Björn Hofmann. 2019. "Why we don't need "Unmet Needs"! on the concepts of unmet need and severity in health-care priority setting." *Health Care Analysis* 27 (1):26-44.
Savaskan, Egemen, Irene Bopp-Kistler, Markus Buerge, Regina Fischlin, Dan Georgescu, Umberto Giardini, Martin Hatzinger, Ulrich Hemmeter, Isabella Justiniano, and Reto W Kressig. 2014. "Recommendations for diagnosis and therapy of behavioral and psychological symptoms in dementia (BPSD)." *Praxis* 103 (3):135-148.
Sciences, Ministry of Health-Treatment and Education of Medical, and Supreme Council of Medical Education Planning. 2022. Non-continuous master's degree course in geriatric nursing. Tehran.
Sciences., Ministry of Health-Treatment and Education of Medical, and Supreme Council of Medical Education Planning. 2022. Continuous undergraduate nursing education program. Tehran.
Senel, G, and M Silbermann. 2017. "Cultural challenges in implementing palliative programs in emerging countries." *Palliat Med Hosp Care Open J* (1):S1-S3.
Services., US Department of Health and Human. 2019. "Admission, transfer, and discharge rights." https://www.govinfo.gov/app/details/CFR-2011-title42-vol5/CFR-2011-title42-vol5-sec483-12 Accessed October08, 2019.
Shaarbafchi Zadeh, Nasrin, Faezeh Akbari, Parinaz Khalili Khouzani, and Asal Sadat Niaraees Zavare. 2020. "Comparative study of elderly care services among Iran, United States of America, and Sweden." *Scientific Journal of Kurdistan University of Medical Sciences* 25 (5):123-140.
Shafei, Najmeh, Gholamhossein Abdeyazdan, Lida Sasani, Hydarali Abedi, and Mohammadreza Najafei. 2017. "Family care giving needs of the elderly with Alzheimer's disease (A phenomenological study)." *Journal of Clinical Nursing and Midwifery* 6 (2):48-58.
Shah, Sunil M, Iain M Carey, Tess Harris, Stephen DeWilde, Richard Hubbard, Sarah Lewis, and Derek G Cook. 2010. "Identifying the clinical characteristics of older people living in care homes using a novel approach in a primary care database." *Age and ageing* 39 (5):617-623.
Shamsi Goshki E, Abbasi M, Mohaghegh Damad M, Sashadina AA. 2014. "A Study of Ethical, Jurisprudential and Legal Aspects of the Medical Order of Non-Cardiopulmonary Resuscitation in the Health System of the Islamic Republic of Iran." Ph.D Medical ethics, School of Traditional Medicine, Shahid Beheshti University of medical science (22434p).
Shin, Jennifer A, Amanda Parkes, Areej El-Jawahri, Lara Traeger, Helen Knight, Emily R Gallagher, and Jennifer S Temel. 2016. "Retrospective

evaluation of palliative care and hospice utilization in hospitalized patients with metastatic breast cancer." *Palliative medicine* 30 (9):854-861.

Silbermann, Michael. 2014. *Palliative care to the cancer patient: The Middle East as a model for emerging countries*: Nova Publishers.

Stieger, Mirjam, and Margie E. Lachman. 2021. "Increases in Cognitive Activity Reduce Aging-Related Declines in Executive Functioning." *Frontiers in Psychiatry* 12. doi: 10.3389/fpsyt.2021.708974.

Stjernswärd, Jan, Frank D Ferris, Samir N Khleif, Walid Jamous, Imad M Treish, Mohammed Milhem, Mohammed Bushnaq, Ahmad Al Khateib, Mohammad Nayef Al Shtiat, and Mary S Wheeler. 2007. "Jordan palliative care initiative: a WHO Demonstration Project." *Journal of pain and symptom management* 33 (5):628-633.

Tible, Olivier Pierre, Florian Riese, Egemen Savaskan, and Armin von Gunten. 2017. "Best practice in the management of behavioural and psychological symptoms of dementia." *Therapeutic advances in neurological disorders* 10 (8):297-309. doi: 10.1177/1756285617712979.

Vachon, Mélanie, Lise Fillion, and Marie Achille. 2009. "A conceptual analysis of spirituality at the end of life." *Journal of palliative medicine* 12 (1):53-59.

Vaingankar, Janhavi Ajit, Siow Ann Chong, Edimansyah Abdin, Louisa Picco, Anitha Jeyagurunathan, YunJue Zhang, Rajeswari Sambasivam, Boon Yiang Chua, Li Ling Ng, and Martin Prince. 2016. "Care participation and burden among informal caregivers of older adults with care needs and associations with dementia." *International psychogeriatrics* 28 (2):221-231.

Valiee, Sina, Reza Negarandeh, and Nahid Dehghan Nayeri. 2012. "Exploration of Iranian intensive care nurses' experience of end-of-life care: a qualitative study." *Nursing in critical care* 17 (6):309-315.

van der Steen, J. T., L. Radbruch, C. M. Hertogh, M. E. de Boer, J. C. Hughes, P. Larkin, A. L. Francke, S. Jünger, D. Gove, P. Firth, R. T. Koopmans, and L. Volicer. 2014. "White paper defining optimal palliative care in older people with dementia: a Delphi study and recommendations from the European Association for Palliative Care." *Palliat Med* 28 (3):197-209. doi: 10.1177/0269216313493685.

van der Steen, Jenny T., Natashe Lemos Dekker, Marie-José H. E. Gijsberts, Laura H. Vermeulen, Margje M. Mahler, and B. Anne-Mei The. 2017. "Palliative care for people with dementia in the terminal phase: a mixed-methods qualitative study to inform service development." *BMC Palliative Care* 16 (1):28. doi: 10.1186/s12904-017-0201-4.

Wang, Xiaoming, Warren Kindzierski, and Padma Kaul. 2015. "Comparison of transient associations of air pollution and AMI hospitalisation in two cities of Alberta, Canada, using a case-crossover design." *BMJ open* 5 (11):e009169.

Weuve, Jennifer, Liesi E Hebert, Paul A Scherr, and Denis A Evans. 2014. "Deaths in the United States among persons with Alzheimer's disease (2010–2050)." *Alzheimer's & dementia* 10 (2):e40-e46.

White, Franklin. 2015. "Primary health care and public health: foundations of universal health systems." *Medical Principles and Practice* 24 (2):103-116.

Wimo, A, L Jönsson, A Gustavsson, David McDaid, K Ersek, J Georges, L Gulacsi, K Karpati, P Kenigsberg, and H Valtonen. 2011. "The economic impact of dementia in Europe in 2008—cost estimates from the Eurocode project." *International journal of geriatric psychiatry* 26 (8):825-832.

Wimo, Anders, Linus Jönsson, John Bond, Martin Prince, Bengt Winblad, and Alzheimer Disease International. 2013. "The worldwide economic impact of dementia 2010." *Alzheimer's & Dementia* 9 (1):1-11.

Wold Health Ranking. 2022. world life expectancy Iran-alzheimers-dementia.

World Health Organization. 2002. "WHO definition of palliative care." *http://www. who. int/cancer/palliative/definition/en/index. html.*

World Health Organization. 2018. "Integrating palliative care and symptom relief into paediatrics: a WHO guide for health-care planners, implementers and managers."

World Health Organization. 2019. "Dementia: a global health priority and World Health Organization report." https://www.who.int/news-room/fact-sheets/detail/dementia.

World Health Organization. 2020a. Global Atlas of Palliative Care 2nd Edition. London, UK.

World Health Organization. 2020b. Global Atlas of Palliative Care 2nd Edition. London: Worldwide Palliative Care Alliance; 2020.

Xu, Jing, Rui Pan, Raymond W Pong, Yudong Miao, and Dongfu Qian. 2016. "Different models of hospital–community health centre collaboration in selected cities in China: a cross-sectional comparative study." *International journal of integrated care* 16 (1).

Yang, Siyuan, Yunmei Zhang, Shiqi Xie, Yanhan Chen, Dengbi Jiang, Yetao Luo, Qinghua Zhao, and Bing Yang. 2020. "Predictors of Perceived Social Support for Patients with Dementia: A Mixed-Methods Study." *Clinical Interventions in Aging* 15:595.

Yektatalab, Shahrzad, Mohammad Hossein Kaveh, Farkhondeh Sharif, KHOSHKNAB MASOOD FALLAHI, and Peyman Petramfar. 2012. "Caring for patients with Alzheimer's disease in nursing homes: A qualitative content analysis."

Yektatalab, Shahrzad, Farkhondeh Sharif, Mohammad Hossein Kaveh, Masood Fallahi Khoshknab, and Peyman Petramfar. 2013. "Living with and caring for patients with Alzheimer's disease in nursing homes." *Journal of caring sciences* 2 (3):187.

Yon, Yongjie, Maria Ramiro-Gonzalez, Christopher R Mikton, Manfred Huber, and Dinesh Sethi. 2019. "The prevalence of elder abuse in institutional settings: a systematic review and meta-analysis." *European journal of public health* 29 (1):58-67.

Zamani, Ahmadreza, Armindokht Shahsanai, Shima Kivan, Simin Hematti, and Fariborz Mokarian. 2011. "Iranian physicians and patients attitude toward truth telling of cancer." *Journal of Isfahan Medical School* 29 (143).

Zarea, Kourosh, Maryam Rassouli, Maryam Hazrati, Shahram Molavynejad, and Samira Beiranvand. 2020. "Comparison of The Hospice Palliative Care Delivery Systems in Iran and Selected Countries." *International Journal of Cancer Management* 13 (6).

Zeinah, Ghaith F Abu, Sadeer G Al-Kindi, and Azza Adel Hassan. 2013. "Middle East experience in palliative care." *American Journal of Hospice and Palliative Medicine®* 30 (1):94-99.

Ziloochi, Mohammad Hosain, Abolghasem Pourreza, Feyzollah Akbari, and FOROSHANI A RAHIMI. 2012. "Evaluating the hospitalization costs for elderly patients in teaching hospitals of Kashan university of medical sciences during 2009-10." *Nursing in critical care* 16 (1):8-94.

Zucchella, Chiara, Elena Sinforiani, Stefano Tamburin, Angela Federico, Elisa Mantovani, Sara Bernini, Roberto Casale, and Michelangelo Bartolo. 2018. "The Multidisciplinary Approach to Alzheimer's Disease and Dementia. A Narrative Review of Non-Pharmacological Treatment." *Frontiers in Neurology* 9 (1058). doi: 10.3389/fneur.2018.01058.

12

PAYING THE DEBT OF LIFE TO LATE-STAGE DEMENTIA PARENTS AND PROVIDING BUDDHIST APPROACH SPIRITUAL CARE AT END OF LIFE

SRIVIENG PAIROJKUL, MD.[1] AND RATTANAPORN SIRIKET, RN, MSC.[2]

Like other developed countries around the world, Thailand is entering the aging society phase[1], with the incidence of dementia expected to increase accordingly. Advanced dementia is a life-limiting illness and requires skillful comprehensive care at end of life. The disease trajectory of advanced dementia is unpredictable, and compared to cancer the trajectory is longer and with a variable survival time that is difficult to forecast.[2] A lack of awareness among health care professionals that dementia is a fatal disease may lead to aggressive treatment—often manifested in life-support treatment—of hospitalized, elderly patients with end-stage dementia, thereby causing suffering to the patients and their families[3, 4].

Caring for people with dementia imposes a huge burden on family caregivers[5,6]. Most elderly people with dementia in Thailand are taken care of in their homes by their children. With Thai society becoming more individualistic and with less children per family, the long-term burden on caregiving families is increasing.[7] A lack of awareness among healthcare professionals and the public about dementia's natural course and end of life is leading to aggressive treatment in the hope of improving the patients condition[2,3,4]. In addition, Thai culture places a high value on parental care, believing that one must not lose hope and do everything possible for one's

---

[1] Karunruk Palliative Care Center, Srinagarind Hospital
[2] Faculty of Medicine, Khon Kaen University, Thailand

parents[8]. This leads to hospital admission in the end-of-life phase and results in aggressive treatment in the ICU and death in the hospital.

Cultural context in palliative care

Holistic and patient-centered care is a core principle of palliative care. Accordingly, palliative healthcare personnel need to be aware of the cultural context of their patients, which may greatly affect the provision of care, especially at end of life. Asian countries are characterized by a collectivist culture with strong family values[8]. People highly respect their parents, and family is considered to be the foundation of social life for most Thais. The Thai family structure is composed of many generations living under the same roof, and often the grandparents help raise their grandchildren. Most Thais still live in their parents' house even when they get married. The men always live with their wives and relatives. Thai children are expected to look after their parents in their old age. A fundamental principle in Thai family culture is that children are required to respect their parents and pay back the debt of life[9]. The virtue of filial piety[10] is the culture of East Asia, which has also influenced Thai culture. It obligates respect for one's parents, elders, and ancestors. The rejection of these family duties and obligations is stigmatized by Asian societies[11].

Buddhism and spirituality

Religion and spirituality play a major role in human society. Many studies on religion and spirituality have found that they are pervasive across the world. Early meta-analyses indicated a significant mean correlation between religious belief and mental health[12]. A recent meta-analysis on components of religion/spirituality and forms of mental health found a correlation with distress, well-being, life-satisfaction, and quality of life[13]. In a large meta-analysis of religion/spirituality and life satisfaction (N = 666,085), five dimensions of religion/spirituality were examined separately to gauge their relationships with life satisfaction. Each dimension of religion/spirituality was significantly and positively associated with life satisfaction: religiosity, spirituality, religious attendance, religious practices, and religious/spiritual experiences. The overall effect was moderated by several variables, with a stronger relationship found in samples with higher average age, in more recent studies, in developing nations, and in countries with a higher percentage of people who consider religion very important in their lives[14].

Buddhism plays a major role in the spirituality of Thai people. Theravada Buddhism is the dominant Buddhist sect in Thailand, and it has a strong influence on Thai people's attitudes, thoughts, and way of life. A national survey study of Thai people aged 15 years or older on religiosity, spirituality, and happiness in Thailand from the perspective of Buddhism[15] revealed that the frequency of religious and spiritual practices was significantly associated with greater levels of happiness. Respondents who abided by the five precepts of Buddhism and meditated on Buddhist holy days reported higher levels of happiness. Those who regularly expressed gratitude, gave an opportunity to serve others before themselves, and made donations were more likely to consider themselves happy compared with those who never or rarely engaged in these Buddhist-inspired practices. These findings support the idea that religiosity and spirituality play a relevant role in the level of happiness of Thai people.

When applied to one's parents, the value of gratitude means to pay the debt of life. This is generalized so that when one's parents get sick, every treatment needs to be attempted in order to make sure that every possible measure has been taken to facilitate recovery. Consequently, palliative care constantly faces the situation of elderly patients who have been aggressively treated to the point of medical futility. Since Thai national health insurance covers all the cost of medical treatment, and doctors fear being sued by the families, most treatments are conducted according to the families' wishes. When nothing can be done anymore, the families will bring their parents back to die at their homes. This is a paradoxical situation. A medical anthropologist who stayed in the northeast region of Thailand expressed his surprise when coming across cases in which the adult children tried to obtain for their parents every possible treatment in the ICU, using all possible means; yet, when the doctors suggested that no benefit would be gained from further treatment, that nothing could be done and the patient is dying, they hired an ambulance to take their parent to die at home[9]. Buddhist rituals play an important role in end-of-life care. When the patient is going to die, the monk will be invited to visit the dying patient for merit-making by giving offerings to the monk and to listen to the last Buddhist chanting. In the northeast region of Thailand, when the patient is dying, the relatives will gather around to pay their respect and perform a forgiveness ritual (Photo# 1).

Buddhism and end-of-life decisions

End-of-life decision-making is a difficult situation for the adult children, who must decide whether to start or withdraw life support from their parents in critical situations. Few Thai elderly have an advance care plan,[16] a situation that is perpetuated by cognitive loss in the elderly with dementia. In Thailand, families are becoming more involved in making decisions for patients in the intensive care unit[17]. Decision-making in this situation involves not only weighting benefits and harms but also ethical and moral issues. Buddhists, despite an apparently clear precept against killing, have some flexibility in decision-making if their intentions are pure and their heart is compassionate. Intention plays such a large role in Buddhist ethics that it can be seen as an "intentionist ethics"[18]. A descriptive research that explored end-of-life decisions of Thai Buddhist patients and their families revealed the values underlying their end-of-life decisions[19]. The results showed that more than half of the Thai Buddhist patients and their families (51.9%) decided to forgo life-sustaining treatment, and almost one-third allowed the physician (18.1%) or family (10.5%) to make the decision for them. Only 19.5% decided to continue the treatment. The most important values for continuing and forgoing the treatment were hope (92.7%) and becoming free from suffering (47.7%). Respect was the most important value for Thai Buddhists who allowed their physician or family to make the decision for them (84.2% and 59.1%, respectively). All these findings suggest that healthcare personnel should recognize the difficulties associated with decision-making at end of life, and provide information and support.

A good death in the Thai and Buddhist context

Most elderly people with terminal illnesses hope for a good death, meaning a death with dignity. A survey of opinions regarding wishes toward the end of life among Thai elderly found that toward the end of life, the majority wanted to know the truth about their illness and to be free from uncomfortable symptoms. Seventy-five percent did not want life-prolonging treatments when the chance of surviving is slim[20]. Thai Buddhist family members described what they meant by a peaceful death, namely preparing for a peaceful state of mind, knowing that one's impending death is not a situation of suffering or being alone, but rather a time of being with family members who are not yet mourning one's death[17].

Thai Buddhist patients who have cancer and are in palliative care process death through three dynamic phases: engaging with suffering, being open-minded about death, and adhering to Buddhist practices for increasing death consciousness[21]. A study from Thailand compared the wishes of cancer patients and the perceptions of their relatives regarding end-of-life care. Respondents in both groups placed importance on the place of death, relationships with family, physical and psychological comfort, and relationships with the medical staff. Relatives underestimated the preferences of the patients in three areas: not being a burden to others, preparation for death, and physical and psychological comfort. Factors associated with preference for home death included being married, having had more than six years of education, having lung cancer rather than colon cancer, duration after cancer diagnosis, previous hospital admission, and life satisfaction[22]. Older adults who had firsthand experience in caring for the terminally ill perceived a good death as including a death without suffering (not suffering from life support devices, dying with care); a natural death (death at end-of-life expectancy, death from illness or ailments); and death without worries (preparation for death, spiritual and belief practice toward preparation for death, family and property management before death); death among family members and in their familiar place[23].

A good death according to terminal chronic patients, their caregivers and the hospital palliative care team in upper northern Thailand was characterized by an absence of physical discomfort, psychological and spiritual tranquility, preparedness for death, ability to determine the place of death, and assurance of post-mortem care[24]. A survey among the nurses who work in the hospital asked how they thought older people would respond to each of the questions and what their own preferences would be if they were terminally ill. They rated relief from suffering as the most important component, both for themselves and for those in their care[25]. A general, population-based study on preferences toward end-of-life care in Southern Thailand found only one difference between the end-of-life preferences of the adult group versus the older adult group, which was the adult group had less preference in involvement of patients in treatment decisions. Furthermore, receiving the full truth regarding their illness, being free from distressing symptoms, having loved ones around, and living with a sense of meaning were important end-of-life care preferences for both groups[26]. A study of Thai Buddhist monks providing care for sick monks until they passed away found six main themes of a good death: freedom from suffering, a natural death with good deeds, awareness of death, one's final spirituality becoming mental charity, resting in peace, and nirvana[27].

Relief from suffering, preparation for death, being with family, and place of death were always mentioned in these studies.

Patients with advanced dementia and their families need essential information and time to reflect on their preferences

The Karunruk Palliative Care Center provides palliative care consultation for all palliative patients, both inpatient and outpatient. We also provide home care and crisis intervention. Many of our elderly patients are very frail and sick after being cared for in the intensive care unit due to serious illness. Most of them were never seen by a palliative care team before and never had a chance to formulate an advance care plan. We present two cases of elderly patients with dementia and compare their outcomes.

Mr. Chareon was an 86-year-old retired teacher who was still active and most enjoyed meeting with friends and relatives. He suffered severe post-stroke dementia that caused him to become bedridden and incognitive. Later, he was admitted several times with aspiration pneumonia; the last admission was complicated with hospital multidrug-resistant infection and septic shock. He developed respiratory failure, which required mechanical ventilation, and his kidney injury required hemodialysis. All the time, the family insisted that everything must be done and that they will accept the results, whatever they be. It seemed that his renal function was not recovering and hemodialysis had to be continued. The primary physician foresaw the difficulties of continuing dialysis and directed the palliative care team to work with the family.

Mr. Chareon had two children, and he was living with his wife and his daughter, who had a 2-year-old son, of which she was the primary caregiver. His other son lived in Bangkok and want the daughter to be major health care proxy. Mr. Chareon was a retired teacher who enjoyed good health and never had an advance care plan. In the first family meeting, both his wife and his daughter stated that they wanted everything to be done, even though they knew that Mr. Chareon was bedridden and had no cognitive function. In their family, the elderly had been looked after by the family; previously, they had taken care of their grandmother, who had lived to the age of 100 years, despite being bedridden. All the family helped take care of the grandmother since it is the duty of children to pay the debt of life to their parents. A month later, Mr. Chareon had stabilized but hemodialysis continued. He was still in an unconsciousness state, breathing with a ventilator. His general condition was run down with poor nutrition. Finally, hemodialysis was difficult to maintain due to catheter malfunction. We conducted several family meetings with his wife and his daughter. Their values required them to do everything for their loved one and not to abandon him. When we asked the daughter what her father's values were, she said that her father is a fighter, he wanted to live as long as possible. We tried to guide the family to realize the suffering of continuing the life-support treatment that their loved one was receiving, and that we needed to relieve him from this suffering. Finally, the nephrologist informed them that he would stop dialysis and that survival would be one to two weeks, and then the family decided to bring Mr. Chareon back to die at their home. At that point, he was wasting severely and his skin broke down all over the body. We helped with the process of transferring the patient back home and provided a home visit. He died two days later at their home.

Ms. Rein was a 75-year-old female who had been diagnosed with early dementia, while her husband was diagnosed with lung cancer at the same time. Their daughter, who was the primary caregiver, and the son-in-law were devoted to taking care of both of them, and consequently, they planned not to have children at that stage since the burden of looking after the parents was unbearable. Ms. Rein saw all the suffering of her husband and therefore had formulated an advance care plan for comfort care. We had been taking care of Ms. Rein for several years and had witnessed the devotion of her daughter and son-in-law. Ms. Rein was taken care of very well by her daughter. She developed several episodes of pneumonia that were treated at home without admission, and finally died peacefully at home.

Both Mr. Chareon and Ms. Rein received the best care from their family, which accepted the burden and provided care with love; the difference was that Ms. Lein and her daughter received palliative care services, which provided them with knowledge on the trajectory of the disease, time for reflection on their values and preferences, and time to prepare their advance care plan.

Patients have control over their lives through advance care planning

Amah, which means "mother" in Chinese, was 82 years old when she was diagnosed with dementia four years ago. When she was first diagnosed, she had written her living will to not use life support, including the nasogastric tube. But in fact, the Advance Directive Act had been in force for more than

15 years in Thailand[28], even though most people are unaware of it. For Thai and Chinese people, talking or thinking about death is bad luck. When people attend a funeral, after they return home they need to sprinkle water with pomegranate leaves on their body to chase the evil spirits away before entering their homes. However, it seems that Amah was a very modernized Chinese who was born in Thailand. Four years after the diagnosis, she could still walk without support and her cognitive function remained intact. The family hired two caregivers to take care of her. Two months before we met her, she had a fall, which resulted in a fracture of her right shoulder. She was admitted to the regional hospital, where she was immobilized, but later a complication with upper gastrointestinal hemorrhage occurred, requiring an esophagogastroduodenoscopy; gastritis was diagnosed. Her recovery was uneventful, but later she refused to eat. All subspecialties were consulted, including a geriatrician, nutritionist, and psychiatrist, but no cause was found. The psychiatrist concluded that cognitively she was fine and not depressed. The nutritionist suggested using a nasogastric tube, but Amah resisted.

The fasting had been going on for several weeks causing concern to the family, at which time Viroon, her son, asked me for an opinion and requested that Amah be referred to our care. We admitted her to our unit. She was thin, fully conscious, and responding to questions. She slept all day, only sipping several spoonfuls of Ensure. There was no pain, and she slept most of the time. However, fasting began once more. An occupational therapist was consulted to test her swallowing function, which was intact. Other subspecialties were consulted, including a geriatrician. A urine exam and culture was recommended to rule out urinary tract infection, which required catheterization. At first she resisted, but with the encouragement of the family, Amah surrendered. The result was negative. Finally, the geriatrician suggested a CT brain scan. At this point a discussion was held with the family. Amah stated that she wanted to go back home, so we decided to discharge her and referred her to our home care team.

After Amah was back home it seemed that she got better. A daughter from Bangkok came to visit; she bought Amah's favorite food and suddenly she started to eat. The family reported that she enjoyed eating and could eat a significant amount of food. Our home care team reported that she seemed to be fine. The family was very happy and regularly sent me Amah's photos while eating. A month later Viroon called me and reported that Amah had reverted to the same situation again, refusing to eat and sleeping most of the time. The daughter from Bangkok visited her every weekend. There was no fever and no other symptoms. We asked the family to keep an eye on her and if she did not improve, we might need to see if she needed admission.

The next morning, Viroon called that they had measured her blood pressure and found that it was low. Therefore, we admitted her to our palliative ward. She had low blood pressure and a blood test revealed an acute kidney injury; her urine output was low. We then provided fluid resuscitation. Amah was drowsy and answered questions by nodding. She sipped only a bit of fluid, looked very weak, and slept all day. Her daughter came from Bangkok and we then held a meeting with the family. We knew that her goal of care was comfort, and that she had chosen to forgo artificial feeding and all types of life support treatment. During the period that we took care of her, whenever we asked her permission to do blood tests or urinary catheterization, she refused at first but when the doctor insisted, she agreed. I felt that she did not want to upset the doctors. After the discussion, the family said that they want to take her back home. They asked for my opinion if it was right that they had brought her back to the hospital. Now they wanted to bring her back home to experience a comfortable death, which I agreed to. She went back home and died peacefully three days later, among her family.

Amah used to state to the family her wish that the they allocate some amount of money for the two caregivers who had been looking after her. I attended her funeral, and Viroon retold the history of Amah, that when she was a teenager she was washing clothes near the river when she saw a boy who was drowning; she jumped into the water and rescued the boy. All the neighborhood respected her very much. Everybody loved her and appreciated that she was kind to everyone. I myself knew that she did not want to continue living; she knew that she had dementia and after suffering a two-month admission and finding that her function was declining, she decided to let go of her life. She did not have any unfinished business; it seems that she decided that she had had enough.

An elderly couple came to consult us concerning the wife's mother who had dementia and who had been placed in a nursing home several years prior. Both of them were retired, and then the husband was diagnosed with ischemic heart disease, which required a bypass operation and several admissions to the hospital. Since both of them were retired, they were then faced with a financial problem. They came to ask us to help remove the mother's feeding tube—they wanted to end their economic burden. In Thai culture, removal of life support is a sensitive problem and generalized as killing. In our consultation work, it is quite common that we are asked to see the elderly who are admitted into the ICU with mechanical ventilation. After the primary physician informs the family that nothing can be done, the family consults the palliative care team. When we conduct family meetings, we try to make the family see the suffering that will occur if we continue the treatment. Some families resist withdrawal of life support and prefer letting their parents die with the ventilator.

The perception that you need to do everything for the parents is linked to the concept of paying the debt of life to their parents. Whenever an elderly person is neglected by their children it is called "akatunyu", which means ungrateful. What we find nowadays is that many families chose to stop mechanical ventilation and let their parents die peacefully at our palliative ward or at their homes. Fifteen years ago, the first case in which we withdrew the ventilator created much distress to the ICU team and was not very well accepted. Nowadays, our team performs withdrawal of life support at least in ten cases a month. Although withdrawal of a feeding tube in a patient in vegetative state is allowed in some countries[29], however we had never withdraw a feeding tube from a stable advanced dementia patient, but withhold feeding tube is quite common in our situation.

It is important that the elderly have a chance to take part in decision-making and formulate their own advance care planning, especially when they have been diagnosed with early dementia. The case of Amah shows how she was able to control her end of life. Most of the elderly do not want to put a huge burden on their children to make a decision, which creates feelings of guilt in their children. Unfortunately, the concept of advance care planning in Thailand is still in the beginning phase.

Recognition of disease trajectory and suffering of patients with advanced dementia

Families should realize that dementia is a fatal disease and that infections are usually a terminal event[30,2]. The CASCADE study[2], which examined the clinical course of advanced dementia in twenty-two US nursing homes, found a six-month mortality rate in patients who developed pneumonia (46.7% of patients), had a febrile episode (44.5%), and eating problems (38.6%). In the last three months of life, dyspnea and pain developed in 46% and 39.1% of the patients, respectively. Forty percent of the patients underwent at least one burdensome intervention such as hospitalization, emergency room visit, intravenous fluid administration, and tube feeding. Proxies who understood the prognosis of advanced dementia had less burdensome interventions. A comparison of end-of-life experiences within 120 days of death between cancer and advanced dementia patients showed that tube feeding, lab investigations, and restraint use were significantly associated with advanced dementia, and that pneumonia and pressure ulcer were more common. Another important finding was that there was less advance care planning in advanced dementia[31].

Concerning tube feeding, a recent study showed no evidence that tube feeding improves survival or quality of life, reduces pain or mortality, decreases behavioral and psychological symptoms of dementia, leads to better nourishment, or improves family or carer outcomes such as depression, anxiety, carer burden, or satisfaction with care. There is some evidence that there is a clinically significant risk of pressure ulcers from internal tube feeding[32]. Pneumonia is a terminal event for patients with late-stage dementia in nursing homes. A study of chart reviews found that one-third of residents had at least one episode of pneumonia. The patients who did not receive antibiotics had a shorter, three-month survival rate, but they were more comfortable. There was no statistical difference in survival between oral, intramuscular, or intravenous treatment routes of antibiotics[33]. A study of the patterns of antimicrobial use among nursing home residents with advanced dementia found that at least one course of antimicrobial therapy was prescribed, and the number of courses per resident was four. Respiratory infection was the most common cause, and among the decedents, nearly half of them received antimicrobials during the two weeks before death, of which nearly half were administered via the parenteral route[34]. Research evidence suggests that antibiotics may improve survival rates but decrease patient's comfort. Decisions about treating pneumonia with antibiotics should depend on the patient's goal of care. For those with a goal of comfort care, antibiotics should either be withheld or only given orally, and for those with a goal of prolonging life, antibiotics should be aggressively administered.

Advance care planning is an important element in spiritual care for dementia patients. The process of advance care plan communication involves exploring one's understanding of the disease prognosis and reflecting on one's values, health care preferences, and setting the scope of treatment. According to the evidence[20], most elderly patients prefer to receive information concerning their own illness and do not want aggressive treatment if the chance of survival is slim. Thus, advance care planning is a tool to control the medical treatment the patients want to receive in the future, when they have lost their cognitive abilities. Advance care planning should be a routine care element for the elderly, especially the elderly with early dementia.

The late-stage dementia palliative program at the Karunruk Palliative Care Center

The Karunruk Palliative Care Center serves palliative patients in the Srinagarind Hospital, the Faculty of Medicine, Khon Kaen University. Karunruk is also a national training center in Thailand and provides support and networking for palliative units throughout Thailand. Srinagarind Hospital is the reference center in the northeast region of Thailand. This region comprises one-third of the country's area and also one-third of the population[35]. The palliative care network in the Northeast is very strong. Palliative home care is made possible due to strong connections between the provincial hospitals and their district hospital networks. The National Health Insurance Office provides reimbursement for palliative home care support. Since our cancer center is the reference cancer center for Northeast Thailand, a large amount of our patients have cancer, making up approximately 60%–70% of all consulting cases. Palliative care has been integrated into oncology as well as into other subspecialties such as chronic kidney diseases, late-stage dementia, severe strokes, and perinatal-neonatal-pediatric care.

The late-stage dementia palliative care program was established in 2018. It is a comprehensive palliative care program for patients who were referred from the Geriatric Department and for patients who use our consultation services. The program provides comprehensive care including a thorough holistic assessment, establish care plan, and advance care planning. Since most cases of dementia that come into our care are in the late stage and have no cognition, information is usually provided to the family, which is educated on the nature and trajectory of advanced dementia. Regular home visits are provided, together with a caregiver empowerment program. The caregiver, too, is educated about the nature and trajectory of advanced dementia and directed to explore the values and preferences of the patient and their family. An advance care plan is established and the patient's and family's values and preferences are recorded. Future medical care and hospital admission are discussed, including antibiotic administration by oral route at home or a systemic route at the palliative ward for pneumonia, fluid and nutrition. The place of care and place of death are also discussed. The patient's advance care plan and advance directive is documented in the hospital's medical history electronic system. Medical instruments necessary for care at home are provided. Telephone consultation is provided 24/7, and if a crisis requires admission, the patient will be admitted directly to the palliative ward without going to the emergency room. The palliative nurse teaches the caregiver how to recognize pain and other symptoms, and how to give medication. Caregiver burden is assessed from time to time, and the nurse provides support. Caregiver empowerment is a key element, and therefore psychosocial and spiritual support as well as bereavement care is provided. The program has been well received, and we have 30–40 patients/year. The program protocol is shown in Table 1.

Table 1. Karunruk comprehensive care program for the elderly with late-stage dementia

Schedule of home visits	Activity	Details	Implement caregiver educational bundle
First visit 1-2 weeks after first consultation if not in crisis	• Thorough assessment by a palliative multidisciplinary team • Care planning	• Review medical history • Patient physical & mental assessment: PINAD for pain assessment Mini Nutritional Assessment (MNA) Neuropsychiatric Inventory Questionnaire (NPI-Q) • Caregiver assessment: The Zarit Burden Interview (ZBI)	**Module 1:** PC concept, natural history of dementia, caregiver's role
Second visit 1-2 weeks later	Further assessment by a doctor and a PC nurse	• Patient and caregiver assessment: - PINAD for pain assessment every visit (as appropriate) - Zarit Burden Interview (ZBI) on second and third visit. - Quality of Life in Late-Stage Dementia (QUALID) Scale (every 6 months)	**Module 2:** Symptom assessment & management, emergency issues; **Module 3:** General & specific nursing care, safety issues
Follow up visit Every 1-2 months if stable	Follow up (a doctor and a PC nurse)	• Patient and caregiver assessment (as appropriate): - PINAD for pain assessment every visit - Zarit Burden Interview (ZBI) on second and third visit. - Quality of Life in Late-Stage Dementia (QUALID) Scale (every 3-6 months)	**module 4:** Advance care planning and advance directive

End-of-life phase	Care in the terminal phase	• Patient and caregiver assessment: - Comfort Assessment in Dying with Dementia (CAD-EOLD) Scale	**Module 5:** Care in the last days of life, good death
Post death 1 month after death	Post death care	• Telephone call - Satisfaction with Care at End of life (SWC-EOLD) Scale. • Recruitment into the "Bereavement Companionship Program" if appropriate	**Module 6:** Self-care and bereavement care

Outcomes of the late-stage dementia palliative care program of the Karunruk Palliative Care Center

Herein we present recent reports of the outcomes of our program:

- **Concordance of patients' preferences with actual outcomes among the elderly with late-stage dementia[16]**
  Profiles of 65 patients recruited from October 1, 2020 to September 30, 2022 were analyzed. Eighty-four percent were age ≥80 year, 76.93% were in Functional Assessment Staging Tool (FAST) stage ≥ 7c, and 43.07% had nasogastric tube feeding/percutaneous endoscopic gastrostomy. Only 10.76% had an advance care plan before referral. Later, all the patients in our program had an advance care plan. Place of death: of the 30 patients who died, 43.33% were at home, 43.33% at the palliative unit, and 10.0% at other medical wards (2 in the COVID-19 ward), and 3.34% at a nursing home. The concordance of patients' preferences and actual outcomes was 72.22%. Six patients changed their place of death to the hospital due to the following reasons: two patients had COVID-19 infection and required admission and isolation, and four patients due to caregiver burden. Overall, the concordance of place of death was 80% and all patients received comfort care. The patient preferences in our program were well respected. A comprehensive palliative care program is essential to improve outcomes and avoid medical futility in these patients.
- **Outcomes of dementia patients receiving the palliative care program[36]**
  Analysis of 47 dementia patients to whom we provided care between March 1 and December 31, 2022. The majority of patients were female (53.19%), aged 80-89 (46.81%), with a min. of 64 and max. of 100 (SD 8.97). More than half of the patients (59.58%) were widowed, of which 31.91% had a FAST dementia severity level of 7F. During the study period, 57.43% of patients did not have any infection, 25.53% had pneumonia, and 8.52% contracted COVID-19. For patients with dysphagia, 77.23% required tube feeding, and 22.73% continued hand feeding. All patients had an advance care plan (ACP) while participating in the PC program, and 91.49% stipulated full comfort care. All 15 patients who died did so in accordance with their ACP (100%). The period of care from the beginning until death was more than 365 days in seven (46.67%) cases (min 68, max 2132, mean 538.6 days). The results of the Scales

for the Evaluation of End-of-Life Care in Advanced Dementia (SWC-EOLD) indicated high satisfaction from care (mean 3.773, min. 3.4, max. 4.0 and SD 2.63).

How to provide spiritual care to a dementia patient who is at the end of life

In Northeast Thailand, the palliative care network is strong, followed by the southern region. Each province has created an internal network, which helps with the seamless referral of palliative patients. Palliative home care can be reimbursed via the National Health Insurance regime, which endorses the home visit system. Most health care professionals lack knowledge regarding the trajectory of advanced dementia and have meager knowledge and skills in providing good care for the elderly with late-stage dementia[37,38]. The Karunruk Palliative Care Center is starting a program to provide awareness, knowledge, and skills to palliative care professionals in order to improve their capacity to provide care for dementia patients who are at the end of life. The spiritual aims of the elderly are to be in control, not to be a burden on their children, and to experience care and death at home[20,22,23,24,25]. We provide care that meets their needs by developing a comprehensive home care program for this group of patients. Advance care planning is an essential process to ensure that their wishes will be honored and should be included in the routine care of the elderly. Professional and public awareness of advanced dementia and advance care planning is essential. Lastly, health professionals in palliative care should realize the impact of culture, religiosity and spirituality, which all have a relevant role in end-of-life care.

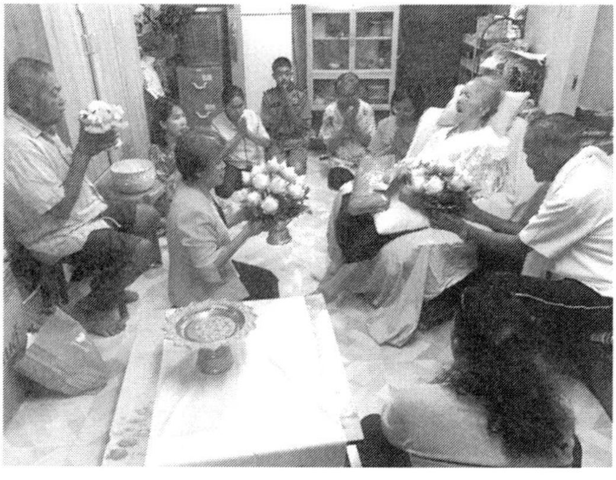

Relatives gather around to pay their respect and perform a forgiveness ritual

References

1. United Nations Department of Economic and Social Affairs (UNDESA) (2019), *World Population Prospects, 2009 Highlights*. New York: United Nations.
https://population.un.org/wpp/Publications/Files/WPP2019_Highlights.pdf
2. Mitchell SL, Teno JM, Kiely DK, Shaffer ML, Jones RN, et al. The Clinical Course of Advanced Dementia. NEJM 2009; 361:1529-1538 DOI: 10.1056/NEJMoa0902234.
3. Alzheimer's Disease International. World Alzheimer Report 2019, Attitudes to dementia.
https://www.alzint.org/u/WorldAlzheimerReport2019.pdf (access Mar 7, 2023)
4. Cahill S, Pierce M, Werner P, Darley A, Bobersky A. A systematic review of the public's knowledge and understanding of Alzheimer's disease and dementia. Alzheimer Dis Assoc Disord 2015;29:255-75.doi:10.1097/WAD.0000000000000102.
5. Cheng AT. Dementia Caregiver Burden: a Research Update and Critical Analysis. Curr Psychiatry Rep. 2017; 19(9): 64. doi: 10.1007/s11920-017-0818-2
6. Liu R, Chi I, Wu S. Caregiving Burden Among Caregivers of People With Dementia Through the Lens of Intersectionality. *The Gerontologist 2022;62:*650–661.
https://doi.org/10.1093/geront/gnab146
7. Teerawichitchanan BP, Pothisiri W, Knodel J, and Prechuabmoh V. Thailand's older persons and their well-being: an update based on the 2017 survey of older persons in Thailand.
https://theactive.net/data/aged-society/ (access Mar 7, 2023)
8. Marcia Carteret, M. Ed. Oct 21,2010
https://www.dimensionsofculture.com/2010/10/cultural-values-of-asian-patients-and-families/ (access Mar 7, 2023)
9. Stonington SD. The Debt of Life-Thai Lessons on a Process-Oriented Ethical Logic. NEJM 2013; 369:1583-1585.
DOI:10.1056/NEJMp1308613
10. Filial Piety. https://en.wikipedia.org/wiki/Filial_piety
11. Zhan HG, Feng Z, Chen Z, Feng X. The role of the family in institutional long-term care: cultural management of filial piety in China. *Int J Soc Welfare 2011:* **20**: S121–S134.
DOI: 10.1111/j.1468-2397.2011.00808.x

12. Bergin AE. (1983). Religiosity and mental health: A critical reevaluation and meta-analysis. Professional Psychology: Research and Practice 1983;14:170.
13. Hackney CH, Sanders GS. (2003). Religiosity and mental health: A meta-analysis of recent studies. Journal for the Scientific Study of Religion, 2003;42:43–55.
14. Yaden DB, Batz-Barbarich CL, Ng V, Vaziri H, Jessica N, et al. A Meta-Analysis of Religion/Spirituality and Life Satisfaction. Journal of Happiness Studies (2022) 23:4147–4163 https://doi.org/10.1007/s10902-022-00558-7
15. Winzer L, Samutachak B, and Gray RS. Religiosity, Spirituality, and Happiness in Thailand from the Perspective of Buddhism. J of Population and Social Studies, 2018;26: 332 – 343. DOI: 10.25133/JPSSv26n4.023
16. Siriket R, Ngamsit T, Buabanbut R, Piasupun P, Pairojkul S. Concordance of the patients' preferences and the actual outcomes in elderly with late-stage dementia in Karunruk advance dementia care program. Abstract. 8th International Advance Care Planning Conference. Singapore, May 24-27, 2023.
17. Kongsuwan W, Chaipetch O, and Matchim Y. Thai Buddhist families' perspective of a peaceful death in ICUs. Nurs Crit Care 2012;17(3):151-9. doi: 10.1111/j.1478-5153.2012.00495.x.Epub 2012 Feb 15.
18. Schlieter J. and Goodman C. Consequences of compassion: An interpretation and defense of Buddhist ethics. New York: Oxford University Press [Book Review]. *Religion*, 40,358-359. [Crossref], [Web of Science ®], [Google Scholar]
19. *Manasurakarn J, Chaowalit A, Suttharangsee W, Isaramalai S, Geden E.* Values underlying end-of-life decisions of Thai Buddhist patients and their families. Songkla Med J 2008;26(6):549-559.
20. Srinonprasert V, Kajornkijaroen A, Na Bangchang P, Wangtrakuldee G, Wongboonsin J, et al. A survey of opinions regarding wishes toward the end-of-life among Thai elderly. J Med Assoc Thai 2014; 97 (Suppl. 3): S216-S222. Full text. e-Journal: http://www.jmatonline.com
21. Upasen R, Thanasilp S, Akkayagorn L, Chimluang L, Tantitrakul W, et al. Death Acceptance Process in Thai Buddhist Patients With Life-Limiting Cancer: A Grounded Theory. Global Qualitative Nursing Research 2022;9: 1–10.
22. Chindaprasirt J, Wongtirawit N, Limpawattana P, Srinonprasert V, Manjavong M, et al. Perception of a "good death" in Thai patients with cancer and their relatives. Heliyon 5 (2019) e02067.

23. Tipwong A, Ruamsook T, Hongkittiyanon T, Kgowsiri K. The perceptions on good death of the older adults in the semi-urban community: A qualitative study. Int J Nurs Sc 2020;9:389-96.
24. Panuthai S, Srirat S, and Wonghongkul T. Characteristics of a Good Death as Perceived by Related People in the Upper Northern Thai Context. Thai Journal of Nursing Council 2020; 35(4) 35-53.
25. Srinonprasert V, Limpawattana P, Manjavong M, Juntararuangtong T, Kuichanuan T. Perspectives regarding what constitutes a "good death" among Thai nurses: A cross-sectional study. Nurs Health Sci. 2019;21:416–421. DOI: 10.1111/nhs.12634
26. Jiraphan A and Pitanupong J. General population-based study on preferences towards end-of-life care in Southern Thailand: a cross-sectional survey. *BMC Palliative Care (2022) 21:36:1-11*
https://doi.org/10.1186/s12904-022-00926-3
27. Sangchart B, Ngamgam SP, Ekwuttiwongsa R, and Sangruangake M. The views of Thai Buddhist monks on a good death. Dise Prev Public Health J 2020;14,107-14.
28. Thai living will. https://www.thailivingwill.in.th
29. Luce JM and Alpers A. Legal aspects of withholding and withdrawing life support from critically ill patients in the United States and providing palliative care to them. Am J Respir Crit Care Med 2001;163:2029-32.
30. Healthline. Can you die from dementia?. https://www.healthline.com/health/dementia/can-you-die-from-dementia
31. Mitchell SL, Kiely DK, and Hamel MB. Dying with advanced dementia in the nursing home. Arch Intern Med 2004;164:321-326. DOI: 10.1001/archinte.164.3.321
32. Davies N, Barrado-Martin Y, Vickerstaff V, Rait G, Fukui A, et al. Enteral tube feeding for people with severe dementia. Cochrane Database of Systematic Reviews 13 August 2021. https://doi.org/10.1002/14651858.CD013503.pub2
33. Givens JL, Jones RN, Shaffer ML, Kiely DK, and Mitchell SL. Survival and comfort after treatment of pneumonia in advanced dementia. Arch Intern Med 2010 Jul 12;170(13):1102-7. doi: 10.1001/archinternmed.2010.181.
34. D'Agata E, Mitchell SL. Patterns of antimicrobial use among nursing home residents with advanced dementia. *Arch Intern Med*, 2008;168:357-62.
35. CEIC. Thailand Population: By Region: Northeastern. https://www.ceicdata.com/en/thailand/population-by-region-and-registration/population-by-region-northeastern

36. Siriket R, Piasupun P, and Pairojkul S. Outcomes of dementia patients receiving palliative care program. Abstract submitted for Asia Pacific Hospice Palliative Care Conference. Inchon October 4-6,2023.
37. Rice H, Howard R, and Huntley J. Professional caregivers' knowledge, beliefs and attitudes about awareness in advanced dementia: a systematic review of qualitative studies. Int Psychogeriatr 2019;31:1599-609. DOI: 10.1017/S1041610218002272
38. Wang Y, Xiao LD, Luo Y, Xiao SY, Whitehead C, and Davies O. Community health professionals' dementia knowledge, attitudes and care approach: a cross-sectional survey in Changsha, China. BMC Geriatrics 2018;122 https://doi.org/10.1186/s12877-018-0821-4

13

OF BONDS, BONDAGE, BONDING, AND BEYOND: TRAJECTORIES IN PERSON-CENTERED PALLIATIVE CARE AMONG FILIPINO PHYSICIANS CAREGIVING FOR A PARENT WITH ADVANCED DEMENTIA

MARIA MINERVA P. CALIMAG, M.D., M.SC., PH.D.[1]

[Alzheimer's] From the moment of diagnosis, it's "a truly long, long goodbye."
—Nancy Reagan, 2005

Abstract

Better healthcare has resulted in the projected aging of the population worldwide thus family caregiving has become a public health priority and a pressing social issue. It is likely that more assistance than ever before will be provided to frail or ill older persons. Older persons afflicted with dementia need special attention. An abundance of family research on dementia has demonstrated that it has consequences for whole families. These studies suggest that certain forms of coping are useful, but it is unclear whether the same coping strategies are applicable to physicians acting as family caregivers coping with the burden of caring for a family member with advanced dementia. To address this gap, the present study was undertaken to answer the central question: How do Filipino physicians, as

[1] Faculty of Medicine and Surgery, the Research Center for Social Science and Education, and the Research Center for the Health Sciences
University of Santo Tomas, Manila, PHILIPPINES

family and professional caregivers, collectively make meaning of their lived experience of trajectories in palliative care while undertaking the caregiver role and providing person-centered patient care for a parent with advanced dementia? Anchored on interpretive phenomenology, this naturalistic inquiry sought to study people in their own environment. After ensuring anonymity, six physicians who cared for a parent with advanced dementia generously shared their stories of caregiving, hoping that their collective narratives can serve as inspiration to others. Guided by the rules of cool and warm analysis, field texts underwent phenomenological reduction, interpretation, and member-checking procedures for validation. Interestingly, four themes representing the caregiving experience of physicians emerged: bonds (reminiscences and reconciliation as the wellspring of caregiving); bondage (restraints restrictions as the boundaries in caregiving); bonding (relations and reconnections as the links in caregiving); and beyond (release and relief as the catharsis in caregiving). Physicians are in the enviable position of knowing the medical implications of dementia on their significant others. Policies in dementia care should continue to emphasize person-centered family care as the cornerstone of assistance to older adults with advanced dementia.

Keywords: palliative care, person-centered care, dementia, Filipino

Introduction

It was the late medical essayist, Lewis Thomas who famously labeled Alzheimer's Disease as the Disease of the Century. In his 1992 essay, Thomas explained that: "Of all the things that can go wrong in aging, the loss of the mind is far and away the worst and most feared. And here I believe, is the greatest of all opportunities for medical science in the improvement of the human condition" (Campbell, 2004). The looming Alzheimer's epidemic is a disease that embodies everything we fear most about aging — weakness and dependence, humiliation, and oblivion. The insidious onset and relentless progression have tremendous implications not only on a societal level but on a family and individual level as well.

Living with dementia until the end of life is a growing challenge that significantly affects not only individuals with dementia but likewise impacts their family caregivers and health care professional. In the advanced stage of dementia, affected individuals are practically fully dependent on caregivers (WHO, 2002). Dementia, one of the most common causes of death (WHO, 2012), has become even more conspicuous given the increasing number of people affected worldwide. It is estimated to double every 20 years (Prince et al., 2016), rising to over 131 million by 2050 (Alzheimer's Disease International, 2015). A new diagnosis of dementia occurs every 3 seconds with 9.9 million new cases reported in 2015 (Prince et al., 2014)

Dementia syndrome is common and is expected to increase significantly among older people and is characterized by the loss of cognitive, psychological, and physical functions. The need for palliative care and an increase in family caregiving in aging people with dementia is expected to increase over the next decades as better healthcare results in the projected "greying" of the population. Older persons afflicted with dementia need special attention, frequently though, they do not receive adequate palliative care which may relate to poor understanding of the natural course of dementia. Thus, family caregiving has become a public health priority and a pressing social issue (Sapkota & Subedi, 2019; WHO, 2012). Understanding that dementia is a progressive, and terminal life-limiting syndrome without curative treatment is fundamental to a focus on comfort care in advanced dementia (WHO, 2002). Palliative care focusing on the quality of life for people with advanced dementia can improve symptom burden, prevent undertreatment of symptoms and overtreatment with unnecessary and burdensome treatment and can also reduce caregiver burden and enhance caregiver quality of life (Mitchel et al., 2009; van Soest-Poortvliet et al., 2015).

Dominguez et al. (2021) provided Philippine data on the incidence, burden, and cost of care for dementia. Results of their study showed the crude incidence rate was 16 (CI: 13–20) cases per 1,000 person-years (pyr) with a higher incidence among females of 17 (CI: 12–21) per 1,000 pyr versus 14 (CI: 9–21) per 1,000 pyr for males. Projections based on this incidence, revealed an estimation of 220,632 new cases in 2030, 295,066 in 2040, and 378,461 in 2050. The disease burden was at 2,876 DALYs per 100,000 persons. The economic burden per patient was around Php 196,000 annually (i.e., ~4,070 USD, or 36.7% of the average family's annual income in the Philippines). Direct medical costs accounted for only 13.48% of this care expense while the rest (86.29%) were attributed to indirect costs of estimated lost potential earnings of unpaid family caregivers. In a country like the Philippines, family members take on the caregiving role naturally and do not consider themselves as such. Literature is replete with research that demonstrates its consequences for whole families. In such instances, a family member regularly and without pay provides support and care to an elderly person who has a significant or persistent health problem, chronic or disabling condition, or loss of autonomy. Studies suggest that certain forms of coping strategies are applicable when physicians act as family caregivers to a parent with dementia.

The implications of dementia for primary caregivers are certainly important. No study was found in the literature which examined the voice of physicians in the role of caregivers trying to cope with the burden of caring for a family member with advanced dementia. Moreover, there are not many studies that focus on person-centered care in the context of the local culture. Douglas et al., (2010) defined person-centered care as care based on the concept of personhood, "a socially created entity established through the action of others." Person-centered care is the maintenance of an individual's personhood, through the context of personal and social relationships (Kitwood 1997), while viewing the world from the perspective of the person with dementia which includes an understanding of their culture. Brooker (2004) posited four elements of person-centered care, i.e., valuing people with dementia and those who care for them; treating people as individuals; viewing the world through the lens of the person with dementia; and providing them with a positive social environment.

In the Philippines, there are now several private and public nursing homes in the country, but it is still somewhat considered taboo for many Filipinos to confine their loved ones in a care facility. Dominant cultural beliefs come into play at the societal level, as people become stigmatized for conditions over which they themselves have no control. The stigma associated with placing an older family member in residential care emerged throughout several studies, with an emphasis on filial piety across several cultures. Stigma negatively impacts family relationships as it is often associated with heightened stress, and shame (Antelius & Kiwi 2015; Kanwar & Whomsley 2011).

Medical school has honed physicians in the science of medicine, while much of the humane aspect of caring has been relegated to the background. To address this gap this study was undertaken to answer the central question: How do Filipino physicians, as family and professional caregivers, collectively make meaning of their lived experience of transitions to palliative care while undertaking the caregiver role and providing person-centered patient care for a parent with advanced dementia?

Methodology

Anchored on interpretive phenomenology, this naturalistic inquiry sought to study people in their own environment.

After ensuring anonymity, six physicians who cared for a parent with advanced dementia generously shared their stories of caregiving, hoping that their collective narratives can serve as inspiration to others. Respondent physicians in this study met several criteria, which include that as family caregivers, they must be the primary source of care and decision-making for their parent who has dementia and currently residing with them. The care recipients were aged 65 or over and in need of assistance with at least one instrumental activity of daily living (IADL), such as cooking or home maintenance, or activity of daily living (ADL), such as bathing, and had received help from family in a non-institutional setting for at least 3 months before the study's onset.

The respondents' demographic information using *robofoto* (a Dutch term that pertains to the delineation of the respondents) (Ketchermans & Ballet, 2002 as cited by Caña et al. 2005) revealed the following baseline characteristics: two were males (33.33 percent) and females comprised 66.67 percent). Their mean age was 42.3 years. All respondents share in the primary caregiving role.

An in-depth interactive interview was conducted to evolve narratives of six physicians acting as caregivers of significant others with dementia and to capture their collective experiences of their caregiving experience. Guided by the rules of cool and warm analysis, field texts underwent phenomenological reduction, interpretation, and member-checking procedures for validation.

Findings

Interestingly, four themes representing the caregiving experience of physicians emerged: bonds (reminiscences and reconciliation as the wellspring in caregiving); bondage (restraints restrictions as the boundaries in caregiving); bonding (relations and reconnections as the links in caregiving); and beyond (release and relief as the catharsis in caregiving).

Bonds: Reminiscences and Reconciliation as the Wellspring in Caregiving

The respondents invariably started their narratives with recollections of their relationships with their significant other. Based on the interviews, the care relationships emerged against a backdrop of attachment and common social history. Our respondents evoked a past constructed on the intimacy of family relationships, shared commitments, admiration felt for the cared-for parent, and the importance held by the cared-for.

> "My father died when I was three years old, my mother is the only parent I knew. Caring for her needs now that she has dementia is the least I can do to repay her." (Respondent 1)

> "I was the well-loved daughter. I modeled myself after Mom and loved her with all my heart. I was her confidant and I listened to her. She taught me how to take care of her. She was so proud when I told her that I wanted to become a doctor." (Respondent 2)

> "I've never had a relationship with my dad and when he developed Alzheimer's, I didn't feel as much hurt as when I lost my mom, but I felt the need to care for him." (Respondent 6)

Caregivers reflect on "what used to be" versus "what is." Through comparison of present and past lifestyles, caregivers express sorrow about lost or changed relationships. In this phenomenological study, our respondents felt "they were essentially grieving for someone they once knew."

> "I pray to God for help and healing, I miss mom so much even though she is still here with us." (Respondent 2)

> "My mother was the gentlest, kindest person I knew. Now she would go into fits and tantrums." (Respondent 3)

> As I transitioned to the role of caregiver, I grieve over the loss of the special bond that I have with my father. He had that quiet kind of love…teaching me how to read, combing my hair and bringing me to school and later when I would sleep late reviewing for my subjects in Medicine, he would bring me home pansit lomi and lumpiang shanghai (Chinese noodles and spring rolls)." (Respondent 4)

> "It is hard for me to remember who my father was before Alzheimer's. The disease has robbed not only my father's memories but also the memories of those who care for him." (Respondent 5)

Bondage: Restraints and Restrictions as the Boundaries in Caregiving

The caregiving experiences of physicians likewise resonated with feelings of physical restraints and functional restrictions in their usual daily activities.

> "When we lost Dad, my Mom's memory started to drift. I was in denial convinced that she might be suffering from depression, melancholia maybe, and not Alzheimer's." (Respondent 2)

> "During eating times, my Mom would sit on the dining table and eat only a few morsels of food after which she would stand up and walk around. It is as if she had difficulty swallowing her food. I have to wait a while until she sits back and takes on a few more of the food on her plate." Sometimes, it would be thirty minutes or maybe an hour, and I have to patiently wait on her." (Respondent 3)

> "I cannot go far…my brother and sisters are not doctors and they need me to look after Dad when his memory started to go. Med[sic] School did not prepare me for this." (Respondent 5)

> "Long periods of silence marked our daily encounters with Dad as he stared back blankly at us." (Respondent 6)

The physician caregivers also felt the need to restrict their parents' mobility outside the house by locking the doors as their loved ones would sometimes get lost while wandering outside.

> "One night, we were shocked to find out that Mom wandered off outside the house and we lost her for three days. All she remembered was my name and people looked me up on social media." (Respondent 1)

> "Dad got lost one time when he went out of the house. He found his way home only after he told people that our phone was under my name in the Yellow Pages." (Respondent 4)

Bonding: Relations and Reconnections as the Links in Caregiving

Bonding refers to opportunities to interact with a supportive network of family and friends, and increased family caregivers' coping by providing a listening presence and perspective. Most of the respondents remembered that they were brought up knowing that they should take care of their elders.

"I would deck, like what we would do in Med[sic] School, with my sister in coming home to bring afternoon snack for our mother. We would arrange our daily schedule so at least one of us would be free to go home for even just an hour, at around three o'clock or thereabouts." (Respondent 1)

"I am just glad that I have brothers and sisters who share the caregiving role with me, I guess each of us just developed our own way of transitioning from the role of son or daughter to one of caregiver. If we didn't do that…(pause), it would be very hard to cope with our dad's condition." (Respondent 4)

Beyond: Release and Relief as the Catharsis in Caregiving

Our respondents experienced intense emotional release as the caring process ended with the death of the loved one. This allowed them to surface repressed emotions, complexes, and feelings. One respondent said that he benefited from having an opportunity to talk about his caregiving experiences to someone else.

"I sighed long and deep as I realized that I am left with nothing, but boxes of photographs and memories of a time gone by." (Respondent 1)

"I trust the Lord has a plan, not only for my father but also for us who cared for him. I know in my heart that it is a good plan." (Respondent 5)

"I waited for my dad to breathe his last, his pulse growing weaker until it stopped. As the doctor in the family, I pronounced him dead." (Respondent 6)

Discussion

Approximately 7% of the Philippines' total population in 2015 is aging and it is projected to increase by 11% in 2025 and 16% in 2045. (Philippine Statistics Authority, 2017). The estimated number of Filipino elderly (60 years and older) will more than double from 9.5 million in 2020 to 19.7 million in 2040 (Ageing Population in the Philippines, 2022). According to Article XV, Section 4 of the Philippine Constitution, "The family has the duty to care for its elderly members although the State may also do so through just programs of social security." The traditional close family ties of Filipinos are exhibited through the usual setup in the household where the elderly live with their children and rely on them for financial support. Geriatric care can be quite difficult to deal with at home, most especially if members of the household are not professionally trained or if they lack experience in caring for the sick elderly. Not to mention, age-related illnesses like dementia and depression can greatly affect the caregiver's daily routine and may possibly strain family ties. By 2015, approximately 301,000 Filipinos with dementia were reported by the Geriatrics Infolink Management Strategies Philippines Inc. (2018). The organization likewise predicted that these cases were expected to reach up to 568,000 and 1.15 million by 2030, and 2050, respectively.

The course of dementia is characterized by a prolonged decline in function with extensive limitations to cognitive, psychological, and physical functioning in advanced stages (Eisenmann et al., 2020). With further progression, it becomes increasingly difficult to predict the course in the individual and in contrast to the diagnosis of malignancy, it is difficult to predict when a person approaches the advanced stage of dementia.

As the disease progresses it becomes difficult to predict the duration of the different stages of dementia, as these can vary widely between individuals. Moderate and advanced stages represent the longest periods of the disease with a mean of 12 months. Women generally live longer in the advanced stage (Rizzuto et al., 2012). People with Alzheimer's disease over the age of 70 were found to spend on average 4 years in the stage of advanced dementia (Arrighi, 2010). The severity of dementia increases with age (Prince, 2014). While half of the people with dementia die from moderate dementia, one-quarter of them die from advanced dementia (Koopmans, 2003).

Bonds: Reminiscences and Reconciliation as the Wellspring in Caregiving

Close and intimate family members can provide essential biographical information to get to know and understand the person with dementia or provide the impetus for person-centered care to meet the individual's needs (Schmidt et al., 2018). Most often, they felt that they have to carry their emotional burdens and are therefore at risk of experiencing prolonged grief. Grief and feeling of loss do not necessarily begin with the death of the affected person, but already earlier in phases of the personality change and when the loved one can no longer recognize their relatives (Sachs et al., 2004; D'Onofrio et al., 2015; Moore et al., 2017). Depression should be addressed during the early stages of dementia as it is often an underrecognized target for the prevention of cognitive decline in dementia (Dafsari & Jessen (2020). In the Philippines where people with dementia are increasingly cared for at home by family members and home care staff, the care of people with dementia is person-centered; however, little is known about how home care staff understands and enact person-centered care in their daily work. Establishing familiarity is essential in continuously fostering person-centered care of people with dementia. When familiarity was in place, the care recipient and those who provide the home care acted as a team to perform the care (Hedman et al., 2022).#

Bondage: Restraints and Restrictions as the Boundaries in Caregiving

Most people with advanced dementia who live and die in institutional care often suffer a range of burdensome symptoms and complications. Shortly before dying, people with advanced dementia may suffer symptoms such as pain, eating problems, breathlessness, neuropsychiatric symptoms, and complications such as respiratory or urinary infections, and often, they would experience burdensome transitions. Caring for people with advanced dementia poses different challenges than caring for people with mild to moderate dementia. There is less evidence of palliative care interventions even with an increase in research.

Over the course of the disease difficulties in eating become more and more manifest with consequently reduced food intake and need for support with eating and drinking. People with advanced dementia have problems swallowing adequately. Moreover, they tend to keep food in their mouths and stop chewing or spitting out food. In the last month of life, patients with advanced dementia exhibit observable weight loss due to difficulty with swallowing (Sampson, 2018). Advanced dementia is often accompanied by deterioration in oral health and oral hygiene with possible subsequent damage to the oral cavity and teeth, and a sore mouth that causes pain thus hindering the use of dental prostheses and leading to reduced food intake (Bedi, 2015). Other acute medical events need to be examined, as possible causes for eating problems, which include acute infections, medication-related side effects, and stroke (Mitchell, 2015). Moreover, advanced dementia is a risk factor for aspiration followed by pneumonia (van der Maarel-Wierink et al., 2011).

As dementia progresses people experience reduced or lost verbal communication abilities (WHO, 2012) with a consequent impact on care. Several authors noted that despite restrictions in verbal communication among people with advanced dementia, they can use other means of nonverbal communication such as body tension or minimal movements, turning their head away, frequency of breath, and paralinguistic signals to express their current wishes or needs (Kuehlmeyer et al., 2015; Eisenmann et al., 2016; Diehl-Schmid et al., 2018). Agreement or rejection reactions in a situation can be observed, although the interpretation of nonverbal communication varies between health professionals (Kuehlmeyer et al., 2015).

Behavior is more correctly interpreted if the caregiver is well acquainted over a longer period of time with the person suffering from dementia (Schmidt et al., 2018). Some patients with dementia may exhibit Behavioral and Psychological Symptoms of Dementia (BPSDs) such as screaming, wandering, resisting care, and acting aggressively, both verbally and physically (Hugo & Ganguli, 2014 as cited by Swall et al., 2020

Wandering represents one of many problematic behavioral disorders occurring in people with dementia associated with a variety of negative outcomes. Wandering includes different types of behavior such as aimless movement without a discernible purpose. The etiology of wandering, an acutely distressing problem worldwide, both for patients and caregivers, is poorly understood and remains an unsolved riddle. It is a major reason for restricting outdoor activities among older persons with dementia. It is possible that management of coexistent psychopathology through pharmacological and non-pharmacological interventions would help to ameliorate this behavioral disorder.

Bonding: Relations and Reconnections as the Links in Caregiving

Emotion-focused coping was the most commonly used strategy among caregivers of patients with dementia. Monteiro et al., 2018 showed that the use and development of coping strategies may ameliorate the depressive symptoms, anxiety, and burden of caregivers. However, cohort studies over time that clearly describe the type of coping strategy are still needed in relation to the outcomes they presented. Advanced care planning allows for establishing and implementing values and preferences and is associated with comfort and decreasing burdensome interventions in a patient-centered approach.

Proxy decision-making is often necessary due to a lack of decisional capacity (Bogaerts et al., 2023). Restricted capacity of communication and cognitive function implies impediments to decision-making that typically requires informed consent. Due to temporal or permanent lack of decisional capacity, surrogate decision-making may become necessary, e.g., by family members and health care professionals. Family carers often found proxy decision-making challenging (Soofi, 2022), however, physicians performing caregiving roles in the home can immediately make important decisions that are beneficial for their loved ones. They can initiate palliative care through the prevention and relief of suffering by means of early identification, assessment, and treatment of pain and other physical, psychosocial, and spiritual problems in order to maintain or improve quality of life.

Beyond: Release and Relief as the Catharsis in Caregiving

In his book *How we die: Reflections on Life's Final Chapter,* Nuland (1995) reminded physicians that disease, not death, is the real enemy, and despite the fact that most deaths are unpleasant, painful, or agonized, to argue otherwise is to cover up the truth. Furthermore, he stressed that the physician should instill in dying patients the hope not for a miraculous cure but for the dignity and high quality of the remainder of their lives as well as of what they have meant—and will continue to mean—to family, friends, and colleagues. Unfortunately, patients with advanced dementia are not aware of their impending death.

The reported median survival from diagnosis, although varying by patient cohort and study setting, is influenced by the dementia type. In a systematic review, Brodaty et al. (2012) reported survival from diagnosis ranging from 1.3 to 7.2 years. Other studies, notably by Brookmeyer et al. (2002) reported median postdiagnosis survival of 3.2–8.3 years among patients with Alzheimer's Disease. Age and severity of dementia at diagnosis also influence survival. Women are disproportionately affected by shortened life span due to dementia apparently because they live longer. In advanced dementia, the median survival time is 1.3 years (Mitchell et al., 2009).

Reliable estimation of the remaining lifetime and recognizing signs of an ending life can contribute to increasing the availability of palliative care in any care setting (Eisenmann et al., 2020). However, it remains difficult to predict the end of life of people with dementia (Sampson et al., 2018). Health professionals often overestimate the remaining lifetime, e.g., only half of the expected deaths coincided with the actual time of death (Lundin & Godskesen, 2021).

Although nursing homes are common places for end-of-life care and many people with dementia die in nursing homes or hospitals, their preferred place to die is their original home (Badrakalimuthu & Barclay, 2014; Dasch et al., 2018). Achieving this is more likely where the goals of treatment are symptomatic relief only, indicating the importance of advance care planning during the early stages of dementia when the patient can share in the decision-making. In the Philippines where home care is preferred throughout the trajectory of dementia care, it behooves physicians living with their loved ones afflicted with dementia to educate their relatives with whom they share the dementia caregiving role about person-centered care and thus provide a positive home environment for both the caregivers and their loved ones with dementia.

Conclusion

Physicians know the medical implications of dementia on their significant others. While providing palliative home care to family members with advanced dementia, they are in an enviable position to provide person-centered care, i.e., valuing people with dementia and those who care for them; treating people as individuals; viewing the world from the perspective of the person with dementia; and providing a positive social environment for their loved one with dementia. Their families can benefit from additional information and support to reinforce and improve their caregiving efforts. Several variables must be targeted when considering programs for caregivers, many of which can be adequately and appropriately addressed through the intervention of a physician who has been through the caregiving experience either through formal education or advocacy. Overall, this chapter reinforces that the individual needs of the person living with dementia and their family must be considered to provide person-centered and comprehensive palliative care, enabling them to live well until death ensues. Policies especially in LMIC that culturally value dementia care at home should continue emphasizing person-centered family care as the cornerstone of assisting older adults with advanced dementia.

References

Ageing Population in the Philippines. *Help Age Network.* Available online at: https://ageingasia.org/ageing-population-philippines/ (accessed December 3, 2022).

Antelius E, Kiwi M (2015) Frankly, none of us know what dementia is: dementia caregiving among Iranian immigrants living in Sweden. Care Management Journals 16(2), 79-94.

Arrighi, H. M., Neumann, P. J., Lieberburg, I. M., & Townsend, R. J. (2010). Lethality of Alzheimer disease and its impact on nursing home placement. *Alzheimer Disease & Associated Disorders*, *24*(1), 90-95.

Bogaerts, J. M., Warmerdam, L. A., Achterberg, W. P., Gussekloo, J., & Poortvliet, R. K. (2023). Proxy Decision-Making for Clinical Research in Nursing Home Residents With Dementia: A Qualitative Analysis. *Journal of the American Medical Directors Association.*

Brodaty, H., Seeher, K., & Gibson, L. (2012). Dementia time to death: a systematic literature review on survival time and years of life lost in people with dementia. *International psychogeriatrics*, *24*(7), 1034-1045.

Brooke, J., Cronin, C., Stiell, M., & Ojo, O. (2018). The intersection of culture in the provision of dementia care: A systematic review. *Journal of Clinical Nursing*, *27*(17-18), 3241-3253.

Brookmeyer, R., Corrada, M. M., Curriero, F. C., & Kawas, C. (2002). Survival following a diagnosis of Alzheimer disease. *Archives of neurology*, *59*(11), 1764-1767.

Brooker D (2004) What is person-centred care for people with dementia? Reviews in Clinical Gerontology 13, 215-222.

Campbell, C. C. (2004). The human face of Alzheimer's. *The New Atlantis*, (6), 3-17.

Dafsari, F. S., & Jessen, F. (2020). Depression—an underrecognized target for prevention of dementia in Alzheimer's disease. *Translational Psychiatry*, *10*(1), 160.

Diehl-Schmid, J., Riedl, L., Rüsing, U., Hartmann, J., Bertok, M., Levin, C., Hamann, J., Arcand, M., Lorenzl, S., Feddersen, B. and Jox, R.J. (2018). Provision of palliative care for people with advanced dementia. *Der Nervenarzt*, *89*, 524-529.

D'Onofrio G, Sancarlo D, Addante F, Ciccone F, Cascavilla L, Paris F, et al.(2015). Caregiver burden characterization in patients with Alzheimer's disease or vascular dementia. *Int J Geriatr Psychiatry* 30(9):891–9. doi: 10.1002/gps.4232

Dominguez, J., Jiloca, L., Fowler, K. C., De Guzman, M. F., Dominguez-Awao, J. K., Natividad, B., Domingo, J., Dominguez, J.D., Reandelar Jr, M., Ligsay, A., Yu, J.R., Aichele, S. & Phung, T. K. T. (2021). Dementia incidence, burden and cost of care: a Filipino community-based study. *Frontiers in Public Health*, *9*, 628700. & Phung, T. K. T.

(2021). Dementia incidence, burden and cost of care: a Filipino community-based study. *Frontiers in Public Health*, *9*, 628700.

Douglass C, Keddie A, Brooker D, Surr C (2010). Cross-cultural comparison of the perceptions and experiences of dementia care mapping "mappers" in the United States and the United Kingdom. Journal of Aging and Health 22(5), 567-588.

Eisenmann, Y., Schmidt, H., Voltz, R., & Perrar, K. M. (2016). Expression and perception of needs in severe dementia: A case study. *Journal of Hospice & Palliative Nursing*, *18*(3), 268-272.

Eisenmann, Y., Golla, H., Schmidt, H., Voltz, R., & Perrar, K. M. (2020). Palliative care in advanced dementia. *Frontiers in psychiatry*, *11*, 699.

Etkind, S. N., Bone, A. E., Gomes, B., Lovell, N., Evans, C. J., Higginson, I. J., & Murtagh, F. E. M. (2017). How many people will need palliative care in 2040? Past trends, future projections and implications for services. *BMC Medicine*, *15*(1), 1-10.

Geriatrics Infolink Management Strategies Philippines Inc. (2018).

Hedman, R., Sandman, P. O., & Edvardsson, D. (2022). Enacting person-centred care in home care services for people with dementia. *Journal of Clinical Nursing*, *31*(11-12), 1519-1530.

Hugo, J., & Ganguli, M. (2014). Dementia and cognitive impairment: epidemiology, diagnosis, and treatment. *Clinics in geriatric medicine*, *30*(3), 421-442 as cited by Swall, A., Hammar, L. M., & Gransjön Craftman, Å. (2020). Like a bridge over troubled water–a qualitative study of professional caregiver singing and music as a way to enable person-centred care for persons with dementia. *International journal of qualitative studies on health and well-being*, *15*(1), 1735092.

Kanwar S, Whomsley S (2011). Working with Pakistani service users and their families. A practitioner's guide. Available at: www.cpft.nhs.uk (accessed 6th April 2023).

Ketchermans, G., & Ballet, K. (2002) as cited by Caña, M. B., Cueto, Q. L. G. G., de Guzman, A. B., Fuchigami, K. B., Manalo, L. R. T., & Yu, J. C. U. (2005). Clientele recognition of library terms and concepts used by librarians: A case of an academic library in the Philippines. Journal of Librarianship and Information Science, 37(4), 195–204.

Kitwood T (1997) Dementia reconsidered: the person comes first. Open University Press: Buckingham.

Koopmans, R. T., Ekkerink, J. L., & Van Weel, C. (2003). Survival to late dementia in Dutch nursing home patients. *Journal of the American Geriatrics Society*, *51*(2), 184-187.

Kuehlmeyer, K., Schuler, A. F., Kolb, C., Borasio, G. D., & Jox, R. J. (2015). Evaluating nonverbal behavior of individuals with dementia during feeding: a survey of the nursing staff in residential care homes for elderly adults. *Journal of the American Geriatrics Society*, *63*(12), 2544-2549.

Lundin, E., & Godskesen, T. E. (2021). End-of-life care for people with advanced dementia and pain: a qualitative study in Swedish nursing homes. *BMC nursing*, *20*, 1-11.

Memorial Services in the Congress of the United States and Tributes in Eulogy of Ronald Reagan, Late a President of the United States. (2005). United States: U.S. Government Printing Office.

Mitchell, S. L. (2015). Advanced dementia. *New England Journal of Medicine*, *372*(26), 2533-2540.

Mitchell SL, Teno JM, Kiely DK, Shaffer ML, Jones RN, Prigerson HG, et al. (2009). The clinical course of advanced dementia. *New Engl J Med* 361(16):1529–38. doi: 10.1056/NEJMoa0902234

Monteiro, A. M. F., Santos, R. L., Kimura, N., Baptista, M. A. T., & Dourado, M. C. N. (2018). Coping strategies among caregivers of people with Alzheimer disease: a systematic review. *Trends in psychiatry and psychotherapy*, *40*(3), 258–268. https://doi.org/10.1590/2237-6089-2017-0065

Moore KJ, Davis S, Gola A, Harrington J, Kupeli N, Vickerstaff V, et al. (2017). Experiences of end of life amongst family carers of people with advanced dementia: longitudinal cohort study with mixed methods. *BMC Geriatr* 17(1):135. doi: 10.1186/s12877-017-0523-3

Murphy E, Froggatt K, Connolly S, O'Shea E, Sampson EL, Casey D, & Devane, D. (2016). Palliative care interventions in advanced dementia. *Cochrane Database Syst Rev* 12: Cd011513. doi: 10.1002/14651858.CD011513.pub2

Nuland, S. B. (1995). *How we die: Reflections on life's final chapter*. Vintage.

Philippine Statistics Authority. *Projected Population, by Age Group, Sex, and by Five-Calendar Year Interval, Philippines: 2010−2045*. (2017). Available online at: https://psa.gov.ph/sites/default/files/attachments/hsd/pressrelease/Table 1_8.pdf (accessed December 22, 2022).

Prince M, Knapp M, Guerchet M, McCrone P, Prina M, Comas-Herrera A, et al. (2014). *Dementia UK: Update*. Alzheimer's Society.

Prince, M., Ali, G. C., Guerchet, M., Prina, A. M., Albanese, E., & Wu, Y. T. (2016). Recent global trends in the prevalence and incidence of dementia, and survival with dementia. *Alzheimer's research & therapy*, *8 (1):23*, 1-13. doi: 10.1186/s13195-016-0188-8

Rizzuto, D., Bellocco, R., Kivipelto, M., Clerici, F., Wimo, A., & Fratiglioni, L. (2012). Dementia after age 75: survival in different severity stages and years of life lost. *Current Alzheimer Research*, *9*(7), 795-800.

Sachs GA, Shega JW, Cox-Hayley D.(2004). Barriers to excellent end-of-life care for patients with dementia. J Gen Internal Med 19(10):1057–63. doi: 10.1111/j.1525-1497.2004.30329.x

Sampson, E. L., Candy, B., Davis, S., Gola, A. B., Harrington, J., King, M., ... & Jones, L. (2018). Living and dying with advanced dementia: a prospective cohort study of symptoms, service use and care at the end of life. *Palliative medicine*, *32*(3), 668-681.

Sapkota, N., & Subedi, S. (2019). Dementia as a public health priority. *Journal of Psychiatrists' Association of Nepal*, *8*(2), 1-3.

Schmidt H, Eisenmann Y, Golla H, Voltz R, Perrar KM (2018). Needs of people with advanced dementia in their final phase of life: A multi-perspective qualitative study in nursing homes. *Palliat Med* 32(3):657–67. doi: 10.1177/0269216317746571

Soofi, H. (2022). Ethical aspects of facilitating the recruitment of people with dementia for clinical trials: A call for further debate. *British Journal of Clinical Pharmacology*, *88*(1), 22-26.

van Soest-Poortvliet MC, van der Steen JT, de Vet HC, Hertogh CM, Deliens L, Onwuteaka-Philipsen BD (2015). Comfort goal of care and end-of-life outcomes in dementia: A prospective study. *Palliat Med* 29(6):538–46. doi: 10.1177/0269216315570409

World Health Organization. (2012). *Dementia: a public health priority*. World Health Organization.

World Health Organization. *WHO Definition of Palliative Care 2002*. (2002) http://www.who.int/cancer/palliative/definition/en/.

14

THE CURRENT PERSPECTIVE OF CARING FOR THE PEOPLE WITH DEMENTIA İN TURKEY

GONCA OGUZ, MD, PROF[1] AND
DENİZ TUNCEL BERKTAS, MD, PROF[2]

Abstract

Dementia is a progressive neurodegenerative disease with a terminal nature. It is one of the major health problems worldwide. The rate of dementia is rapidly increasing in Turkey along with the aging population. Palliative care is an interdisciplinary approach that focuses in improving quality of life of patients facing problems associated with life-limiting diseases. Early integration of palliative care into dementia care is supposed to provide benefit by addressing the physical, psychosocial and spiritual needs of people with dementia. In Turkey, the legislations and regulations are usually designed for the care of the elderly and disabled. Besides, some barriers exist against the diagnosis and care of dementia patients. National strategies must be developed for dementia awareness, appropriate palliative care provision and education of the patients, families and healthcare professionals.

Keywords: Aging, Culture, Dementia, Palliative Care, Turkey

---

[1]Department of Anesthesiology, Palliative Care Unit,
Dr AY Ankara Oncology Training and Research Hospital, University of Health Sciences, Ankara
[2]Department of Neurology, Kahramanmaras Sutcu Imam University, Kahramanmaras

Introduction

Dementia can be defined as a clinical syndrome characterized by a series of symptoms and signs manifested by impairment in memory, language and other cognitive functions (such as attention, direction finding, recognition, decision making), behavioral changes and impairment in daily living activities. Alzheimer's disease is the most common cause of dementia, accounting for an estimated 60% to 80% of all dementia cases (1, 2). Dementia is a rapidly growing public health problem and one of the leading causes of disability and dependency among older people around the world. It is estimated that about 55 million people live with dementia worldwide and this number will rise to 139 million by 2050 (3). Over the age of 85, almost 32 out of every 100 people develop dementia. At the individual level, dementia reduces life expectancy and quality. Physical, psychological, social and spiritual symptoms increase with the advanced disease and can deteriorate family and patient experiences during the end of life (4). Therefore, a comprehensive assessment and care is needed throughout the disease trajectory, including grief support after the decease of the patient.

Palliative care is a holistic approach that supports the improvement of the quality of life of patients and families who encounter problems arising from life-threatening disease. It aims at optimal management of distressing symptoms while incorporating psychosocial and spiritual care according to their needs, values, beliefs and cultures (5,6). It can be delivered concurrently with disease directed therapies starting at the time of diagnosis and becomes the main focus of care when they are no longer effective or desired. Providing a dignified life by facilitating the patient's autonomy, access to information and the right to make choices are among the main principles of the palliative care approach (7).

Along with the aging population and rise in the prevalence of chronic diseases in the world, the importance of palliative care and its priority in global health policies are also increasing. It has been estimated that over 56.8 million people require palliative care worldwide every year, including 31.1 million prior to and 25.7 million near the end of life (8). Although palliative care is predominantly delivered to patients with advanced cancer in many European countries, it is now well recognized that patients with other chronic life-limiting diseases like HIV/AIDS, neurological, cardiac, pulmonary or renal diseases may also experience similar symptoms and require need for palliative care. According to Global Atlas of Palliative Care by Worldwide Hospice Palliative Care Alliance (WHPCA), dementia makes up 12.2% of the disease groups accounting for adult palliative care (8). In the revised recommendations on standards and norms for palliative care in Europe from the European Association for Palliative Care (EAPC), geriatric and dementia services are highlighted as emerging new areas of specialization in palliative care (4).

Dementia Care in Turkey and Need for a Palliative Care Integration

Populations around the world are ageing at a faster pace than in the past and this demographic transition will have an impact on almost all aspects of society. There are more than 1 billion people aged 60 years or older, with most living in low- and middle-income countries (9). The elderly population has been increasing rapidly in Turkey since the 1990s. According to the data of the Turkish Statistical Institution; the number of elderly population aged 65 and over was 6 million 651 thousand 503 in 2016; it increased by 24.0% in the last five years and reached 8 million 245 thousand 124 people in 2021 (10).

The high proportion of the elderly in the total population is an indicator of the aging and a ratio over 10% shows that the relevant population is 'very old.' In Turkey, the proportion of the elderly population in the whole country was 8.3% in 2016, it increased to 9.7% in 2021. According to statistical projections, it was predicted that the proportion would be 11.0% in 2025, 12.9% in 2030 and 16.3% in 2040. In 2021, 44.3% of the elderly population was male, 55.7% female and 64.7% was in the 65-74 age groups. The elderly dependency ratio, which expresses the number of elderly people per hundred people of working age, was 12.3% in 2016 and this rate increased to 14.3% in 2021. It is estimated that the elderly dependency ratio will be 16.4% in 2025, 19.6% in 2030, and 25.3% in 2040. Turkey ranks 68th among 167 countries in terms of elderly population ratio (10).

In line with the general trend in the world, the number of elderly people living alone in our country is also increasing. Although aging in Turkey is not yet perceived as a big "problem" as in advanced industrial societies, it has the potential to become a problem in the near future with the prolongation of the average life expectancy. There is an increase in health conditions, especially dementia, in the elderly, and a change in the position of the family in elderly care in Turkey as well as in the rest of the world. In addition, elderly dependency rates also show an upward trend (11). The national studies regarding the frequency of dementia in Turkey are limited.

They are conducted in cities with different geographical regions, using the hospital databases or community based input. It is estimated that there are between 600 thousand and 1 million dementia patients in Turkey at the moment and it is expected to be the country with the 4th highest number of Alzheimer's patients in the world in 2050 (12). The results of one of the two large scale community based studies reveal that the prevalence of dementia among individuals older than 70 years in Istanbul, the city with the biggest population, was 20% (13). The other study which was conducted in an Anatolian city demonstrated a prevalence of 8.4%, vascular and Alzheimer's dementia being the prevalent types (14). According to death and cause of death statistics, the number of elderly people who died from Alzheimer's disease increased from 12 thousand 59 in 2015 to 13 thousand 498 in 2019 (10). The risk factors for dementia reported by the studies in Turkey include older age, low level of education, female gender, living in a rural area, having a physical disorder, polypharmacy, comorbidities, and having a history of smoking and alcohol use (15).

Dementia is regarded as a progressive life limiting disease with a terminal nature. The diagnosis of dementia is frequently late in Turkey as the early symptoms of dementia are usually mistaken for signs of aging. The exposure to health professionals are usually at the end of the first stage or at the beginning of the middle stage. In the early stages of dementia, spiritual and social symptoms are very common associated with dementia stigma, uncertainty about the future and declining functional capacity (16). The management focuses on slowing the symptom onset, helping the patient to remain active and independent and planning the future care options. In the advanced stages, care shifts to the control of behavioral and psychological symptoms of dementia and maximizing quality of life. Recognizing the eventual terminal characteristic of dementia is the basis for anticipating future problems and an impetus for the provision of adequate palliative care (4). The unmet palliative care needs like communication, eating difficulties, dyspnea, pain, complex psychosocial and spiritual problems or talking about advance care planning may require specialist palliative care interventions. A person-centered approach that addresses the physical, psychological, spiritual and cultural needs is fundamental to the provision of palliative care. In dementia patients, advanced care planning should start as soon as the diagnosis is made, when the patient can still be actively involved and patient preferences, values, needs and beliefs can be elicited. As a result of late diagnosis in Turkish population and referral after the onset of cognitive decline and behavioral symptoms, it is not always possible to communicate adequately with the patient. The families with the traditional cultural structure also want to withhold the distressing diagnosis from the patient. Decisions and care plans are often made with the family or caregiver on the behalf of the dementia patient.

In the early and middle stages of dementia, 80-90% of the elderly are cared for at home by adult children or spouses. Women and daughters are usually regarded as natural caregivers and take the responsibilities in the care of family members with dementia. The studies have demonstrated that 80% of the caregivers are women in Turkey (17). They are also supposed to care for their children and daily housework. Although there is a tendency for older individuals to traditionally live with their families and children in the country, the recent change from extended family structure to the nuclear family has increased the number of elderly requiring institutional care. Family elders who cannot find a place in the nuclear family are exposed to living alone. In Turkey, 1 million 561 thousand 398 elderly people live alone, 74.9% of these households are elderly women and 25.1% are elderly men. According to Turkish Statistical Institute data, 83.1% of individuals think that children should look after their parents at an advanced age. When it is examined how elderly individuals (65 years and over) prefer to live when they are too old to take care of themselves; 46.0% of them want to stay with their children, 31.6% of them want to receive home care services and 10.3% of them want to go to a nursing home (10). Although nuclear families are increasing in number, the strong familial bonds in the Turkish society still maintain their importance and care giving to the elderly at home continues to be accepted as normal.

Caring for a close relative with dementia entails various psychological and physical restraints for the family carers (18). The quality of life significantly deteriorates with increased care giving burden. The caregivers may experience stress, anxiety, depression, social isolation or socio-economic problems during the course of the illness. In a recent study, polypharmacy, cognitive function, age of the caregiver and having limited space at home were found to be as predictors of caregiver burden in Turkish population (19). Among caregiver characteristics advanced age, female gender, lower education, being spouse, being married, having a chronic disease, living with the patients and having a limited space were associated with burden and quality of life in caregivers. In another study examining Turkish family decision making process for placing a loved one with dementia in long-term care, it was found that they experience difficulty and mention despair, ambivalent emotions, social pressures, and anxieties. Some of them stated that making a decision of institutionalizing their loved ones with dementia resulted in a stigma in the society and they were interpreted as 'getting rid of' the patient (20).

The legislation and legal framework for elderly care are complex both in quality and quantity in Turkey. The regulations are designed for the elderly and disabled care, and not specified for the dementia population. Although the government released standards and certification system for the persons who will work in the area of elderly and disabled care, the standards do not adequately address the needs of demented patients. Services for dementia are also limited in the country. Long-term institutional care services are provided by the Ministry of Family and Social Policies, municipalities, public institutions, non-governmental organizations and private sector care organizations. The care services provided to the elderly by the General Directorate of Disabled and Elderly Services of the Ministry of Family and Social Policies are "Home Care Support Services, Nursing Homes, Rehabilitation Services and Day Care Services". Home care services are provided for free by the home healthcare units of the hospitals or local governments. Although according to Home Health Data, approximately 50% of the 65 years and older population served by a home care center in a city in Turkey were diagnosed with Alzheimer's disease and other types of dementia, the teams are not educated professionally for dementia or palliative care. In families where all individuals have to work or unable to take care of the patient, paid caregivers are hired to care for the dementia patient in his own environment. Family caregivers of the elderly with dementia are provided with monthly financial support called as home care payment after assessment of the disability rate of the elderly and income level of the family.

Barriers for Provision of Palliative Care for Quality Dementia Care

Dementia is a major health problem worldwide significantly impacting the quality of life of patients, family caregivers and health professionals. WHPCA and World Health Organization (WHO) have recognized advanced dementia as a life-limiting condition and a disease that requires palliative care at the end of life (21). Nevertheless, palliative care needs of patients with dementia are often unmet and underassessed in many parts of the world as well as in Turkey.

There are several barriers that have been suggested to be associated with the provision of timely and effective palliative care. Dementia diagnosis can be challenging in the early phases of the disease and first symptoms of dementia are usually attributed to aging in many different cultures. Besides, dementia is often not recognized as a terminal life limiting illness despite its progressive nature. Disease trajectories of dementia are different from cancer patients who may experience a substantial decline in function in the last months or weeks of life and disease progression is relatively well defined (22,23). It is difficult to predict the duration of disease and make a realistic prognostication in dementia. Uncertainty about the duration or its anticipated course impedes early integration of palliative care. Issues about the end of life care are usually not taken into consideration timely and addressed inadequately.

The symptom burden of people with dementia is similar to cancer patients, but the course of the disease is prolonged and severe disability may persist for years (23). The communication restrictions at the advanced stages of dementia make it difficult to reliably recognize distressing symptoms such as pain, and create additional barriers to effective provision of palliative care. The prevalence of pain has been reported to vary from 29% to 83% among residents in long term care facilities (24, 25). Another study indicated that more than 40% of patients in nursing homes endure persistent pain, 6.4% of which were untreated and 32% undertreated (26). In a sample of Norwegian nursing home residents with dementia, about one-third (36%) had clinically significant pain intensity at admission and half of them used medication to reduce pain, mostly paracetamol (27). Communicating with patients and families of people with dementia requires special skills and assessment tools. At the end of life, dementia patients may experience pain, fear, agitation and confusion that they cannot express. Diminished cognitive functions, being unable to communicate wishes and to make decisions for treatment options challenges both the health professionals and family carers at providing optimal care. The ambiguity about the treatment may lead to aggressive, burdensome and futile interventions with no favorable effect on prognosis and patient comfort. Most of the family members are unaware of patient-centered dementia care and there is a stigma about the misconceptions associated with palliative care. Uninformed family members and untrained healthcare staff are also defined as barriers for timely access to palliative care. Lack of sufficient time to care for the patient and insufficient staff sources in care facilities may also constitute limitations contributing to inadequate palliative care in dementia.

The complex legislations not specifically designed for dementia, lack of diversity of the accessible dementia care facilities, funding and financial problems both for the family and organizations, unawareness about the role of early palliative care integration to dementia care in the community and healthcare system can be counted among the other barriers for provision of palliative care for quality dementia care in Turkey.

Future perspectives

The prevalence of dementia is increasing in Turkey with aging of the population. Palliative care is recognized as a key component of care to improve quality of life of people living with dementia and their families. The person-centered care, communication and shared decision making, optimal treatment of symptoms and providing comfort are the important domains of palliative care. Although the significance of early integration of palliative care in oncology practice has been well established, high quality evidence for palliative care in dementia is not yet available (28, 29).

Dementia is regarded as a major health problem throughout the world, but the diagnosis is usually late in the disease course. While executing programs for raising awareness of dementia and sharing information at all levels of the society, research about early diagnosis, developing dementia specific assessment tools and treatment should be encouraged. The health care professionals must have the competency of basic skills of palliative care approach and adapt it to the needs of dementia population. Palliative care is best given with the collaboration of interdisciplinary teams to manage the total symptom burden optimally. When complex symptoms are experienced, the patients and the families must easily get access to specialized palliative care.

In Turkey, 'National Aging Action Plan' is under consideration for the aging population, but national policies developed for management and care of dementia patients are not prevalent. The legislations are generally for the elderly and disabled, not completely addressing the needs of people with dementia. The WHPCA requests ministers to ensure that national dementia strategies are developed which include explicit reference to palliative care. Palliative care must be included in all health and social care workforce-training curricula to ensure that all health professionals and carers in dementia are trained in palliative care. Appropriate pain medications including opioids should be made available and accessible to manage pain and suffering throughout the disease course. Allocation of funding for more new research in the relevant area, and development and provision of dementia services in diverse settings is essential. Increasing public awareness about dementia will reduce barriers against the diagnosis and treatment, also preventing stigmatism for dementia in the society. Financial and psychosocial support for the family caregivers in distress must be among the priorities of national dementia care strategies.

Conclusion

Dementia is a life-limiting syndrome with uncertainty in the course of the disease. Along with the aging population in the world, it seems that it will be one of the major public health concerns in the future. A comprehensive palliative care approach beginning from the time of diagnosis is the integral part of dementia care. There is a need for evidence based interventions to evaluate the effects of palliative care integration in dementia care and organization of care facilities sensitive to physical, psychological, spiritual and cultural perspectives.

References

1. Gale SA, Acar D, Daffner KR. Dementia. Am J Med. 2018; 131(10):1161-1169
2. Alzheimer’s Association Report 2020. Alzheimer's disease facts and figures. Alzheimer’s Dement. 2020; 16: 391-460
3. Alzheimer's Disease International. World Alzheimer Report 2022. Life after diagnosis: Navigating treatment, care and support. London, England. Available from https://www.alzint.org/resource/world-alzheimer-report-2022/
4. van der Steen JT, Radbruch L, Hertogh CM, et al. European Association for Palliative Care (EAPC). White paper defining optimal palliative care in older people with dementia: a Delphi study and recommendations from the European Association for Palliative Care. Palliat Med. 2014 Mar;28(3):197-209
5. Hui D, Mori M, Parsons HA, et al. The lack of standard definitions in the supportive and palliative oncology literature. J Pain Symptom Manage. 2012;43(3):582-92
6. Seaman JB, Lakin JR, Anderson E, et al. Interdisciplinary or Interprofessional: Why Terminology in Teamwork Matters to Hospice and Palliative Care. J Palliat Med. 2020;23(9):1157-1158
7. National Comprehensive Cancer Network Guidelines, Version 1, 2022; Palliative Care
8. Global Atlas of Palliative Care. London: Worldwide Hospice and Palliative Care Alliance; 2020

9. Alzheimer's Disease International. World Alzheimer Report 2015. The Global Impact of Dementia An analysis of prevalence, incidence, cost and trends. London, England. Availabe from https://www.alzint.org/u/WorldAlzheimerReport2015.pdf
10. TURKSTAT. Elderly with Statistics 2021. Retrieved from http//www.tuik.gov.tr.
11. Kurtkapan H. Türkiye'de Demografik Dönüşümün Sosyal Yansimalari VeYaşlılık (Social Reflections of Demographic Transformation and Aging in Turkey). Sosyal Güvence Dergisi (Journal of Social Insurance). 2019; 15: 27-46
12. GBD 2019 Dementia Forecasting Collaborators. Estimation of the global prevalence of dementia in 2019 and forecasted prevalence in 2050: an analysis for the Global Burden of Disease Study 2019. Lancet Public Health 2022; 7: e105–25
13. Gurvit H, Emre M, Tinaz S, et al. The prevalence of dementia in an urban Turkish population. Am J Alzheimers Dis Other Demen 2008; 23(1):67-76
14. Arslantaş D, Ozbabalik D, Metintaş S, et al. Prevalence of dementia and associated risk factors in Middle Anatolia, Turkey. J Clin Neurosci 2009; 16(11):1455-9
15. Lök N, Öncel S, Özer Z, Buldukoğlu K. Institutional Services for Dementia Care in Turkey. Current Approaches in Psychiatry 2017;9(4):464-473
16. Timmons S, Fox S, Drennan J, GuerinS, Kernohan WG. Palliative care for older people with dementia—we need a paradigm shift in our approach. Age and Ageing 2022;51:1-4.
17. Karlikaya G, Yukse G, Varlibas F, Tireli H. Caregiver burden in dementia: a study in the Turkish population. The Internet Journal of Neurology 2005; 4:2
18. Eisenmann Y, Golla H, Schmidt H, Voltz R, Perrar KM. Palliative Care in Advanced Dementia. Front Psychiatry 2020; 21;11:699
19. Tulek Z, Baykal D, Erturk S, Bilgic B, Hanagasi H, Gurvit IH. Caregiver Burden, Quality of Life and Related Factors in Family Caregivers of Dementia Patients in Turkey. Issues Ment Health Nurs 2020;41(8):741-749.
20. Kucukguclu O, Mert H, Soylemez BA. Turkish Family Decision Making Process for Placing a Loved One with Dementia in Long-Term Care. IJCS 2018; 11(3):1722
21. Connor S, Bermedo M. Global Atlas of Palliative Care at the End of Life. Lancaster, England: The Worldwide Hospice Pallaitve Care Alliance, 2014

22. Lunney JR, Lynn J, Foley DJ, Lipson S, Guralnik JM. Patterns of functional decline at the end of life. JAMA 200; 289(18):2387-92
23. Gill TM, Gahbauer EA, Han L, Allore HG. Trajectories of disability in the last year of life. N Engl J Med 2010; 362(13):1173-80
24. Weiner DK, Hanlon JT. Pain in nursing home residents: management strategies. Drugs Aging 2001;18(1):13-29
25. Tang MM, Wollsen MG, Aagaard L. Pain monitoring and medication assessment in elderly nursing home residents with dementia. J Res Pharm Pract 2016;5(2):126-131
26. Hunnicutt JN, Ulbricht CM, Tjia J, Lapane KL. Pain and pharmacologic pain management in long-stay nursing home residents. Pain 2017;158(6):1091-1099
27. Helvik AS, Bergh S, Šaltytė Benth J, Selbaek G, Husebo BS, Tevik K. Pain in nursing home residents with dementia and its association to quality of life. Aging Ment Health 2022; 26(9):1787-1797
28. Temel JS, Greer JA, Muzikansky A, et al. Early palliative care for patients with metastatic non-small-cell lung cancer. N Engl J Med 2010;363:733-42
29. Bakitas MA, Tosteson TD, Li Z, et al. Early versus delayed initiation of concurrent palliative oncology care: patient outcomes in the ENABLE III randomized controlled trial. J Clin Oncol 2015; 33(13);1438-45

15

UNMET NEEDS OF FAMILY CAREGIVERS OF PEOPLE LIVING WITH DEMENTIA: FROM CONCEPTUALIZATION TO INTERVENTION

PERLA WERNER, PH.D.[1],
AVIAD TUR-SINAI, PH.D.[2]
AND HANAN ABOJABEL, PH.D.[3]

Introduction

Dementia is a syndrome characterized by a progressive deterioration of cognitive functioning severe enough to limit a person's ability to perform daily activities independently. Although the reasons for dementia vary, 60-70% of cases are caused by Alzheimer's disease (AD). Recent epidemiological studies estimate that even taking into account new advances in the understanding of risk factors, the number of people living with AD worldwide will continue to increase considerably (Nichols et al. 2022). The greatest burden of this is endured by family members who are the main providers of physical, emotional, social, spiritual and financial care to people living with AD. Informal, unpaid caregivers are usually close family members or friends of the person with AD, who are assuming the main responsibility for the health and wellbeing of their relative (Kimura et al. 2019).

[1] Department of Community Mental Health, University of Haifa, Israel
[2] Department of Health Systems Management, The Max Stern Yezreel Valley College, Yezreel Valley, Israel & University of Rochester Medical Center, School of Nursing, NY, USA
[3] Department of Community Mental Health ,University of Haifa, Israel

Caregiving is a complex and highly demanding function, associated with some positive, but mainly negative consequences, such as objective and subjective burden, depression, low levels of life satisfaction and wellbeing, poor social functioning, and increased risk of morbidity (Tatangelo et al. 2018). The care provided by informal caregivers makes up 70% of the total cost of AD at the US national level (Alzheimer's Association 2022). Recognizing and responding to caregivers' care-related needs is therefore of utmost importance for the wellbeing of people living with dementia and of their informal caregivers, but also for clinicians, policy makers, and researchers. Consequently, in the last decade, we witnessed an increasing number of publications from western and non-western countries reporting about the unmet needs of family caregivers of people living with AD in the community (AboJabel and Werner 2018; Ashrafizade et al. 2021; Black et al. 2013; Campione and Zebrak 2020; Denham et al. 2020; Desin et al. 2016; Mansfield et al. 2022; Park et al. 2017; Sun et al. 2022; Zwingmann et al. 2019).

Despite the importance of these studies, the literature on caregivers' unmet needs is still in its developing stages. A better understanding of how AD caregivers' unmet needs are defined, measured, and managed can guide the development of interventions to respond appropriately to these needs. This chapter summarizes current knowledge on the conceptualization, operationalization, characteristics, and interventions associated with AD caregivers' unmet needs. It is not a systematic review of the literature but an overview aimed at advancing knowledge, future research, and clinical studies on the topic. We start with a brief summary of the conceptual definition of needs and unmet needs, then describe and critically discuss measurement issues. Next, we describe the main findings regarding the dimensions, prevalence, and correlates of unmet needs. After presenting various interventions to manage AD caregivers' unmet needs, we conclude by suggesting future research, practice, and policy steps.

1. Defining AD caregivers' unmet needs

The literature differentiates between various kinds of needs in healthcare by type, stakeholder, and whether or not they are met.

1.1 Healthcare needs

Using a sociological approach, Bradshaw (1972) discerned four types of healthcare needs: (a) *normative,* defined by experts as the minimum standards of care required to attain an acceptable health status; (b) *comparative,* based on the objective comparison of services provided to different groups; (c) *expressed,* reflecting the actual use of services, and (d) *felt or subjective* needs, referring to the services that individuals state they need, want, or desire.

1.2 Unmet healthcare needs

There is no consensus on the definition of unmet needs in the literature but the most widely accepted one denotes *unmet healthcare needs* as the perception of differences between resources, services, or interventions judged necessary to deal appropriately with health problems and the services being received in practice (Carr and Wolfe 1976). Allin and colleagues (2010) expanded this definition by specifying five types of unmet needs: (a) *unperceived*, which are not evident to individuals; (b) *perceived but not requested*, referred to as subjective or chosen unmet needs; (c) *perceived but not fulfilled* because of accessibility problems, referred to as subjective, not chosen unmet needs; (d) *perceived and accessed* by the individual but ultimately not received, referred to as subjective, clinician-validated; and € perceived and accessed but judged inappropriate. This classification combines for the first time the type of unmet need with its reason, which falls into three categories (Chen and Hou 2002; Sibley and Glazier 2009): *availability* of services (waiting time, not available when required, and not available in the area), *acceptability* (feeling it will be inadequate, deciding not to seek care, too busy to seek, not knowing where to go, disliking providers or being afraid of them, personal or family responsibilities, and language problems), and *accessibility* (cost and transportation).

Based on these definitions, Smith and Connolly (2019) have recently introduced the need to differentiate conceptually between needs and demands or requests for help. This is an important distinction because the healthcare system cannot attend to perceived needs that are not expressed and transformed into explicit demands. Smith and Connolly's innovative thinking provides a more dynamic view of the concept making it possible to examine the process or trajectory of how and why some healthcare needs are perceived but not expressed or transformed into help-seeking while others are not perceived at all.

1.3 AD caregivers' unmet needs

As in the case of unmet needs in general, there is no agreed definition of the unmet needs of informal caregivers of people living with AD. Studies on the topic usually infer the presence of unmet needs from subjective evaluations about an unfulfilled healthcare need that can affect the wellbeing and quality of life of caregivers, care receivers, or both (Bangerter et al. 2017; Bressan, Visintini, and Palese 2020). The lack of specificity and clarity in the definition of the concept is especially problematic when trying to compare studies. For example, a recent review examining tools to assess unmet caregiver needs (Kinchin et al. 2022) included instruments measuring close but different concepts such as "caregivers' activation" (Sadak, Korpak, and Borson 2015) or "caregiver burden" (Charlesworth, Tzimoula, and Newman 2007). To the best of our knowledge, only three studies have used a theoretical perspective for understanding AD caregivers' unmet needs: Black et al. (2013) and Werner and Tur-Sinai (2021) used Andersen's Behavioral Model of Health Services Use (Andersen and Davidson 2007) to assess correlates of unmet needs, and Park et al. (2017), using Pearlin's Stress Model (Pearlin et al. 1990), conceptualized unmet needs as a stressor factor of caregivers' burden.

2. Measuring AD caregivers' unmet needs

Five reviews examining instruments for assessing AD caregivers' unmet needs were published in the last few years. Two were systematic reviews (Novais et al. 2017; Kipfer et al. 2020), two were descriptive critical reviews (Bangerter et al. 2017; Mansfield et al. 2016), and one was a meta-review (Kinchin et al. 2022). Except Novais and colleagues (2017), all reviews included quantitative measures only. Because of differences in the conceptualization of unmet needs, the reviews varied in the number of instruments identified (39 quantitative measures in Novais et al. (2017), 26 in Bangerter et al. (2017), 4 in Mansfield et al. (2016), and 18 in Kipfer et al. (2020) despite covering similar periods. The main characteristics of the reviewed instruments are presented in Appendix 1.

The tools reviewed contained between two and 70 items aimed to assess caregivers' needs, either in addition to the assessment of care receivers' needs or focusing on caregivers only. The majority were developed for use in clinical settings and only four for research purposes. Psychometric characteristics (mainly internal consistency and content validity) were examined and found adequate for the majority of instruments. Finally, only a few studies examined construct validity by exploring how different items in the assessment instrument are tapping different dimensions of the concept. Finally, the majority of the studies relied on items created *ad hoc* and on dimensions derived descriptively.

3. Dimensions and prevalence of AD caregivers' unmet needs

Despite the lack of strong empirical evidence regarding the presence of underlying dimensions, and although the number of items assessed varied greatly, all quantitative studies included, as recently defined by Clemmensen and colleagues (2021), two types of unmet needs: those originating with the care receivers and those originating with the caregivers. The latter are further divided in the majority of the studies into *emotional, spiritual and social support needs* (including help with caregiving tasks, financial support, psychological support, spiritual support, support from social services) and *information and communication needs* (including access to personalized information about the disease in the present and in the future, information about available services, and information and knowledge about appropriate communication with professionals, family members, and the person living with dementia) (Bressan et al. 2020; Cova et al. 2018; Khanassov et al. 2021; Millenaar et al. 2017; Soong et al. 2020; Queluz et al. 2019). Other commonly mentioned types of unmet needs were those related to caregivers' personal health (Soong et al. 2020; Queluz et al. 2019) and housing (Queluz et al. 2019). Ducharme and colleagues (2014), in the only study examining the needs of partners of people with young onset dementia, found psycho-educational needs (e.g., receiving more information) as one of the most common unmet needs.

Few studies have examined the prevalence of AD caregivers' unmet needs. Those that did found that 76-97% of participants reported experiencing at least one unmet need. Emotional support and information needs were found consistently to be the dimensions with the highest percentage of participants expressing unmet needs (Black et al. 2013; Zwingmann et al. 2017; Mansfield et al. 2022).

4. Correlates

Studies on AD caregivers' unmet needs examined a large number of correlates. Although the studies were based on cross-sectional designs, we will divide the correlates into those that can be understood as antecedents and those that are consequences of unmet needs.

4.1 Antecedents of AD caregivers' unmet needs included care receiver characteristics (severity of the disease, difficulties in the performance of basic activities of daily living, and behavioral problems) (Campione and Zebrak 2020; Cova et al. 2018; Fjaer et al. 2017; Hwang 2018; Park et al. 2017; Zwingmann et al. 2017); caregiver characteristics (low educational level, low-income status, young age, and belonging to a minority group) (Campione and Zebrak 2020; Cova et al. 2018; Fjaer et al. 2017).

4.2 Consequences of AD caregivers' unmet needs included high levels of caregivers' burden and depression and low levels of caregiving satisfaction and quality of life (Black et al. 2013; Campione and Zebrak 2020; Cova et al. 2018; Hughes et al. 2014; Park et al. 2017).

5. Interventions

Advances in understanding AD caregivers' unmet needs in the last years have not been matched by the development of interventions designed to address these needs despite the consistent association of increasing numbers of unmet needs with negative caregiver outcomes, such as burden and stress, and despite evidence from interventions conducted with informal caregivers of people living with cancer of the importance of assessing and meeting unmet needs to reduce caregivers depression and stress (Carey et al. 2011; Heckel et al., 2018; Lambert and Girgis 2017). The few studies describing interventions to reduce AD caregivers' needs show that attending to the personalized needs of caregivers and providing person-centered coordinated care is a promising model for improving caregiving experiences (Bass et al. 2013; Klein et al., 2021; Teles et al. 2020; Zwingmann et al. 2019).

6. Conclusion and recommendations

This chapter provided an overview of the state of knowledge about the definition, assessment, and management of AD caregivers' unmet healthcare needs. As the number of people living with AD increases and informal caregivers continue to provide the bulk of care in the community (WHO 2022), understanding what family caregivers need to fulfill their role appropriately is essential for reducing the high burden and stress associated with caregiving and improving the quality of life and care of the person with dementia. A main objective of healthcare systems worldwide is to provide access to high-quality care for the entire population, including those caring for people living with dementia. Understanding unmet needs may provide valuable criteria for resource allocation decisions, identifying priorities and guiding the development of interventions. This is especially important at times of crisis, such as the COVID-19 pandemic, when resources are scarce and must be prioritized.

These goals can be achieved successfully only if there are clear definitions, valid measures, and effective interventions for assessing and managing unmet needs. The overview provided in this chapter demonstrates that despite the increase in public health attention to the topic of unmet needs in the last years, conceptual, methodological, and strategic limitations continue to obstruct the successful translation of this interest into productive research and intervention initiatives. Below are several research and practice recommendations:

Recommendations for research: Research in the area of AD caregivers' unmet needs must move from descriptive, cross-sectional studies to longitudinal designs, to better guide the development of evidence-based interventions. The validity and reliability of available measures must be compared, and the most rigorous, feasible, and shortest instrument selected. The development of programs aimed at meeting unmet needs must be based on theory to identify its elements, outcomes, and efficacy. Similarly to other types of intervention (Cao, Feng, and Luo 2022), we suggest considering the use of multi-component curricula, involving caregivers in the development phase, and exploring the increased use of technological advances, such as telehealth, as a means to respond to some of the needs. Some mixed method designs with both qualitative and quantitative measurement is probably the best way to assess the needs.

Recommendations for practice: We suggest that healthcare professionals meet family caregivers of people with AD to conduct short systematic assessments of their unmet needs. This can guide and improve treatment recommendations, providing clinical responses that address the unique individual needs of both caregiver and care receiver. Professionals should also be sensitive to discern the type of unmet need being expressed: is it one that can be fulfilled, for example, directing caregivers expressing information needs to sources of information). Or is it one that cannot be fulfilled, such as the need to find a treatment or a cure for their relatives' condition? Futile hope that the situation could be reversed may increase caregivers' stress, frustration, and grief.

In sum, increasing the conceptual, methodological, practical, and clinical clarity of AD caregivers' unmet needs is important for several reasons. First, it adheres to the relationship-centered approach, supporting a holistic care framework and acknowledging the views, preferences, and needs of the person with dementia and the caregiver (Mohr et al. 2021). Second, a clear assessment and understanding of caregivers' unmet needs may provide important information in times of scarcity, when it is necessary to make clinical and ethical priority decisions. A recent study examining the unmet needs of 76 caregivers of people with dementia during one of the lockdowns in Israel showed that about half the participants reported that they had forgone the services of a family or expert physician despite the need for such services both for themselves and for their relative with dementia (Werner, Tur-Sinai, and AboJabel 2021). We expect these efforts to result in an improvement in the quality of life and quality of care of people with dementia and their caregivers, and to reduce healthcare expenses at the individual, organizational, and national levels.

Appendix A – Main characteristics of most common unmet need instruments

Name	Target	Dimensions/sections (number of items)	Response type (scoring range)	Psychometric characteristic
CADI	PwD, CG	8 (30)	3-point scale (30-90)	Internal consistency Structural validity
CARENAP	PwD, CG	5	Dichotomy 3-point scale (18-54)	Inter-rater and internal reliability Content validity
CNA-D	PwD, CG	18 (18)	3-point scale (0-18)	Test-retest, inter-rater, and internal reliability Content validity
CNCD	CG	5 (26)	5-point scale recoded into 3-point scale (0-52)	Internal reliability Content validity, hypothesis testing
JHDCNA	PwD, CG	4 (12)	Dichotomy	Hypothesis testing
NAS	CG	3 (39)	3-point scale	-
PBH-LCI:D	CG	6 (32)	5-point scale (0 – 128)	Reliability and validity
RAM	CG	6 (16)	Varies	Internal reliability, hypothesis testing
QCNE	CG	4 (19)	Dichotomy	Internal reliability, structural validity
QNP	CG	14 (30)	Varies	Internal reliability
SIDECAR	CG	(70)	Dichotomy	Content validity
Tayside	PwD, CG	3 (31)	-	-
UNM	CG	7 (34)	Dichotomy	Internal reliability, hypothesis testing

References

Alzheimer's Disease and Dementia. "Alzheimer's Disease Facts and Figures," 2022. Accessed December 6, 2022. https://www.alz.org/error-pages/500?aspxerrorpath=/alzheimers-dementia/facts-figures.

AboJabel, Hanan, and Perla Werner. "Examining Israeli Arab dementia family caregivers' perceptions regarding services for persons with dementia" Poster presented at the International Conference of Health Policy. (2018) Tel Aviv, Israel.

Allin, Sara, Michel Grignon, and Julian Le Grand. "Subjective Unmet Need and Utilization of Health Care Services in Canada: What Are the Equity Implications?" *Social Science & Medicine* 70, no. 3 (2010): 465–72. https://doi.org/10.1016/j.socscimed.2009.10.027.

Andersen, Ronald M., and Pamela L. Davidson. "Improving access to care in America: Individual and contextual indicators." *Changing the US Health Care System: Key Issues in Health Services Policy and Management* (2007): 3-31.

Ashrafizadeh, Hadis, Mahin Gheibizadeh, Maryam Rassouli, Fatemeh Hajibabaee, and Shahnaz Rostami. "Explaining Caregivers' Perceptions of Palliative Care Unmet Needs in Iranian Alzheimer's Patients: A Qualitative Study." *Frontiers in Psychology* 12 (2021). https://doi.org/10.3389/fpsyg.2021.707913.

Bangerter, Lauren R., Joan M. Griffin, Steven H. Zarit, and Rachel Havyer. "Measuring the Needs of Family Caregivers of People with Dementia: An Assessment of Current Methodological Strategies and Key Recommendations." *Journal of Applied Gerontology* 38, no. 9 (2017): 1304–18. https://doi.org/10.1177/0733464817705959.

Bass, David M., Katherine S. Judge, A. Lynn Snow, Nancy L. Wilson, Robert Morgan, Wendy J. Looman, Catherine A. McCarthy, et al. "Caregiver Outcomes of Partners in Dementia Care: Effect of a Care Coordination Program for Veterans with Dementia and Their Family Members and Friends." *Journal of the American Geriatrics Society* 61, no. 8 (2013): 1377–86. https://doi.org/10.1111/jgs.12362.

Black, Betty S., Deirdre Johnston, Peter V. Rabins, Ann Morrison, Constantine Lyketsos, and Quincy M. Samus. "Unmet Needs of Community-Residing Persons with Dementia and Their Informal Caregivers: Findings from the Maximizing Independence at Home Study." *Journal of the American Geriatrics Society* 61, no. 12 (2013): 2087–95. https://doi.org/10.1111/jgs.12549.

Bradshaw, Jonathan. *"Taxonomy of Social Need". Problems and progress in medical care: essays on current research,* 7th series, (1972): 71-82. http://eprints.whiterose.ac.uk/118357/

Bressan, V., Chiara Visintini, and Alvisa Palese. "What Do Family Caregivers of People with Dementia Need? A Mixed-method Systematic Review." *Health & Social Care in the Community* 28, no. 6 (2020): 1942–60. https://doi.org/10.1111/hsc.13048.

Campione, Joanne R., and Katarzyna A. Zebrak. "Predictors of Unmet Need Among Informal Caregivers." *The Journals of Gerontology: Series B* 75, no. 10 (2020): 2181-92. https://doi.org/10.1093/geronb/gbz165

Cao, Yang, Yuxin Feng, and Yaling Luo. "Relationship between Unmet Needs for Assistance and Healthy Aging among Disabled Older Adults in China." *Frontiers in Public Health* 10 (2022). https://doi.org/10.3389/fpubh.2022.914313.

Carey, Mariko, Sylvie Lambert, Rochelle Smits, Chris Paul, Rob Sanson-Fisher, and Tara Clinton-McHarg. "The Unfulfilled Promise: A Systematic Review of Interventions to Reduce the Unmet Supportive Care Needs of Cancer Patients." *Supportive Care in Cancer* 20, no. 2 (2011): 207–19. https://doi.org/10.1007/s00520-011-1327-1.

Carr, Willine, and Samuel Wolfe. "Unmet Needs as Sociomedical Indicators." *International Journal of Health Services* 6, no. 3 (1976): 417–30. https://doi.org/10.2190/mcg0-uh8d-0ag8-vfnu.

Charlesworth, G. M., X. M. Tzimoula, and S. P. Newman. "Carers Assessment of Difficulties Index (CADI): Psychometric Properties for Use with Carers of People with Dementia." *Aging & Mental Health* 11, no. 2 (2007): 218–25. https://doi.org/10.1080/13607860600844523.

Chen, Jiajian, and Feng Hou. "Unmet needs for health care." *Health Reports* 13, no. 2 (2002): 23-34.

Cova, Ilaria, Nicole Travi, Laura Maggiore, Valentina Cucumo, Claudio Mariani, and Simone Pomati. "What Are the Caregivers' Needs on Dementia Care? An Integrated Qualitative and Quantitative Assessment." *Neurological Sciences* 39, no. 6 (2018): 1085–91. https://doi.org/10.1007/s10072-018-3332-3.

Denham, Alexandra M., Olivia Wynne, Amanda L. Baker, Neil J. Spratt, Alyna Turner, Parker Magin, Kerrin Palazzi, and Billie Bonevski. "An Online Survey of Informal Caregivers' Unmet Needs and Associated Factors." *PLOS ONE* 15, no. 12: e0243502 (2020). https://doi.org/10.1371/journal.pone.0243502.

Desin, P. J., Allison M. Caban-Holt, Erin Lynn Abner, Linda J. Van Eldik, and Frederick A. Schmitt. "Factors Associated with Unmet Needs among African-American Dementia Care Providers." *Journal of Gerontology & Geriatric Research* 05, no. 01 (2016). https://doi.org/10.4172/2167-7182.1000267.

Ducharme, Francine, Marie-Jeanne Kergoat, Renée Coulombe, Louise Lévesque, Pascal Antoine, and Florence Pasquier. "Unmet Support Needs of Early-Onset Dementia Family Caregivers: A Mixed-Design Study." *BMC Nursing* 13, no. 1 (2014). https://doi.org/10.1186/s12912-014-0049-3.

Fjær, Erlend L., Per Stornes, Liubov V. Borisova, Courtney L. McNamara, and Terje A. Eikemo. "Subjective Perceptions of Unmet Need for Health Care in Europe among Social Groups: Findings from the European Social Survey (2014) Special Module on the Social Determinants of Health." *European Journal of Public Health* 27, no. suppl_1 (2017): 82–89. https://doi.org/10.1093/eurpub/ckw219.

Heckel, Leila, Kate M. Fennell, John Reynolds, Anna Boltong, Mari Botti, Richard H. Osborne, Cathrine Mihalopoulos, et al. "Efficacy of a Telephone Outcall Program to Reduce Caregiver Burden among Caregivers of Cancer Patients [PROTECT]: A Randomised Controlled Trial." *BMC Cancer* 18, no. 1 (2018). https://doi.org/10.1186/s12885-017-3961-6.

Hughes, Travonia B., Betty S. Black, Marilyn Albert, Laura N. Gitlin, Deirdre M. Johnson, Constantine G. Lyketsos, and Quincy M. Samus. "Correlates of Objective and Subjective Measures of Caregiver Burden Among Dementia Caregivers: Influence of Unmet Patient and Caregiver Dementia-Related Care Needs." *International psychogeriatrics* 26, no. 11 (2014): 1875-83. https://doi.org/10.1017/S1041610214001240

Hwang, Jongnam. "Understanding Reasons for Unmet Health Care Needs in Korea: What Are Health Policy Implications?" *BMC Health Services Research* 18, no. 1 (2018). https://doi.org/10.1186/s12913-018-3369-2.

Khanassov, Vladimir, Laura Rojas-Rozo, Rosa Sourial, Xin Qiang Yang, and Isabelle Vedel. "Needs of Patients with Dementia and Their Caregivers in Primary Care: Lessons Learned from the Alzheimer Plan of Quebec." *BMC Family Practice* 22, no. 1 (2021). https://doi.org/10.1186/s12875-021-01528-3.

Kimura, Hiromi, Midori Nishio, Hiromko Kukihara, Kayoko Koga, and Yuriko Inoue. "The Role of Caregiver Burden in the Familial Functioning, Social Support, and Quality of Family Life of Family Caregivers of Elders with Dementia." *Journal of Rural Medicine* 14, no. 2 (2019): 156–64. https://doi.org/10.2185/jrm.2999.

Kinchin, Irina, Layla Edwards, Emily Adrion, Yaohua Chen, Aya Ashour, Iracema Leroi, Anna Brugulat-Serrat, Jane Phillips, Fiona Masterson, and Slavica Kochovska. "Care Partner Needs of People with Neurodegenerative Disorders: What Are the Needs, and How Well Do the Current Assessment Tools Capture These Needs? A Systematic Meta-review." *International Journal of Geriatric Psychiatry* 37, no. 7 (2022). https://doi.org/10.1002/gps.5764.

Kipfer, Stephanie, and Sandrine Pihet. "Reliability, Validity and Relevance of Needs Assessment Instruments for Informal Dementia Caregivers: A Psychometric Systematic Review." *JBI Evidence Synthesis* 18, no. 4 (2020): 704. https://doi.org/10.11124/JBISRIR-2017-003976.

Klein, Olga A., Melanie Boekholt, Dilshad Afrin, Christina Dornquast, Adina Dreier-Wolfgramm, Armin Keller, Bernhard Michalowsky, et al. "Effectiveness of a Digitally Supported Care Management Programme to Reduce Unmet Needs of Family Caregivers of People with Dementia: Study Protocol for a Cluster Randomised Controlled Trial (GAIN)." *Trials* 22, no. 1 (2021). https://doi.org/10.1186/s13063-021-05290-w.

Lambert, Sylvie D, and Afaf Girgis. "Unmet Supportive Care Needs among Informal Caregivers of Patients with Cancer: Opportunities and Challenges in Informing the Development of Interventions." *Asia-Pacific Journal of Oncology Nursing* 4, no. 2 (2017): 136–39. https://doi.org/10.4103/2347-5625.204485.

Mansfield, Elise, Allison W Boyes, Jamie Bryant, and Rob Sanson-Fisher. "Quantifying the Unmet Needs of Caregivers of People with Dementia: A Critical Review of the Quality of Measures." *International Journal of Geriatric Psychiatry* 32, no. 3 (2016): 274–87. https://doi.org/10.1002/gps.4642.

Mansfield, Elise, Emilie C. Cameron, Allison W. Boyes, Mariko L. Carey, Balakrishnan Nair, Alix E. Hall, and Rob W. Sanson-Fisher. "Prevalence and Type of Unmet Needs Experienced by Carers of People Living with Dementia." *Aging & Mental Health* (2022). https://doi.org/10.1080/13607863.2022.2053833.

Millenaar, Joany K., Christian Bakker, Deliane van Vliet, Raymond T.C.M. Koopmans, Alexander Kurz, Frans R.J. Verhey, and Marjolein E. de Vugt. "Exploring Perspectives of Young Onset Dementia Caregivers with High versus Low Unmet Needs." *International Journal of Geriatric Psychiatry* 33, no. 2 (2017): 340–47. https://doi.org/10.1002/gps.4749.

Mohr, Wiebke, Anika Rädke, Adel Afi, David Edvardsson, Franka Mühlichen, Moritz Platen, Martina Roes, Bernhard Michalowsky, and Wolfgang Hoffmann. "Key Intervention Categories to Provide Person-Centered Dementia Care: A Systematic Review of Person-Centered

Interventions." *Journal of Alzheimer's Disease* 84, no. 1 (2021): 343–66. https://doi.org/10.3233/jad-210647.

Nichols, Emma, Jaimie D Steinmetz, Stein Emil Vollset, Kai Fukutaki, Julian Chalek, Foad Abd-Allah, Amir Abdoli, et al. "Estimation of the Global Prevalence of Dementia in 2019 and Forecasted Prevalence in 2050: An Analysis for the Global Burden of Disease Study 2019." *The Lancet Public Health* 7, no. 2 (2022): e105–25. https://doi.org/10.1016/s2468-2667(21)00249-8.

Novais, T., V. Dauphinot, P. Krolak-Salmon, and C. Mouchoux. "How to Explore the Needs of Informal Caregivers of Individuals with Cognitive Impairment in Alzheimer's Disease or Related Diseases? A Systematic Review of Quantitative and Qualitative Studies." *BMC Geriatrics* 17, no. 1 (2017). https://doi.org/10.1186/s12877-017-0481-9.

Park, Myonghwa, Sora Choi, Song Ja Lee, Seon Hwa Kim, Jinha Kim, Younghye Go, and Dong Young Lee. "The Roles of Unmet Needs and Formal Support in the Caregiving Satisfaction and Caregiving Burden of Family Caregivers for Persons with Dementia." *International Psychogeriatrics* 30, no. 4 (2017): 557–67. https://doi.org/10.1017/s104161021700196x.

Pearlin, Leonard I., Joseph T. Mullan, Shirley J. Semple, and Marilyn M. Skaff. "Caregiving and the Stress Process: An Overview of Concepts and Their Measures." *The Gerontologist* 30, no. 5 (1990): 583–94. https://doi.org/10.1093/geront/30.5.583.

Queluz, Francine N. F. R., Emily Kervin, Lori Wozney, Pamela Fancey, Patrick J. McGrath, and Janice Keefe. "Understanding the Needs of Caregivers of Persons with Dementia: A Scoping Review." *International Psychogeriatrics* 32, no. 1 (2019): 35–52. https://doi.org/10.1017/s1041610219000243.

Sadak, Tatiana, Anna Korpak, and Soo Borson. "Measuring Caregiver Activation for Health Care: Validation of PBH-LCI:D." *Geriatric Nursing* 36, no. 4 (2015): 284–92. https://doi.org/10.1016/j.gerinurse.2015.03.003.

Sibley, Lyn, and Richard Glazier. "Reasons for Self-Reported Unmet Healthcare Needs in Canada: A Population-Based Provincial Comparison." *Healthcare Policy* 5, no. 1 (2009): 87–101. https://doi.org/10.12927/hcpol.2009.20934.

Soong, Aijia, Shu Ting Au, Bhone Myint Kyaw, Yin Leng Theng, and Lorainne Tudor Car. "Information Needs and Information Seeking Behaviour of People with Dementia and Their Non-Professional Caregivers: A Scoping Review." *BMC Geriatrics* 20, no. 1 (2020). https://doi.org/10.1186/s12877-020-1454-y.

Smith, Samantha, and Sheelah Connolly. "Re-Thinking Unmet Need for Health Care: Introducing a Dynamic Perspective." *Health Economics, Policy and Law* 15, no. 4 (2019): 440–57. https://doi.org/10.1017/s1744133119000161.

Sun, Tongda, Rangcheng Jia, Jodie-Ann Clarke, Mingze Zhu, Debra Dobbs, Yuntong Di, Xiaoxin Dong, and Hongdao Meng. "Perceived and Unmet Needs for Health and Social Services among Families Coping with Dementia in China: A Descriptive Study." *Dementia* 21, no. 5 (2022): 1699–13. https://doi.org/10.1177/14713012221094979.

Tatangelo, Gemma, Marita McCabe, Ashley Macleod, and Emily You. "'I Just Don't Focus on My Needs.' The Unmet Health Needs of Partner and Offspring Caregivers of People with Dementia: A Qualitative Study." *International Journal of Nursing Studies* 77 (2018): 8–14. https://doi.org/10.1016/j.ijnurstu.2017.09.011.

Teles, Soraia, Constança Paúl, Milaydis Sosa Napolskij, and Ana Ferreira. "Dementia Caregivers Training Needs and Preferences for Online Interventions: A Mixed-methods Study." *Journal of Clinical Nursing* 31, no. 13–14 (2020): 2036–54. https://doi.org/10.1111/jocn.15445.

Werner, Perla, and Aviad Tur-Sinai. "Prevalence and Correlates of Forgone Care among Adult Israeli Jews: A Survey Conducted during the COVID-19 Outbreak." *PLOS ONE* 16, no. 11 (2021): e0260399. https://doi.org/10.1371/journal.pone.0260399.

Werner, Perla, Aviad Tur-Sinai, and Hanan AboJabel. "Examining Dementia Family Caregivers' Forgone Care for General Practitioners and Medical Specialists during a COVID-19 Lockdown." *International Journal of Environmental Research and Public Health* 18, no. 7 (2021): 3688. https://doi.org/10.3390/ijerph18073688.

World Health Origination (WHO). "Dementia." 2022. Accessed October 30, 2022. https://www.who.int/news-room/fact-sheets/detail/dementia,

Zwingmann, Ina, W. Hoffmann, B. Michalowsky, A. Dreier-Wolfgramm, J. Hertel, D. Wucherer, T. Eichler, et al. "Supporting Family Dementia Caregivers: Testing the Efficacy of Dementia Care Management on Multifaceted Caregivers' Burden." *Aging & Mental Health* 22, no. 7 (2017): 889–96. https://doi.org/10.1080/13607863.2017.1399341.

Zwingmann, Ina, Bernhard Michalowsky, Alexander Esser, Anika Kaczynski, Jessica Monsees, Armin Keller, Johannes Hertel, et al. "Identifying Unmet Needs of Family Dementia Caregivers: Results of the Baseline Assessment of a Cluster-Randomized Controlled Intervention Trial." *Journal of Alzheimer's Disease* 67, no. 2 (2019): 527–39. https://doi.org/10.3233/jad-180244.

II

Palliative Care for the Patient with Dementia

16

PALLIATIVE CARE FOR PATIENTS WITH ADVANCED DEMENTIA: INSIGHT FROM AN AFRICAN EXPERIENCE

JOHN WERU[1]

Abstract

Dementia is becoming a common disease in the aging population in Africa and is a major burden for patients and families. Due to its multiple symptoms and incurability, palliative care is a significant service that can lead to good quality of life while reducing care givers burden and burnout. However, there is paucity of skilled manpower in this field in the African context.

Further, there are multiple challenges to the provision of palliative care for patients with dementia which includes but not limited to: health care system, beliefs, negative views and stigma towards patients with dementia, lack of clarity on goals of care, poor communication skills coupled with lack of timely patient and family education, lack of appreciation of the role of palliative care for patients with dementia.

This chapter will highlight the status of palliative care provision for patients with dementia in Africa. It will outline the challenges and the strategies that can be used to mitigate them.

Keywords: Palliative care, advanced dementia, Africa, end of life care

[1] Aga Khan University Hospital, Nairobi, Kenya

Introduction

Dementia is currently the seventh leading cause of death and one of the major causes of disability and dependency among older adults globally and in its final stages many symptoms occur that cause immense suffering not only to the patient but a lot of distress to family members. The hallmarks of dementia diagnoses include evidence of significant cognitive decline from a previous level of functioning in at least one cognitive domain such as learning and memory, language, executive functioning, complex attention, perceptual-motor capabilities, or social cognition.[1]

In tandem with the increasing aging population, the burden of dementia is rising on the African continent with prevalence varying from 2.3% to 20.0% and incidence rates as high as 13.3 per 1000 person-years with increasing mortality in parts of Africa.[2] As the burden of non–communicable diseases increase in Africa, there is significant economic burden due to dementia. Thus, dementia and related disorders are areas of increasing public health concern in African countries. To worsen matters, Africa has the fastest growing population in the world while at the same time, dementia is normally dismissed as a part of normal ageing. This means that many patients are suffering from dementia related complications and symptoms without ever them or the family knowing the diagnosis.[3]Sub-Saharan Africa will soon face an important challenge for the management of these patients.[4] However, there are challenges to the provision of palliative care to these patients.

Challenges

Belief systems and traditional medicine

In Africa, 80 per cent of the population still uses traditional remedies, fully or partially, rather than modern medicine for primary healthcare. This is even more in the context of dementia where it is believed that it is equal to schizophrenia, curse or a wrong committed to the ancestors by the sick person or the family. By the time the patient and family seek hospital care, the disease is usually advanced. According to World Health Organization (WHO), Traditional medicine is the sum total of the knowledge, skill, and practices based on the theories, beliefs, and experiences indigenous to different cultures, whether explicable or not, used in the maintenance of health as well as in the prevention, diagnosis, improvement, or treatment of physical and mental illness.[5] Peoples' reaction to illnesses is linked to their values which have social and cultural meanings. Lack of understanding of the traditional, cultural, and social norms of a people can be detrimental to provision of quality health care due to the limited acceptance and buy in by the community.[6]

Health care systems

Although the African Palliative Care Association recommends palliative care for all patients facing life limiting illnesses, palliative care for patients with dementia in Africa is limited generally because of limited and poor health infrastructure in the continent. The appreciation for the role of palliative care for patients with dementia is also limited.[7] On issues palliative care for patients and families facing dementia, there is minimal literature. The possible reasons for these findings are considered: differential survival rates, the hiding of cases by relatives because of stigma, reluctance to seek medical assistance as inappropriate, poor access to medical care, the feeling that the old person has come to the end of his useful life and defective case-finding techniques. Further, there is paucity of polices, guidelines and standardized tools.[8] With many competing lines of care and infrastructure in the background of meager resources, palliative care provision is not a priority.

Further, there is a general paucity of skilled palliative care practitioners in the African continent. Brooke et al. in 2018 while assessing palliative care in Kenya and Uganda, noted that despite efforts to improve palliative care education and training, there remain insufficient numbers of specialists which may be due to lack of funding for specialist palliative care training, low HCP-to-patient ratio, and organizational constraints related to insufficient numbers of qualified instructors in the field to mentor other physicians.[9] There is limited palliative care budgetary support in the public sector. Poudel et al. in a review article on access to palliative care in low income and high-income countries in 2019 concluded that palliative care service provision in LMICs is limited in the public sector because there is no allocation of public funds or institutional resources and no reimbursement for services rendered through health insurance programs.[10] My interpretation would be that palliative care services are resource intensive and there is priority in the public sector to direct resources to people who can be cured and thus continue being productive in the society.

Negative view and stigma

As mentioned before, there is a dissonance in the community between the presentation of people with dementia and supporting them not only in palliative care and end of life but also throughout the trajectory of the illness. Negative stereotyping by family members, carers and health care providers that people with dementia will disturb others, require extra aggressive care such as restraining is a significant ethical issue and a limitation to the provision of palliative care. The fact that dementia is equated to schizophrenia and major depressive disorders lead not only to the castigation of the patient and families but also their stigmatization. When a disease is as prevalent as dementia, yet still poorly understood, it's easy for false beliefs to spread. Left unchallenged, these beliefs perpetuate stigmatizing attitudes against people living with dementia, reducing their quality of life. These attitudes extend to the families and caregivers of people living with dementia, affecting them as well.[11] This is more so likely in communalistic societies such as the African context and worsened by the poor understanding of dementia and late diagnosis.

Therapeutic goals

As dementia is a long-term illness with no likelihood of cure, there is need for setting goals of care and therapies in the early stages of care. Early on, the goal may be to preserve functional status, and undertake activities of daily living. However, as the disease progresses, goals should shift to activities such as maintaining ability to live at home within the social circle, maintaining mobility if possible, reducing caregiver burden and working towards a comfortable, respectful, and dignified death. This therefore means that in dementia care, decisions need to be considered within the context of the stage of the disease, the patient's goals and preferences.[12] However, in a setting where the diagnosis is mostly unknown, there is associated stigmatization and discrimination against people with dementia, this is unlikely to happen. The patients thus die in indignity. It is even impossible to pick goals that are important to specific patients and families eg going back to upcountry where one was born.[13]This leads to eventual poor quality of care, lack of continuity of care and care plans and thus no goals of care for the given patients.

Findings indicate that, given the necessary resources, persons with Alzheimer's can live meaningful, purposeful lives and creatively manage to protect and preserve identity. In contrast to previous research, participants did not reveal a great deal of concern about potential loss of self.[14]

Clinicians might use these results to consider what their goals of care are, when and in what ways their goals are convergent or divergent with the goals of patients and families, whether or not aspects of divergence are problematic, and what they should discuss with patients and families in order to arrive at shared goals.[15]

Communication

As dementia is a progressive illness, it is important to hold frequent clinician-patient and family conversations about end-of-life goals and preferences early in the trajectory of the disease. This is because dementia will gradually affect the way a person communicates and their ability to present rational ideas and to reason clearly will change. However, this process rarely occurs in the context of dementia care in the African context due to the fact that end of life care is still associated largely with cancer and also due to the stigma associated with dementia. There is thus lack of clear goals of care and advance directives discussions. This is contrary to the generally recommended approach that patients and families need to be offered options and to be asked their opinions.[5]

Identification of Palliative Care (PC) needs

It is critical that those caring for patients with dementia have the right attitude, interest and are able- to recognize special needs on how to bring comfort and quality palliative care for patients and families facing dementia. These needs should be holistic- spiritual, social, physical, emotional and familial. For contextual palliative care needs to be identified, the support system should be intact both clinically and socially. However, in dementia this is not the case due to paucity of knowledge in regard to palliative care for this group and also due to the fact that it is nor accepted as a medical diagnosis in most settings.[5]

End of life care

The European Association for Palliative Care (EAPC) dementia white paper asserts that although the palliative approach may be applied from the time of diagnosis, it becomes increasingly important for people with more severe dementia, for those who are at the point when quality of life is a more relevant care goal than the length of life.[16] During the literature review for this chapter, I did not come across any African guidelines or policies geared towards or guiding palliative care for patients with dementia. At Aga Khan University Hospital, Nairobi, palliative care for patients with dementia is outlined in the palliative care referral criteria.[17]

Strategies

Polices, guidelines and respect for patients' wishes

Palliative care for dementia patients should be part and parcel of quality health care provision. These should include public as well as clinicians' education on the principles of palliative care for dementia. The diagnosis and risk factors for this disease also need to be well stipulated so that the myth and beliefs are dealt with. The wishes and preferences of people with dementia should inform decisions on future care Professionals must explore and recognize the individual perspectives of people with dementia and family carers.[18] However, this is only possible if palliative care for patients with dementia is entrenched in polices, guidelines and protocols both nationally and institutional wise. These should encompass referral criteria, scope of symptom management, person-centered care, various levels of care and communication strategies.[19] A good example can be the EAPC Delphi study, based on both consensus and evidence that identified the avoidance of treatment that is inappropriate or futile in dementia care, and a new or renewed focus on comfort. It emphasizes on the need for a focus on comfort in order to professionalize the care with the right attitude, mix of medical and social care, skills and tools.[19] Beneficial effects can be expected if requirements of staff time, sensitive attitude and skills are met. This calls for management, local and national policy, academics and society to facilitate the basis for good terminal care for people with dementia.[19]

Clinical care system improvement

Part of a clinical continuum of care should be availing support of good practice and offer those with dementia the opportunity to live well until the end and give their families a more positive experience in the last days of their lives together as well as be part and parcel of the care provision process.[20] As suggested, there are important knowledge gaps that need urgent action, in order to prepare the continent for the anticipated local surge not only in dementia but also other neurodegenerative diseases.[21] An optimal approach should combine availability of medical care especially trained and dedicated nursing staff with compatible social and community environment.

For the clinal care aspect, the use of dementia assessment specific tools and protocols should be utilized so as to standardize care and ensure quality improvement as evaluations are done regularly. In regard to care funding, palliative care not only for patients with dementia should be funded by national budgets so as to ease the burden on families who have to pay out of pocket. The funding of specialist palliative care services should also be assured. Training of health care providers interested in the field of palliative care should also be considered.

End of life and place of death

This is a critical element of quality end of life care needed by patients and families facing dementia. Families should be able to express their preferred continuity in care and living arrangements as the patient approaches end of life. The complex support needs at end of life requires engagement of multidisciplinary teams. It is important that families are prepared early on regarding this scenario. The care team should at least comprise of a person well known to the family so as to avoid mistrust and ensure communication continues uninterrupted. Families need to know that it is important to consider the goals of care and weigh the benefits, risks, and side effects of any treatment. Family education thus suffices to make sure that they make a treatment decision based on the patient's comfort rather than trying to extend their life or maintain their abilities for longer. This is because Family carers are important for people with advanced dementia they also experience distress and are in need for support.[22]

Advance Care Planning and Advance Directives

Wishes and preferences of people with dementia and their family carers may differ. To ensure the wishes of people with dementia are respected, their views should be ascertained early in the disease before their ability to consider the future is compromised. Thus, advance care planning and advance directives documentation is a critical component of respect of persons with dementia. However, in a continent where advance directives uptake is very low, this might not be possible in most cases.[23] Due to this and also the fact that at the time of diagnosis most patients lack decisional capacity, proxy decision making is often necessary. Thus, discussion with family members should be an opportunity of establishing values and preferences in the best interest of the patient with the aim of comfort care and decrease of burdensome interventions. The support offered at this time must be in keeping with a person's wishes, their spiritual views, culture and life history.

Research and education

It cannot be overemphasized that quality palliative care will only be possible if contextualized approach is used. This will be possible if research studies are done within the setting of the African continent instead of copy and pasting the western models of care. However, it is unfortunate that most studies on dementia in Africa are epidemiological with few population-based studies to guide care itself. The onus is on the palliative care practitioners in Africa to be in the frontline in conducting scientific studies on the patients within their jurisdiction of practice.

Conclusion

In conclusion, due to the terminal nature of dementia and complex needs, people with dementia and their families can and should benefit from access to palliative care. This will address the priorities of families and patients for continuity of care, place of care, place of death and what entails comfort. This will also enable families deal with anticipatory grief and avoid pathological grief when their loved one dies. For this to be actualized, all stakeholders have a role to play starting from policy makers, institutional leaderships, health care providers, communities, and patients & families.

References

1 Osvaldo, N and Lori Anne, C. Palliative care for patients with advanced dementia. {Internet}. 2022. Accessed 20 Oct 2022. Available from: https://journals.lww.com/nursing/Fulltext/2022/03000/Palliative_care_for_patients_with_advanced.6.aspx

2 Akinyemi, r; et al. Dementia in Africa: Current evidence, knowledge gaps, and future directions. {Internet}. 2022. Accessed 20 Oct 2022. Available from: https://alz-journals.onlinelibrary.wiley.com/doi/10.1002/alz.12432#:~:text=Abstract,parts%20of%20rapidly%20transforming%20Africa.

3 George- Carey, R, et al. An estimate of the prevalence of dementia in Africa: A systematic analysis. {Internet}. Accessed 14 Feb 2023. Available from: https://www.ncbi.nlm.nih.gov/pmc/articles/PMC3529309/

4 Preux, M. Epidemiolocy of dementia in sub-Saharan Africa. {Internet}. 2015. Accessed 11 Feb 2023. Available from: https://pubmed.ncbi.nlm.nih.gov/29879338/

5 Che C and Andrae-Marobela K. Traditional Medicine. 2017. {Internet}. Accessed 22 Aug 22. Available from: https://www.sciencedirect.com/topics/agricultural-and-biological-sciences/traditional-medicine

6 Nchinda T. Traditional and Western Medicine in Africa: Collaboration or Confrontation? 1976. {Internet}. Accessed 22 Aug 22. Available from: https://journals.sagepub.com/doi/abs/10.1177/004947557600600315

7 African Palliative Care Association APCA Standards for Providing Quality Palliative Care Across Africa. {Internet}. 2010. Accessed 10 Jan 2023. Available from: https://www.thewhpca.org/images/resources/npsg/APCA_Standards_Africa.pdf

8 Ineichen, B. The epidemiology of dementia in Africa: a review. {Internet}. 2000. Accessed 12 Feb 2023. Available from: https://pubmed.ncbi.nlm.nih.gov/10795972/

9 Fraser B, et al. Palliative Care Development in Africa: Lessons From Uganda and Kenya. {Internet}. 2017. Accessed 24 Dec 2022}. Available from: https://ascopubs.org/doi/10.1200/JGO.2017.010090

10 Poudel A, et al. Access to palliative care: discrepancy among low-income and high-income countries. {Internet}. 2019. Accessed 23 Jan 2023. Available from: https://www.ncbi.nlm.nih.gov/pmc/articles/PMC6812938/

11 Rewerska-Juśko, M and Rejdak K. Social Stigma of People with Dementia. {Internet}. 2020. Accessed 13 Feb 2023. Available from: https://pubmed.ncbi.nlm.nih.gov/33185610/

12 Case et al. Older Adults' Recognition of Tradeoffs in Healthcare Decision Making. {Internet}. Accessed 28 Dec 2022. Available from: https://www.ncbi.nlm.nih.gov/pmc/articles/PMC4892363/

13 Jennings, L. Patient and Caregiver Goals for Dementia Care. {Internet}. 2018. Accessed 15 Jan 2023. Available from: https://www.ncbi.nlm.nih.gov/pmc/articles/PMC5382930/#:~:text=Some%20of%20the%20goals%20identified,and%20eventually%20dying%20with%20dignity.

14 Macrae H. Managing identity while living with Alzheimer's disease. {Internet}. 2010. Accessed 11 Jan 2023. Available from: https://pubmed.ncbi.nlm.nih.gov/19940091/
15 Bogardus, S, et al. A Taxonomy for Goal Setting in the Care of Persons with Dementia. {Internet}. Accessed 10 Jan 2023. Available from: https://www.ncbi.nlm.nih.gov/pmc/articles/PMC1500896/
16 Van der Steen- J, et al. Palliative care for people with dementia in the terminal phase: a mixed-methods qualitative study to inform service development. {Internet}. 2017. Accessed 30 Jan 2023. Available from: https://bmcpalliatcare.biomedcentral.com/articles/10.1186/s12904-017-0201-4
17 The Aga Khan University Hospital, Nairobi. Clinical services. {Internet}. 2022. Accessed 10Feb 2023. Available from: https://hospitals.aku.edu/nairobi/ServicesAndFacilities/Pages/PatientServiceCentres.aspx
18 Poole, M; et al. End-of-life care: A qualitative study comparing the views of people with dementia and family carers. {Internet}. 2017. Accessed 7 Feb 2023. Available from: https://pubmed.ncbi.nlm.nih.gov/29020864/
19 Brayne, C, et al. Dementia before death in ageing societies--the promise of prevention and the reality. {Internet}. 2006. Accessed 01 Feb 2023. Available from: https://pubmed.ncbi.nlm.nih.gov/17076551/
20 Fleming R, et al. 'I want to feel at home': establishing what aspects of environmental design are important to people with dementia nearing the end of life. {Internet}. 2015. Accessed 05 Feb 2023. Available from: https://pubmed.ncbi.nlm.nih.gov/25962895/
21 Lekoubou A; et al. Epidemiology of neurodegenerative diseases in sub-Saharan Africa: a systematic review. {Internet}. 2014. Accessed 14 Feb 2023. Available from: https://pubmed.ncbi.nlm.nih.gov/24969686/
22 Eisenmann, Y; et al. Palliative Care in Advanced Dementia. {Internet}. 2020. Accessed 12 Dec 2022. Available from: https://www.ncbi.nlm.nih.gov/pmc/articles/PMC7394698/
23 Omondi S, et al. Factors that influence advance directives completion amongst terminally ill patients at a tertiary hospital in Kenya. {Internet} 2017. Accessed 13 Dec 2022. Available from: https://www.ncbi.nlm.nih.gov/pmc/articles/PMC5264302/

17

PALLIATIVE CARE FOR PEOPLE WITH DEMENTIA IN THE MIDDLE EAST: CHALLENGES AND OPPORTUNITIES

MANAL ABDUL MAJEED HUSSAIN AL ZADJALI[1], ANNA E BROWN[1], HAMED AL SINAWI[2], SALIM KHAMIS ZAHRAN AL ISMAILI[1], AND NOORA ABDUL HAKEEM AL ZADJALI[1]

Abstract

Dementia is an incurable progressive illness, and some people can live with it for several years. People with dementia experience a wide range of multi-faceted and complex care needs and as caregivers play an important role in managing the progress of the disease, these needs can have a major impact on the quality of life of affected individuals and their caregivers. To address these needs a palliative care approach is advocated. Palliative care aims to improve the quality of life for patients and their caregivers through the early detection, assessment and treatment of pain and other problems by taking their physical, psychosocial, and spiritual needs into account. Palliative care has been shown to be most effective when considered early in the course of the illness; therefore, early diagnosis of the disease is essential for the provision of appropriate care.

Dementia is a significant problem in the Middle East. Reports from the World Health Organization (WHO) highlight a staggering increase in

[1] Higher Institute of Health Specialties
[2] Department of Behavioral Medicine, Sultan Qaboos University

people with dementia in this region. This increase calls for action to ensure the early diagnosis, care, and management of people with dementia and their caregivers. However, although studies have demonstrated that early access to palliative care may have positive benefits, access to palliative care in the Middle East is limited and varies greatly across these countries, where some countries have more developed services for the diagnosis and management of people with dementia, and some other countries have no known palliative care services. This chapter provides an insight into the challenges related to providing palliative care to patients with dementia in Middle East and highlights some opportunities to address these challenges in these countries.

Keywords: Dementia, palliative care, access to palliative care, challenges in palliative care, Middle East, caregiver burden, cultural beliefs.

Introduction

The world's older adult population (aged 65 and above) is experiencing a net increase of 1.2 million each month and is estimated to reach 976 million by the year 2050 with 72% living in developing countries. In the Arab countries, Middle East and North Africa (MENA) region, the older adult population makes 5.1% of the total population and is expected to reach 19% by the year 2050 (The World Bank 2022).[1] Ageing is one of the risk factors for dementia (World Health Organization 2022).[2]

Dementia is a syndrome that causes group of neurocognitive disorders characterized by deficits in multiple brain functions such as memory, thinking, orientation, comprehension, learning, language, and judgment. These impairments are associated with difficulties in emotional regulation, social behavior, or motivation (World Health Organization 2022).[2] These diseases undoubtedly have a significant negative impact on the lives of patients, families, and the whole society. According to the World Health Organization, there are around 50 million people worldwide living with dementia and almost 10 million new cases diagnosed annually. This number is projected to rise to 139 million by 2050. Dementia is a leading cause of disability and dependency and the 7th leading cause of death globally (World Health Organization 2022).[2]

The World Health Organization's Dementia report reveals a staggering increase in dementia across the Middle East and North Africa Region (MENA) region with its prevalence likely to increase by 125% in 2050. This increase calls for special attention from health and social care stakeholders to develop dedicated services for early diagnosis and management to improve the quality of lives of people with dementia and their caregivers (Zhou et al. 2021).[3]

Palliative Care and Dementia

Palliative care is defined as "an approach that improves the quality of life of patients (adults and children) and their families who are facing problems associated with life-threatening illness. It prevents and relieves suffering through the early identification, correct assessment and treatment of pain and other problems, whether physical, psychosocial or spiritual" (World Health Organization 2020).[4] In the Middle East, palliative care training started in 1992 in Saudi Arabia (Zeinah, Al-Kindi, and Hassan 2012).[5] Generally, there were sporadic efforts by all Middle Eastern countries to train healthcare professionals in palliative care. However, due to the political situation and lack of resources, many are making limited progress, if any, in palliative care in general (Zeinah, Al-Kindi, and Hassan 2012). [5] Middle East countries are reported to have a shortage of palliative care resources and local laws (Al-Zadjali and Silbermann 2015).[6] In most countries, palliative care services are not widely recognized as a separate specialty and when it is offered, it is typically dispersed and underfunded (Osman et al. 2017). [7]

People with Dementia often experience a gradual worsening of their symptoms that makes them unable to perform basic daily living activities and need help and support from a caregiver. The complexity of their needs requires palliative care similar to those with terminal illnesses; however, such needs are less likely to be recognized, let alone addressed by the health care providers. This progression is made worse by the fact that people with dementia are usually of old age and have other medical comorbidities that impact their functioning.

In addition, in providing care for patients with dementia, lack of skills in managing the problem often leads to mismanagement of it and further complications. For instance, toward the end stages of dementia, a person may experience pain but due to their inability to communicate, they might exhibit distress in the form of behavioral disturbance such as agitation, screaming or aggression (Schnelli et al. 2021).[8] Such behavioral disturbance may be under-detected or improperly managed with antipsychotic medications instead of pain medication which may not be available or limited to tertiary care centers in these countries. Therefore, healthcare professionals must be trained in palliative care to provide holistic culturally relevant palliative care for these patients.

Public Awareness of Dementia

It is stated that awareness of dementia is the ability to recognize deficit and cognitive impairments related to the nature of the disease and how this may affect the person (Dourado et al. 2016).[9] Dementia in the Middle East is often a hidden condition because there are few, if any, efforts done to raise public awareness about this disorder (de Cent 2015).[10] It is considered as a part of ageing process. Older adults often do not seek preventive care or seek care for memory issues (Javaid, Al-Zahmi, and Abbas 2021; Yaghmour, Bartlett, and Brannelly 2018). [11, 12] Moreover, Middle Easterners link several diseases such as dementia to fate, evil eye or even evil spirit (Yaghmour, Bartlett, and Brannelly 2018).[12] They use the word *Kharaf* to refer to Dementia. This word refers to someone who has lost their mind giving an undesirable implication to it (Cipriani and Borin 2014).[13] Thus, increasing public awareness and understanding dementia is significant.

Governments should increase the accessibility of public spaces by creating community places where older adult can meet and perform social activities (World Health Organization 2021).[14] These places can be used to raise awareness regarding dementia in the community encouraging older adult to seek medical advice whenever appropriate. Furthermore, a dementia action plan is highly recommended to help people to develop a positive attitude towards dementia in the community by sharing different experiences with other people with dementia and this can be achieved through training and education programs on dementia for the community support groups (World Health Organization 2021). [14]

In order to do so, the Middle Eastern governments must put efforts to empower healthcare professionals with knowledge and skills to raise awareness regarding dementia and the associated risk factors to encourage the public to visit their physicians about their mental health status (Lakey et al. 2012).[15] All healthcare professionals and social care staff should have access to dementia care training programs that are consistent with their responsibilities to improve awareness among people and their families and caregivers (Lakey et al. 2012).[15] This only can be achieved by providing a range of information services, resources and training for healthcare providers that are culturally relevant to the Middle East population.

Prevention of Dementia

Prevention is the key for protecting oneself from more serious complications (Dourado et al. 2014). [16] Livingston et al. (2020)[17] specified 12 modifiable risk factors, including excessive alcohol consumption, head injury, air pollution, low literacy, hypertension, hearing impairment, smoking, obesity, depression, physical inactivity, diabetes, and infrequent social contact, that can prevent or delay approximately 40% of worldwide dementias (Livingston et al. 2020; Winblad et al. 2016).[17, 18] These are thought to have higher impact on the prevention of dementia in low- and middle-income countries (Livingston et al. 2020; Thorsen, Dourado, and Johannessen 2020).[17, 19] As one can observe most of these risk factors are growing in most Middle Eastern countries due to modernization and globalization. Nevertheless, public awareness must be raised about dementia, emphasizing the importance of these factors as risk factors. It is through prevention, governments can significantly reduce the individual and socioeconomic burdens of dementia (Musyimi et al. 2021).[20]

Early Detection and Diagnosis of the Disease

Diagnosis is the first step to accessing dementia care and support (Dourado et al. 2014).[16] The early symptoms of dementia can include memory problems, difficulties in word finding and thinking processes, changes in personality or behavior, a lack of initiative and changes in day-to-day function at home (Alsebayel et al. 2022).[21] Therefore, early detection of dementia is critical for preventing its complications. It is the first step in designing management strategies (Alsebayel et al. 2022).[21] In addition, as the first sign of cognitive decline might or might not develop into dementia, it is important to train healthcare workers on diagnosis and early detection. Early detection and diagnosis helps people with dementia and their family to get help in understanding and adjusting to the diagnosis and to prepare for the future in an appropriate way. It allows the person to actively participate in planning care and choosing management strategies on their own. Furthermore, it will allow families the time to learn how to communicate with patients with dementia (Alsebayel et al. 2022).[21] However, as mentioned earlier, in Middle East, many think that dementia is part of ageing and there is no cure for it. Therefore, it is difficult to detect it in early stages (Alsebayel et al. 2022).[21]

Management of Dementia on the Middle East Countries

Dementia is a vast challenge to any community, both in terms of providing good care for people living with dementia and their family caregivers, as well as in looking for medical solution (Mukadam, Cooper, and Livingston 2010).[22] It is found that dementia is a significant health problem in the Middle Eastern countries. The sociocultural and political factors have shaped the concept of health in the Middle East (Lakey et al. 2012).[15] Therefore; these factors have a direct impact on care. The belief that dementia is part of the normal ageing process and like any other diseases is thought to be the act of "fate", lead them not to seek any medical care. If at all they seek help, they tend to use traditional and religious healers to treat dementia (Okasha and Boutros 2010; Al Abed, Davidson, and Hickman 2013).[23,24] This further complicates the problem and hinders them from seeking medical care that might often be more beneficial.

Similarly, due to the cultural and religious obligations, people with dementia are often taken care of at home until towards the end stages (Zaidi et al. 2018).[25] Their management of their care falls on the shoulders of family members, domestic workers, and hired individual e.g. a nurse (Javaid, Al-Zahmi, and Abbas 2021).[11] Often the caregivers at home have very little or lack of knowledge to deal with dementia (Balouch et al. 2020; Phung et al. 2017; Kane et al. 2021).[26,27,28] This further increases the burden on the caregivers who are already taking the burden of caring for a patient who is having behavioral disturbances and is gradually deteriorating towards dependence on the caregiver for their activities of daily living.

Further, most of the people in Middle East reside in rural areas where there is a challenge of telecommunications, availability of roads or access to professional care which might affect the access to care (Javaid, Al-Zahmi, and Abbas 2021).[11] This will hinder the availability of professional care for these people who are in need for management.

Palliative Care Status in Middle East Countries

Palliative care aims to alleviate suffering and to promote well-being and quality of life for patients with progressive, incurable disease or injury; this includes taking their physical, psychological, social, and spiritual needs into account (World Health Organization 2020).[4] Although studies have demonstrated that early access to palliative care may have positive benefits (Zeinah, Al-Kindi, and Hassan 2012; Love and Liversage 2013),[5, 29] access to palliative care in the Middle East is a major challenge (Fadhil, Lyons, and Payne 2017)[30] where it is estimated that only 5% of adults who need this care receive it (Worldwide Palliative Care Alliance 2014)[31].

Access to palliative care in the Middle East varies greatly for while some countries have more developed services than others, generally the level of palliative care is basic, and some countries have no known palliative care services (Fadhil, Lyons, and Payne 2017; Sánchez-Cárdenas et al. 2022).[30,32] Even countries where palliative care is well developed still face several challenges and barriers. These barriers include lack of national strategies to integrate palliative care into the health system, shortage of healthcare professionals to provide palliative care, insufficient palliative care education for health professionals and volunteers, low public awareness (Sánchez-Cárdenas et al. 2022)[32] and strict regulations that govern accessibility and use of essential analgesics, and limitations on who can prescribe opioids (Nasser et al. 2016).[33] Fadhil et al. (2017)[30] suggested that addressing these barriers will improve palliative care delivery (Fadhil, Lyons, and Payne 2017).[30] In addition, Sanchez-Cardenas et al. (2022)[32], emphasized that policy improvements present an opportunity to improve access to palliative care services in the Middle East.

Importance of Palliative Care in Dementia

With a growing world population, a longer life expectancy, and more deaths due to chronic diseases, the need for palliative care is increasing (Are, McIntyre, and Reddy 2017).[34] The main aim of this care is to improve the quality of life of the patients and reduce the sufferings of them and their families by identifying, assessing, and treating pain and other physical, psychosocial, and spiritual problems (Khan, Gomes, and Higginson 2013).[35]

Dementia is a progressive, life-altering, and incurable illness and some individuals can live with the disease for many years (Curnow et al. 2019).[36] Patients with dementia experience a wide range of intense physical, psychosocial, and spiritual care needs (Curnow et al. 2019),[36] and the psychological and economic strain on caregivers is substantial (Prince et al. 2015).[37] To address these needs a palliative care approach is recommended (van der Steen et al. 2013).[38] Access to quality palliative care helps minimize unnecessary suffering, improves the quality of life for people with dementia and is most effective when considered early in the course of the illness. However, although dementia is a significant problem in the Middle East and there is an urgent need to increase care and support for individuals living with dementia and their caregivers (Javaid, Al-Zahmi, and Abbas 2021),[11] access to dementia care is limited (Phung et al. 2017)[27] and people with dementia receive a diagnosis late in the course of the disease, if at all (Prince et al. 2015).[37] With an increase in life expectancy and an older population, dementia has become one of the most prevalent public health issues; therefore, palliative care is crucial in addressing the care needs of people with dementia (Are, McIntyre, and Reddy 2017).[34]

Challenges in palliative care related to dementia

Personal Challenges

Dementia is a progressive illness that grows worse over time, and the symptoms associated with dementia progress differently and affect each person in a different way. As the illness progresses, people with dementia often develop behavioral and psychological symptoms such as wandering, delusions, anxiety, depression, and aggression at some point (Huang et al. 2012).[39] These symptoms add challenges for caregivers to manage daily care activities and are associated with higher levels of caregiver burden, higher rates of morbidities, mortality, and hospitalization. The progression of the illness falls into stages depending on the severity of the illness (Hanson et al. 2016).[40] The severity of symptoms as the illness progresses, is one of the main factors contributing to caregiver burden (Chiao, Wu, and Hsiao 2015).[41]

Pain is the highest reported symptom among older people with dementia, with prevalence rates as high as 83% and it is often undertreated (Zwakhalen, van't Hof, and Hamers 2012).[42] The assessment of pain in older adults with dementia can be challenging as their ability to self-report pain becomes more difficult as the illness progresses. Therefore, the identification and management of pain in dementia patients is essential to maintaining function and quality of life (Zwakhalen, van't Hof, and Hamers 2012).[42]

Socio-cultural Challenges

Cultural and religious believes are major influencing factors to help seeking and caring for a person with dementia. In the Middle East region, the majority of people are Muslims and according to the Islamic perspective one is expected to take full care of his or her parent when they reach old age and ensure their dignity is maintained. This is reflected in the strong support systems provided by extended families that involves multiple generations of children and grandchildren (Hammad et al. 2022).[43] A high value and respect is placed for older people and the duty and responsibility of caring for older people are placed on the family members (Abyad 2015) [44] or domestic workers, and hired individuals (Javaid, Al-Zahmi, and Abbas 2021).[11] Despite recent move toward a nuclear family system in some Arabic communities, family members still live in proximity and are actively involved in supporting the person with dementia. Published studies from the region described the family in the Middle East as an "inherent hierarchical structure of authority and kinship relations within this traditional extended family structure" (Hammad et al. 2022)[43] where decision-making is made regarding care of a person with dementia is typically made by the eldest male member of the family (DeFrain et al. 2018).[45] Placement outside of the family home (e.g., in care facilities) is considered an abandonment of family duty which is unacceptable. Consequently, the region has few care facilities, access to dementia care is limited (Abyad 2015)[44] and the care provided to people with dementia depends on the family caregiver's own knowledge and skills (Al Abed, Davidson, and Hickman 2013).[24] Evidences suggest that older people with dementia had more care needs than those without and that caregivers for people with dementia had higher levels of burden compared to those caring for people without dementia (Phung et al. 2017).[27] Additionally, as the illness progresses, people with dementia often need special care; which can be difficult for caregivers and can affect their physical and mental health, family life, job, and finances (Javaid, Al-Zahmi, and Abbas 2021; Abyad 2015).[11,44] Other stressors may include role strains, family conflicts, pressure from the social environment (Sun 2013)[46], negative images and feelings and stigma (Low and Purwaningrum 2020).[47] Stigma and stereotyping can alter dementia care and treatment (Javaid, Al-Zahmi, and Abbas 2021),[11] including help seeking (Xiao, Habel, and De Bellis 2015)[48]. It is associated with increased caregiver burden (Kahn et al. 2016),[49] caregiving stress (Sun 2013)[46] and social isolation (Stokes, Combes, and Stokes 2012).[50]

Moreover, caregiver burden and burnout is term used to describe the physical, psychological, emotional, social and financial stressors associated with the caregiving role for a person with dementia. A study from Oman showed 70% of caregivers who participated in the study, demonstrated high degree of burden as quantified by Zait Burden Interview (ZBI). Factors such as patient's age, duration and severity of dementia, level of dependency and female gender of the caregiver were associated with higher burden (Al Maqbali and A-Sinawi 2016).[51]

A study by Granbo et al. (2019)[52] exploring the perspectives of dementia caregivers about the quality of care provided to their loved ones the care given was described as "passive care and a lack of individualization. Those with experiences with home care services reported a service characterized by unpredictability, with too many employees and unstable staff teams" (Granbo et al. 2019).[52] Caregivers reported that health care services did not meet their needs or the needs of the person with dementia, focusing more on the diagnostic aspect but failing to provide personalized care plans. Palliative care was not commonly offered (Granbo et al. 2019).[52] A Scopus review by Kane et al (2021)[28] about caregivers' perspectives in the MENA region demonstrated that despite the impact of the caregivers or so called "invisible second patients" role on the person's quality of life, there are not many studies that looks at the insight of the caregivers or the value of psychosocial and religious support in the Middle Eastern context (Kane et al. 2021).[28] Additionally, there are not enough support groups, and services for people with dementia and their caregivers in the Middle Eastern region. However, given the growth of the aging population in the Middle East with expected multiple chronic illnesses including dementia, the traditional system of care by the family will require much greater support (Javaid, Al-Zahmi, and Abbas 2021).[11] Therefore, there is a need for intermittent or continuous long term care services to become an important part of health care planning (Abyad 2015).[44] Moreover, there is a need for studies that explore and encourage in depth understanding of experience of the caregivers in this culture (Javaid, Al-Zahmi, and Abbas 2021; Yaghmour, Bartlett, and Brannelly 2018; Kane et al. 2021; Abyad 2015).[11,12, 28, 44]

Financial Challenges

As dementia is an irreversible and progressive illness, the symptoms might get worse over time and in different ways in different individuals. As the numbers of patients are growing in the Middle East, the disease will pose a financial challenge on the healthcare system in these countries. Qassem et al. (2022)[53] studied the cost per individual patient with dementia and the resources that are used for their care management considering the Gross Domestic Product per capita in year 2020 in Arab world. The total direct cost was approximately 16 462.5 million dollars and 15 463.8 million dollars for patients with dementia who are above 50 and those above 60, respectively. Also, when they calculated the indirect cost for caregiver support in the best and worst cases, they found that in patients who were above 50 years of age, the cost was 2 699.2 million dollars and 6 241.9 million dollars, respectively. In patients who were above 60 years of age, the indirect cost was 2 502.1 million dollars and 5 786.0 in best and worst-case scenarios, respectively (Qassem et al. 2022).[53] These numbers are alarming and are calling for attention of governments to allocate specific resources for this growing problem.

Furthermore, as it is clear due to the nature of dementia, one can imagine the burden that it can put on individuals and families. Taking care of a patient at home may require the caregiver to reduce their number of working hours or leave their job or allocate resources to hire a worker who can support in caring for the patient. Children often help in funding the care of their parents and they might not be able to fully fund care which may lead them to find alternative resources such as personal loans (Kane et al. 2021).[28] Many families might experience bankruptcy and they may decide to discontinue medical care due to the financial burden of the disease on the person and their family. Therefore, it is recommended that governments must provide financial support to extend homecare services and to support the construction of formal care facilities (Kane et al. 2021).[28]

Training and Education

Providing palliative care to individuals affected by dementia and their families is imperative in order to improve their quality of life. Therefore, healthcare professionals must be trained on providing palliative care to these individuals. Palliative care education is not fully included into medical and nursing school curricula; consequently, there are very few specialists in palliative care who are qualified to provide high-quality care (Kolmar et al. 2019).[54] This is creating one of the major challenges affecting early detection, symptom management and caring for the patients and their caregivers.

In addition, it is also important to educate the caregivers who are often forgotten from the situation despite their importance. Training caregivers can increase the chance of moving the patients to their own home reducing the economic burden that is placed on the healthcare system (Kane et al. 2021).[28] Religious scholars can work closely with the health care professionals to develop guidelines in dealing with difficult situations which would help the caregivers make the right decision. Besides, communities must be educated on dementia and accepting patients with dementia in community. This will improve the quality of life of the patient and their caregivers.

Policy and procedure (Administrative challenges)

Due to the often thought provider being the family, Middle Eastern governments seldom have policies or guidelines, if any, related to care provision and support provided for the patient with dementia and the caregivers. Therefore, when providing care for patients with dementia, healthcare workers face several challenges in finding policies and guidelines governing aspects of end of life such as resuscitation, insertion of a feeding tube or pain management. In these situations, a surrogate decision maker, who is often a family member i.e. the caregiver, is involved in the decision making. They might often be reluctant to make a decision due to fear of blame from other family members or feeling of guilt. Consequently, there is a need for policies facilitating formal care provision for patients and their caregivers in order to support them especially in critical circumstances (Kane et al. 2021).[28]

Opportunities Available

As mentioned earlier, dementia is a growing health problem in Middle East countries. Several opportunities for improving healthcare delivered to patients with dementia exist. These include opportunities related to the growing educated new generations and better opportunities for prevention, research, policies and care.

Growing Educated New Generations

Growing educated new generations are considered as an opportunity for prevention. Communication plays an important role in providing care to patients with dementia. However, due to illiteracy and language barrier, this can be affected. Patients, their families and the caregivers might not be able to find the right information if information are not presented in a way that is understandable by the patients and their caregivers. This might not be the case in the populations where literacy is growing and people are becoming more educated. Therefore, thinking about creating accessible awareness programs using technology such as the using social media in educating the caregivers regarding providing care. The systems should provide the caregivers learning and training opportunities as well as social support and the available resources (World Health Organization 2019).[55]

Communities must be educated in order for them to accept dementia as one of the chronic diseases so that patients with dementia and their families can live and express their fear and concerns without fear of stigma and rejection from others (Hamieh et al. 2019; Erskine 2018).[56,57] This is important as patients often seek medical advice when the symptoms are more advanced (Prince et al. 2011; Ghalib 2012).[58,59] Also, families suffer from lack of support. Therefore, as the generations become more educated, there is an opportunity for new Non-governmental organizations (NGOs) or support groups to evolve and support these families. Evidence based events or offering consultations to caregivers is much needed (Javaid, Al-Zahmi, and Abbas 2021).[11] These can be done through webinars or online meetings as done in some Middle East countries such as Lebanon (Hayek et al. 2020).[60] Simultaneously, in order to encourage the public to seek medical care for dementia, it is advised to change the terminology that is used to describe it, as mentioned earlier; therefore, it is recommend to use the term mild cognitive impairment for diagnoses other than Alzheimer's Disease, as it is considered more acceptable (Okasha and Boutros 2010).[23] In addition, the healthcare providers need to think about the support that needs to be provided to the career of these individuals including training as well as physical and emotional support.

Research

Although growing, research related to dementia and related aspects of care are still scarce in Middle Eastern countries. Despite the complications of the problem, there is often lack of information regarding prevalence of dementia. Very few publications exist that discusses the incidence and prevalence of dementia in Middle Eastern countries (Yaghmour, Bartlett, and Brannelly 2018; Al Sinawi 2018).[12,61] There is a need for studies that "determine epidemiological parameters of dementia" (Bhalla et al. 2018) [62] in the Middle East. There is a need to assess the trends and traits of dementia based on sociocultural factors.

Additionally, there are several areas of research in caring for patients with dementia including: assessment, diagnosis, management and the needs of caregivers. More research is needed to assess the modifiable risk factors that are associated with dementia (Alsebayel et al. 2022).[21] Further, despite the differences in culture, level of literacy or resources availability, the healthcare workers in low and middle income countries including Middle East countries use the same instruments as in Western countries, either in translated or adopted versions. These instruments might not be applicable for the Middle Eastern countries (Yaghmour, Bartlett, and Brannelly 2018; Al Sinawi 2018).[12,61] Despite the development of several new promising instruments that have good reliability and validity, their properties, applicability and discriminative accuracy need to be studied in Middle Eastern countries (Magklara, Stephan, and Robinson 2018; Ghalib 2012).[63,59]

An important area of research that might need to be thought about is studying the needs of caregivers in the Middle East. These might include assessing their training, emotional, physical, and other needs that are required for them to continue providing care for individuals with dementia (Hamieh et al. 2019).[56] This is especially important as there is a strong association between the caring for patients with dementia and chronic stress, physical illness, mental illness and poor quality of life (Erskine 2018).[57]

In addition, it is imperative that the Middle East countries work on promoting evidence based research on dementia (Yaghmour, Bartlett, and Brannelly 2018; Kane et al. 2021)[12,28] paying a special attention to designing culturally relevant frameworks for caring for patients with dementia in Middle East countries (Yaghmour, Bartlett, and Brannelly 2018; Halabi and Zafar 2010).[12,64]

Further, more studies are needed to understand the socio-cultural factors that form the attitudes and perceptions of the public to decrease dementia burden on the healthcare system and guide future interventions and policies (Hamieh et al. 2019).[56] There is a clear lack of information base related to dementia in the Middle Eastern countries that needs an immediate action for it to be revived.

Policies

Looking at the growing problem of Dementia in the Middle Eastern countries, it should be considered as a political priority. However, policies and guidelines regulating care for patients with dementia, the caregivers and the communities are scarce. There is a need for policies and guidelines that are based on the situation of the Middle Eastern communities, their values and lifestyle rather than applying policies based on the western culture. For instance, in the Middle Eastern countries, the often thought care provider for the patient is the family but there is seldom any policy that supports the patient and their caregivers (Ghalib 2012).[59] It is highly recommended that countries work on developing these policies especially in cases where the patient becomes dependent on the caregiver who is also a breadwinner of the family. The early introduction of palliative care would add a significant impact on the quality of life of people with dementia and their caregivers

(Granbo et al. 2019).[52] Hence, guidelines about providing palliative care and end-of-life care for people with dementia are highly needed.

Furthermore, with the availability of well documented evidences that supports the control of cardiovascular risk factors, healthy lifestyle and education as factors preventing or delaying the onset of dementia (Hamieh et al. 2019; Ghalib 2012),[56,59] countries need to create national programs to prevent dementia or improve care outcomes of patients with dementia and the economic burden on the individuals, the caregivers and the community (Hamieh et al. 2019).[56] In doing so, they might need to work together with NGOs in order to raise public awareness regarding dementia and find resources for patients and their caregivers (Ghalib 2012).[59]

Moreover, a special emphasis needs to be made on providing training opportunities for healthcare professionals and enhancing their competencies in assessing, diagnosing, and managing dementia. Governments must direct universities and colleges to add content related to these aspects of dementia care and palliative care into their health education programs. This will ensure the availability of experts in the field when needed.

Nursing Homes and Home Care Nursing

Due to the sociocultural, religious and economic factors, homes are the preferred setting for taking care of the patients with dementia (Yaghmour, Bartlett, and Brannelly 2018; Al Abed, Davidson, and Hickman 2013).[12,24] The stigmatization of moving an older adult from home to a nursing home or a long-term facility for the above mentioned reasons is high. It is considered negligence of the familial obligations (Yaghmour, Bartlett, and Brannelly 2018; Kane et al. 2021; Ghalib 2012).[12,28,59] However, due to changing of the socio-demographic factors such as longevity, globalization, working women, changing life circumstances and migrations, more communities are starting to think about moving care from homes to nursing homes (Kane et al. 2021).[28] Therefore, although few; however, these nursing homes or care facilities exist. They are often located in urban areas where due to the service demands and lack of space availability, they are considered expensive and are crowded and can lead to high infection rates, loss of privacy and patient dignity (Kane et al. 2021).[28] In communities where home care is provided to the population, it is wise to expand the service and create an interdisciplinary team, if it does not exist already, to visit the patient and the family on a regular basis, assess the patient's health status and provide care and caregiver training as needed.

Training is needed for healthcare workers who are providing home care for patients with dementia (Yaghmour, Bartlett, and Brannelly 2018; Hayek et al. 2020).[12,60] The colleges and universities are required to broaden their programs or have exchange and research programs to prepare a new generation of healthcare professionals for caring for patients with dementia (Erskine, 2018).[57] They need to prepare multidisciplinary teams that can provide comprehensive culturally related family centered care to the patients. Training them through providing palliative care programs with special emphasis on symptom management is imperative (Erskine, 2018).[57]

Conclusion

The Middle East is unique in its all values and beliefs. Dementia in Middle East countries is a growing health problem. However, when studying dementia, several risk factors can be prevented through community-based initiatives. Better outcomes can be achieved in managing care for patients with dementia through better understanding the culture, early diagnosis programs, providing culturally relevant care, obtaining support from the government, and providing holistic palliative care to the patient and their caregivers at the time of diagnosis.

Bibliography

Abyad, Abdulrazak. 2015. "Alzheimer's in the Middle East." *JSM Alzheimer's Disease and Related Dementia*, 2, 1012.

Al Abed, Naser A, Patricia M Davidson, and Louise D Hickman. 2013. "Healthcare Needs of Older Arab Migrants: A Systematic Review." *Journal of Clinical Nursing* 23 (13-14): 1770–84. https://doi.org/10.1111/jocn.12476.

Al Maqbali, M., and H. A-Sinawi. 2016. "Burden of Care among Relatives of People with Dementia Attending Tertiary Care in Oman." *European Psychiatry* 33 (S1): S184–84. https://doi.org/10.1016/j.eurpsy.2016.01.403.

Al Sinawi, Hamed. 2018. "Dementia in the Arab World." *Middle East Journal of Age and Ageing* 15 (2): 25–25. https://doi.org/10.5742/mejaa.2018.93440.

Alsebayel, Faisal M, Abdulaziz M Alangari, Fakhriya H Almubarak, and Rana Alhamwy. 2022. "Prevalence of Dementia and Its Associated Risk Factors among Geriatric Patients Visiting Primary Healthcare Centers in Riyadh, Saudi Arabia: A Cross-Sectional Study." *Cureus* 14 (4). https://doi.org/10.7759/cureus.24394.

Al-Zadjali, Manal and Michael, Silbermann. 2015. "The Fight against the 'Human Disaster' of Cancer in the Middle Eastern Countries." *Palliative Medicine and Hospice Care - Open Journal* 1 (1): 4–7. https://doi.org/10.17140/pmhcoj-1-102.

Are, Madhuri, Amanda McIntyre, and Suresh Reddy. 2017. "Global Disparities in Cancer Pain Management and Palliative Care." *Journal of Surgical Oncology* 115 (5): 637–41. https://doi.org/10.1002/jso.24585.

Balouch, Sara, Asghar Zaidi, Nicolas Farina, and Rosalind Willis. 2020. "Dementia Awareness, Beliefs and Barriers among Family Caregivers in Pakistan." *Dementia*, March, 147130122091506. https://doi.org/10.1177/1471301220915066.

Bhalla, Devender, Elham Lotfalinezhad, Fatemah Amini, Mohsen Salmannejad, Vahid Reza Borhani Nezhad, Seyedeh Fatemeh Rezai Kooshalshah, Ahmed Delbari, et al. 2018. "Incidence and Risk Profile of Dementia in the Regions of Middle East and North Africa." *Neuroepidemiology* 50 (3-4): 144–52. https://doi.org/10.1159/000487761.

Chiao, C.-Y., H.-S. Wu, and C.-Y. Hsiao. 2015. "Caregiver Burden for Informal Caregivers of Patients with Dementia: A Systematic Review." *International Nursing Review* 62 (3): 340–50. https://doi.org/10.1111/inr.12194.

Cipriani, Gabriele, and Gemma Borin. 2014. "Understanding Dementia in the Sociocultural Context: A Review." *International Journal of Social Psychiatry* 61 (2): 198–204. https://doi.org/10.1177/0020764014560357.

Curnow, Eleanor, Robert Rush, Donald Maciver, Sylwia Górska, and Kirsty Forsyth. 2019. "Exploring the Needs of People with Dementia Living at Home Reported by People with Dementia and Informal Caregivers: A Systematic Review and Meta-Analysis." *Aging & Mental Health* 25 (3): 1–11. https://doi.org/10.1080/13607863.2019.1695741.

de Cent, Nick. 2015. "Tackling Dementia Awareness in the Middle East Reuters Events Pharma." Www.reutersevents.com. February 23, 2015. https://www.reutersevents.com/pharma/digital/tackling-dementia-awareness-middle-east.

DeFrain, John, Sylvia Asay, Abdallah Badahdah, Azza Abdelmoneium, Ibn khaldun Center for Research & Studies, and Ahmed Abdennadher. 2019. *The Arab Family Strength in Qatar, Jordan, and Tunisia*. Edited by Doha International Family Institute (DIFI). Hamad bin Khalifa University Press (HBKU Press). https://doi.org/10.5339/difi_9789927137839.

Dourado, Marcia C., Maria F. de Sousa, Raquel L. Santos, José P. Simões

Neto, Marcela L. Nogueira, Tatiana T. Belfort, Bianca Torres, Rachel Dias, and Jerson Laks. 2016. "Quality of Life in Mild Dementia: Patterns of Change in Self and Caregiver Ratings over Time." *Revista Brasileira de Psiquiatria* 38 (4): 294–300. https://doi.org/10.1590/1516-4446-2014-1642.

Dourado, Marcia C.N., Daniel C. Mograbi, Raquel L. Santos, Maria Fernanda B. Sousa, Marcela L. Nogueira, Tatiana Belfort, Jesus Landeira-Fernandez, and Jerson Laks. 2014. "Awareness of Disease in Dementia: Factor Structure of the Assessment Scale of Psychosocial Impact of the Diagnosis of Dementia." *Journal of Alzheimer's Disease* 41 (3): 947–56. https://doi.org/10.3233/jad-140183.

Erskine, Wendy. 2018. "Caring for Those Who Care for Others : Finding a Unique Arab Vision to Lead Care for Family Carers of People with Dementia." *Middle East Journal of Psychiatry and Alzheimers* 9 (2): 36–39. https://doi.org/10.5742/mepa.2018.93591.

Fadhil, Ibtihal, Gemma Lyons, and Sheila Payne. 2017. "Barriers To, and Opportunities For, Palliative Care Development in the Eastern Mediterranean Region." *The Lancet Oncology* 18 (3): e176–84. https://doi.org/10.1016/s1470-2045(17)30101-8.

Ghalib, Saad. 2012. "Dementia in the Developing World: No Place for Complacency." *The Arab Journal of Psychiatry* 23 (1): 23–27.

Granbo, Randi, Elisabeth Boulton, Ingvild Saltvedt, Jorunn L. Helbostad, and Kristin Taraldsen. 2019. "My Husband Is Not Ill; He Has Memory Loss - Caregivers′ Perspectives on Health Care Services for Persons with Dementia." *BMC Geriatrics* 19 (1). https://doi.org/10.1186/s12877-019-1090-6.

Halabi, Abdul Kenj, and Javed Mumammad Zafar. 2010. "Care of the Elderly in United Arab Emirates." *International Journal of Geriatric Psychiatry* 25 (9): 925–27. https://doi.org/10.1002/gps.2600.

Hamieh, Nadine, Eman Sharara, Noura Salibi, Pamela Mrad, and Monique Chaaya. 2019. "Public Knowledge Of, Perceptions about and Attitudes towards Dementia: A Cross-Sectional Survey among Lebanese Primary Health Care Attenders." *Community Mental Health Journal*, July. https://doi.org/10.1007/s10597-019-00436-2.

Hammad, Suzanne H., Suhad Daher-Nashif, Tanya Kane, and Noor Al-Wattary. 2022. "Sociocultural Insights on Dementia Care-Giving in Arab and Muslim Communities: The Perspectives of Family Care-Givers." *Ageing and Society*, March, 1–28. https://doi.org/10.1017/s0144686x22000277.

Hanson, Elizabeth, Amanda Hellström, Åsa Sandvide, Graham A Jackson, Rhoda MacRae, Anna Waugh, Wilson Abreu, and Debbie Tolson. 2016.

"The Extended Palliative Phase of Dementia – an Integrative Literature Review." *Dementia* 18 (1): 108–34. https://doi.org/10.1177/1471301216659797.

Hayek, Samer El, Mohamad Ali Cheaito, Marwa Nofal, Doaa Abdelrahman, Ali Adra, Siham Al Shamli, Mansour AlHarthi, et al. 2020. "Geriatric Mental Health and COVID-19: An Eye-Opener to the Situation of the Arab Countries in the Middle East and North Africa Region." *The American Journal of Geriatric Psychiatry* 28 (10). https://doi.org/10.1016/j.jagp.2020.05.009. https://doi.org/10.1177/1049909112439619.

Huang, Si-Sheng, Meng-Chih Lee, Yi-Cheng Liao, Wen-Fu Wang, and Te-Jen Lai. 2012. "Caregiver Burden Associated with Behavioral and Psychological Symptoms of Dementia (BPSD) in Taiwanese Elderly." *Archives of Gerontology and Geriatrics* 55 (1): 55–59. https://doi.org/10.1016/j.archger.2011.04.009.

Javaid, Syed Fahad, Aishah Al-Zahmi, and Munir Abbas. 2021. "Carer Empowerment Is Key to Reduce Dementia Care Inequalities in the Middle East." *International Journal of Environmental Research and Public Health* 18 (8): 4378. https://doi.org/10.3390/ijerph18084378.

Kahn, Phoebe V., Heather A. Wishart, Jennifer S. Randolph, and Robert B. Santulli. 2016. "Caregiver Stigma and Burden in Memory Disorders: An Evaluation of the Effects of Caregiver Type and Gender." *Current Gerontology and Geriatrics Research* 2016: 1–5. https://doi.org/10.1155/2016/8316045.

Kane, Tanya, Suzanne H. Hammad, Nazmul Islam, Noor Al-Wattary, Justin Clark, and Suhad Daher-Nashif. 2021. "Dementia Caregiving in the Middle East and North Africa: A Scoping Review." *Transcultural Psychiatry* 58 (6): 844–58. https://doi.org/10.1177/13634615211036404.

Khan, Shaheen A., Barbara Gomes, and Irene J. Higginson. 2013. "End-of-Life Care—What Do Cancer Patients Want?" *Nature Reviews Clinical Oncology* 11 (2): 100–108. https://doi.org/10.1038/nrclinonc.2013.217.

Kolmar, Amanda, Megan Jordan, Yu-Lin Amy Lee, David Turner, and Arif Kamal. 2019. "416: A Systematic Review of Provider, Experiences with Palliative Care in Muslim Patient Populations" *Critical Care Medicine* 47 (January): 189. https://doi.org/10.1097/01.ccm.0000551169.37983.0d.

Lakey, Louise, Karishma Chandaria, Chris Quince, Martina Kane, and Tess Saunders. 2012. "Dementia 2012: A National Challenge." https://www.alzheimers.org.uk/sites/default/files/migrate/downloads/alzheimers_society_dementia_2012-_full_report.pdf.

Livingston, Gill, Jonathan Huntley, Andrew Sommerlad, David Ames, Clive Ballard, Sube Banerjee, Carol Brayne, et al. 2020. "Dementia Prevention, Intervention, and Care: 2020 Report of the Lancet Commission." *The Lancet* 396 (10248): 413–46.

Love, Anthony William, and Laura Maher Liversage. 2013. "Barriers to Accessing Palliative Care: A Review of the Literature." *Progress in Palliative Care* 22 (1): 9–19. https://doi.org/10.1179/1743291x13y.0000000055.

Low, Lee-Fay, and Farah Purwaningrum. 2020. "Negative Stereotypes, Fear and Social Distance: A Systematic Review of Depictions of Dementia in Popular Culture in the Context of Stigma." *BMC Geriatrics* 20 (1). https://doi.org/10.1186/s12877-020-01754-x.

Magklara, Eleni, Blossom C.M. Stephan, and Louise Robinson. 2018. "Current Approaches to Dementia Screening and Case Finding in Low- and Middle-Income Countries: Research Update and Recommendations." *International Journal of Geriatric Psychiatry* 34 (1): 3–7. https://doi.org/10.1002/gps.4969.

Mukadam, Naaheed, Claudia Cooper, and Gill Livingston. 2010. "A Systematic Review of Ethnicity and Pathways to Care in Dementia." *International Journal of Geriatric Psychiatry* 26 (1): 12–20. https://doi.org/10.1002/gps.2484.

Musyimi, Christine W, David M Ndetei, Sara Evans-Lacko, Déborah Oliveira, Elizabeth Mutunga, and Nicolas Farina. 2021. "Perceptions and Experiences of Dementia and Its Care in Rural Kenya." *Dementia* 20 (8).https://doi.org/10.1177/14713012211014800.

Nasser, Soumana C., Jeanette G. Nassif, and Aline Hanna Saad. 2016. "Physicians' Attitudes to Clinical Pain Management and Education: Survey from a Middle Eastern Country." *Pain Research and Management* 2016: 1–9. https://doi.org/10.1155/2016/1358593.

Okasha, Tarek, and Nash N. Boutros. 2010. "A Synopsis of Recent Influential Papers Published in Psychiatric Journals from the Arab World." *Asian Journal of Psychiatry* 3 (4): 244–48. https://doi.org/10.1016/j.ajp.2010.08.011.

Osman, Hibah, Alaa Rihan, Eduardo Garralda, John Rhee, Juan Pons, Liliana De Lima, Arafat Tfayli, and Carlos Centeno. 2017. "Atlas of Palliative Care in the Eastern Mediterranean Region." https://www.iccp-portal.org/system/files/resources/UN%20PALIATIVOS%20Atlas%20EMRO%20TABLET%20OK.pdf.

Phung, Kieu T.T., Monique Chaaya, Martin Prince, Samir Atweh, Khalil El Asmar, Georges Karam, Rose Mary Khoury, et al. 2017. "Dementia Prevalence, Care Arrangement, and Access to Care in Lebanon: A Pilot

Study." *Alzheimer's & Dementia* 13 (12): 1317–26. https://doi.org/10.1016/j.jalz.2017.04.007.

Prince, Martin, Anders Wimo, Maëlenn Guerchet, Gemma-Claire Miss, Ali, Yu-Tzu Wu, Matthew Prina, and Yee Kit. 2015. "World Alzheimer Report 2015, the Global Impact of Dementia: An Analysis of Prevalence, Incidence, Cost and Trends." https://www.alz.co.uk/research/WorldAlzheimerReport2015.pdf.

Prince, Martin, Renata Bryce, and Cleusa Ferri. 2011. "World Alzheimer Report 2011." London, UK: Alzheimer's Disease International (ADI). https://www.alzint.org/u/WorldAlzheimerReport2011.pdf.

Qassem, Tareq, Lynn Itani, Dania Al-Ayyat, Syed Fahad Javaid, and Hamed Al-Sinawi. 2022. "Prevalence and Economic Burden of Dementia in the Arab World," May. https://doi.org/10.21203/rs.3.rs-1658762/v1.

Sánchez-Cárdenas, Miguel Antonio, Nasim Pourghazian, Eduardo Garralda, Danny van Steijn, Slim Slama, Edgar Benítez, Marie-Charlotte Bouësseau, and Carlos Centeno. 2022. "Palliative Care in the Eastern Mediterranean: Comparative Analysis Using Specific Indicators." *BMC Palliative Care* 21 (1). https://doi.org/10.1186/s12904-022-01047-7.

Schnelli, Angela, Stefan Ott, Hanna Mayer, and Adelheid Zeller. 2021. "Factors Associated with Aggressive Behaviour in Persons with Cognitive Impairments Using Home Care Services: A Retrospective Cross-Sectional Study." *Nursing Open* 8 (3). https://doi.org/10.1002/nop2.751.

Steen, Jenny T van der, Lukas Radbruch, Cees MPM Hertogh, Marike E de Boer, Julian C Hughes, Philip Larkin, Anneke L Francke, et al. 2013. "White Paper Defining Optimal Palliative Care in Older People with Dementia: A Delphi Study and Recommendations from the European Association for Palliative Care." *Palliative Medicine* 28 (3): 197–209. https://doi.org/10.1177/0269216313493685.

Stokes, Laura A, Helen Combes, and Graham Stokes. 2012. "Understanding the Dementia Diagnosis: The Impact on the Caregiving Experience." *Dementia* 13 (1): 59–78. https://doi.org/10.1177/1471301212447157.

Sun, Fei. 2013. "Caregiving Stress and Coping: A Thematic Analysis of Chinese Family Caregivers of Persons with Dementia." *Dementia* 13 (6): 803–18. https://doi.org/10.1177/1471301213485593.

The World Bank. 2022. "Population Ages 65 and Above, Total - Middle East & North Africa Data." Data.worldbank.org. 2022. https://data.worldbank.org/indicator/SP.POP.65UP.TO?locations=ZQ.-ZQ.

Thorsen, Kirsten, Marcia C. N. Dourado, and Aud Johannessen. 2020. "Awareness of Dementia and Coping to Preserve Quality of Life: A Five-Year Longitudinal Narrative Study." *International Journal of Qualitative Studies on Health and Well-Being* 15 (1): 1798711. https://doi.org/10.1080/17482631.2020.1798711.

Winblad, Bengt, Philippe Amouyel, Sandrine Andrieu, Clive Ballard, Carol Brayne, Henry Brodaty, Angel Cedazo-Minguez, et al. 2016. "Defeating Alzheimer's Disease and Other Dementias: A Priority for European Science and Society." *The Lancet. Neurology* 15 (5): 455–532. https://doi.org/10.1016/S1474-4422(16)00062-4.

World Health Organization. 2020. "Palliative Care." World Health Organization. August 5, 2020. https://www.who.int/news-room/fact-sheets/detail/palliative-care.

World Health Organization. 2021. "Global Status Report on the Public Health Response to Dementia." *World Health Organization*. https://apps.who.int/iris/bitstream/handle/10665/344701/9789240033245-eng.pdf.

World Health Organization. 2022. "Dementia." World Health Organization: WHO. September 20, 2022. https://www.who.int/news-room/fact-sheets/detail/dementia.

World Health Organization. iSupport for dementia. Training and support manual for carers of people with dementia. Geneva: World Health Organization; 2019. Licence: CC BY-NC-SA 3.0 IGO.

Worldwide Palliative Care Alliance. 2014. "Global Atlas of Palliative Care 2nd Edition Global Atlas of Palliative Care at the End of Life Global Atlas of Palliative Care 2nd Edition." https://cdn.who.int/media/docs/default-source/integrated-health-services-(ihs)/csy/palliative-care/whpca_global_atlas_p5_digital_final.pdf?sfvrsn=1b54423a_3.

Xiao, Lily Dongxia, Lesley Habel, and Anita De Bellis. 2015. "Perceived Challenges in Dementia Care by Vietnamese Family Caregivers and Care Workers in South Australia." *Journal of Cross-Cultural Gerontology* 30 (3): 333–52. https://doi.org/10.1007/s10823-015-9264-y.

Yaghmour, Sara Mahmoud, Ruth Bartlett, and Tula Brannelly. 2018. "Dementia in Eastern Mediterranean Countries: A Systematic Review." *Dementia* 18 (7-8): 147130121775377. https://doi.org/10.1177/1471301217753776.

Zaidi, Asghar, Rosalind Willis, Nicolas Farina, Sara Balouch, Hussain Jafri, Irfan Ahmed, and Rubina Draft. 2018. "Understanding, Beliefs and Treatment of Dementia in Pakistan: Interim Findings." https://blog.ageinternational.org.uk/wp-content/uploads/2018/04/understanding_challenges_dementia_pakistan_interim_findings_report_2018.pdf.

Zeinah, Ghaith F. Abu, Sadeer G. Al-Kindi, and Azza Adel Hassan. 2012. "Middle East Experience in Palliative Care." *American Journal of Hospice and Palliative Medicine®* 30 (1): 94–99.

Zhou, Bin, Pablo Perel, George A. Mensah, and Majid Ezzati. 2021. "Global Epidemiology, Health Burden and Effective Interventions for Elevated Blood Pressure and Hypertension." *Nature Reviews Cardiology* 18 (18). https://doi.org/10.1038/s41569-021-00559-8.

Zwakhalen, Sandra MG, Charlotte E van't Hof, and Jan PH Hamers. 2012. "Systematic Pain Assessment Using an Observational Scale in Nursing Home Residents with Dementia: Exploring Feasibility and Applied Interventions." *Journal of Clinical Nursing* 21 (21-22): 3009–17. https://doi.org/10.1111/j.1365-2702.2012.04313.x

18

CURRENT INTEGRATION AND CHALLENGES OF PALLIATIVE CARE INTO DEMENTIA PRACTICE: EVIDENCE AND EXPERIENCE FROM ASIA, EUROPE, AND AFRICA

CHENG-PEI LIN[1], PING-JEN CHEN[2], EVE NAMISANGO[3], SEGGANE MUSISI[4], ALISON GAYTON[5], NIKOLAOS EFSTATHIOU[6] AND PING GUO[7]

---

[1] RN, MSc, PhD Assistant Professor, Institute of Community Health Care, College of Nursing, National Yang Ming Chiao Tung University, Taipei, Taiwan; Cicely Saunders Institute of Palliative Care, Policy and Rehabilitation, Florence Nightingale Faculty of Nursing, Midwifery, and Palliative Care, King's College London, United Kingdom

[2] MD, PhD, FRCP, Edin Department of Family Medicine and Division of Geriatrics and Gerontology, Kaohsiung Medical University Hospital and School of Medicine, Kaohsiung Medical University, Kaohsiung, Taiwan; Marie Curie Palliative Care Research Department, Division of Psychiatry, University College London, London, United Kingdom

[3] PhD, Programmes, Research and Development Manager, African Palliative Care Association, Dr Gibbons Road, Kampala, Uganda

[4] MD, FRCP(C), Department of Psychiatry, School of Medicine, Makerere University College of Health Sciences, Kampala, Uganda

[5] MSc, BSc, RN, FHEA, Lecturer in Mental Health Nursing, School of Nursing and Midwifery, Institute of Clinical Sciences, College of Medical and Dental Sciences, University of Birmingham, Birmingham, United Kingdom

[6] PhD, Associate Professor, School of Nursing and Midwifery, Institute of Clinical Sciences, College of Medical and Dental Sciences, University of Birmingham, Birmingham, United Kingdom; Adjunct Professor, School of Nursing, University of Ottawa, Canada

[7] PhD, Associate Professor, School of Nursing and Midwifery, Institute of Clinical Sciences, College of Medical and Dental Sciences, University of Birmingham, Birmingham, United Kingdom; Visiting Senior Lecturer, Cicely Saunders Institute of

Keywords: Dementia, needs, symptoms, palliative care, person-centred care, caregivers

Introduction

Based on the World Health Organization (WHO) estimation, the proportion of elderly population aged over 60 years old will double from 12% to 22% globally between 2015 to 2050. The number of people living with dementia is expected to reach 139 million in 2050 (Gauthier et al., 2022). The highest proportional increase is projected to occur among those with dementia who experience serious health-related suffering (i.e., 6 million people, 264% increase between 2016 and 2060) (Sleeman et al., 2019). Therefore, palliative and end of life care needs will increase for people with dementia to manage pain, agitation, pressure ulcers, and so on (Timmons et al., 2022). In addition, the majority of rapidly increased palliative care needs (>80%) concentrate in low- and middle-income countries (Sleeman et al., 2019, World Health Organization, 2022a). In this chapter, we provide a brief overview of current evidence on the integration of palliative care into dementia practice from Asia, Europe, and Africa, explore challenges and issues we have faced, and highlight major implications for future work.

Providing palliative care for people living with dementia in Asia

Although some programmes with essential components of palliative care for people living with dementia have been developed (Chen et al., 2018, Hum et al., 2020, Nakanishi et al., 2018), palliative care has not yet been systematically embedded into the healthcare system in many Asian countries because the care provision of palliative care and its associated policies still mainly focus on cancer patients (Yamaguchi et al., 2017). In a documentary analysis of national dementia plans, 33 countries across the globe addressed palliative care in national policies by 2019, of which only five were identified from Asia-Pacific regions including Australia, Japan, Korea, Taiwan, and Indonesia (Nakanishi and van der Steen, 2020).

Given the available literature, Taiwan is the first Asian country to adopt palliative care for people living with dementia in its single-payer national health insurance (NHI) scheme in 2009 (Chen et al., 2018). After the launch

Palliative Care, Policy and Rehabilitation, King's College London, London, United Kingdom of the NHI scheme in 1995, it has reimbursed nationwide palliative care including home-based services since 1996, inpatient services since 2000, and liaison services since 2004. In 2009, the eligible recipients for palliative care expanded to people with non-cancerous major diseases such as dementia, brain injury, and liver and renal failure. According to the Quality of Death Index (Finkelstein et al., 2022, The Economist Intelligence Unit, 2010, The Economist Intelligence Unit, 2015), Taiwan ranked first in Asia consecutively due to its good accessibility to palliative care and coverage of diverse populations.

During the first 5-year period of integrating palliative care into dementia practice in Taiwan, palliative care is rarely provided to national dementia cohort (1.64% in 239,633 people living with dementia) even though its association with reducing life-sustaining treatments (except for tube feeding and non-invasive ventilators) is evident (Chen et al., 2018). In 2016, the national clinical guideline for dementia palliative care was developed and published by the domestic scientific committee in order to improve the quality of care, facilitate advance care planning, and increase public awareness (Chen, 2016). In a subsequent mortality follow back survey, ratio of palliative care utilisation in people living with dementia increased year by year, ranging from 2.3% in 2007 to 16.1% in 2017 (Chen et al., 2022). The eligibility criteria for dementia palliative care in NHI-reimbursed services were modified based on the 2016 national guideline and started to adopt more needs-based triggers for service initiatives at the end of 2022.

Culture shapes dementia palliative care in different ways. In Asia, family caregivers' and healthcare professionals' perceptions on dementia disease trajectory and corresponding treatments differ from those in the Western culture (i.e., North America and Europe), leading to challenges on service provision. Four main challenges informed by the literature and our clinical experience are summarised below:

- **Not considering advanced dementia as a life-threatening and terminal illness**: Unlike cancer patients who might have clearer disease trajectory to inform their function decline for palliative care initiative, the function status of people living with dementia fluctuates lasting for many years in the disease trajectories (Murray et al., 2005). Dementia is therefore considered a chronic disease but not a life-threatening illness by clinicians and relatives, which results in a lower probability of withholding or withdrawing life-sustaining treatments, in particular artificial nutrition (i.e., tube feeding) (Chen et al., 2018). It is recognised that people living with dementia and cancer are more likely to receive palliative care and have less life-sustaining treatments than people living with dementia without cancer (Chen et al., 2017).

- **Life-sustaining treatment choices and utilisation (enteral feeding at the end of life stage):** Different from Western evidence reporting low proportion of dementia patients receiving tube feeding at their end of life stage, in Asia, more than half of the patients with dementia had ever been enterally fed (Clarfield et al., 2006, Kwok et al., 2007). This could be explained by the traditional custom that people believe artificial nutrition is essential to avoid patients to become "hungry ghosts" after death (Chen et al., 2018).
- **Unfamiliarity of mental capacity assessment and presence of surrogate decision-making**: Lack of culturally adapted measurement and unfamiliar knowledge and skills of mental capacity assessment for people living with dementia among healthcare professionals, result in misleading perceptions on patient inability to make all kind of decisions, regardless of their residual function and matters to be decided (Tilburgs et al., 2018). Furthermore, in Asia, family substitute decision-making for patients is prevalent, therefore, no opportunity is available for the patients themselves to be involved in palliative care discussions and voice their preferences (Kwok et al., 2007).
- **Unmet need for community and home-oriented palliative care**: In Asia, the majority of people living with dementia are cared for at home in the community due to social structure and resource allocations (Hum et al., 2018). Family caregivers play key roles in dementia care and share numerous care responsibilities. Therefore, primary palliative care is essential to provide community-based care with the support from specialist palliative care teams in hospitals.

The pressure on global budgets in each healthcare system drives the need to promote community-based models of dementia care, especially in countries where care homes or institutions are less available (World Health Organization, 2015). Establishing a continuum of integrated home-based care with sufficient medical and social care services could be the backbone to support people living with dementia and their families. While focusing on increasing input of specialist palliative care (Kupeli, 2020), we should also develop the generalist palliative care through the development and improvement of primary care system. Evidence demonstrates the potential benefits of the capacity, continuity, or home delivery of primary care services in terms of better end-of-life outcomes among people living with dementia (Chen et al., 2020, Leniz et al., 2022, Nakanishi et al., 2020). It is a value-based healthcare initiative to tailor appropriate home-based services throughout the disease trajectory and reform the strategies and payment system to facilitate the integration of a primary care continuum.

Advance care planning has been suggested to be embedded into dementia routine care, especially for the end-of-life care, in case the patients cannot speak for themselves in the future (Dening et al., 2019). We endorse the UK Mental Capacity Act 2005 (UK legislation, 2005), assuming that people living with dementia can perform the right of self-determination unless it is proved otherwise. Furthermore, people living with dementia should be given all practicable help and support to make their own decisions. By doing so, goal concordant palliative care provision could be facilitated for better end-of-life care outcomes for people with dementia and their families in Asia.

Current integration of palliative care into dementia practice in Europe

Europe's population is ageing. Age is one of the risk factors for developing dementia, and with life expectancy increasing, we expect to see an increase in the number of people with dementia in the future. The prevalence of dementia in Europe is estimated to be more than 10 million, with a projected increase to 14 million by 2050 (Alzheimer Europe, 2019, Mura et al., 2010). Dementia is a life-limiting condition necessitating palliative care interventions for patients and their families (Fox et al., 2017). Person-centred care, shared decision-making, symptom control and psychosocial/spiritual support, advance care planning, continuity of care, family care, and healthcare professional education are all important domains for optimal dementia palliative care, according to the European Association for Palliative Care (van der Steen et al., 2014).

Palliative care is not uniform across Europe due to differences in cultural contexts and policies. In some countries, for example, family members are mostly involved in caring for people with advanced dementia at home, with some palliative care support near the end of life, whereas hospitalisation near the end of life may be common in others. A large cohort study in Belgium discovered that palliative care at home for people with dementia can improve dying quality while also lowering end-of-life care costs (Miranda et al., 2021a). A systematic review found that home palliative care interventions like symptom management, continuity of care, and psychosocial support resulted in better end-of-life care for people with dementia, but the majority of the evidence was of poor quality (Miranda et al., 2019). Although hospitalisation for people with advanced dementia is not preferred, it is quite common, with some countries reporting that up to 20% of people with dementia spend the last month of their lives in hospital (Houttekier et al., 2014). A Swedish study discovered that, despite good symptom management and communication of care plans, death in a hospital was associated with poorer quality of end-of-life care for people with dementia (Martinsson et al., 2020).

People with dementia in Western European countries tend to spend the majority of their final years in long-term care facilities (Houttekier et al., 2014). Palliative care is not well established in most long-term care facilities, such as nursing homes. According to a study conducted in five European countries (Belgium, England, Italy, the Netherlands, and Poland), palliative care typically begins two weeks before death in long-term care facilities (ten Koppel et al., 2019). A research team from seven European countries that developed, implemented, and evaluated a multi-component palliative care intervention for long-term care facilities [PACE Steps to Success (Smets et al., 2018)] [8] concluded that the programme did not improve comfort in dying patients, but it did improve the quality of dying in the final four weeks of life for dementia residents (Miranda et al., 2021b).

Healthcare professionals across Europe recognise that optimal communication and shared decision making are important interventions for delivering person-centred palliative care in dementia (Brazil et al., 2017). These interventions can be actualised through advance care planning. A systematic review has identified that advance care planning interventions appear to increase documentation of advance directives and discussions about goals of care that may lead to improved person-centred care for people with dementia and increase the chances of achieving preferred place of care and death at the end of life (Walsh et al., 2021).

One of the challenges across Europe is the understanding of the difference between palliative and end of life care for people with dementia (Sharp et

[8] The six PACE Steps includes: 1) advance care planning with residents and families; 2) assessment, care planning, and review of resident needs and problems; 3) coordination of care via monthly multidisciplinary palliative care review meetings; 4) high-quality palliative care with a focus on pain and depression; 5) care in the last days of life; and 6) care after death.

al., 2020). There is also a lack of awareness amongst policy makers, health care professionals and members of the public about the benefits of palliative care for people with dementia (World Health Organization, 2020). Pathways of palliative care are inconsistent across countries, resulting in people with dementia having variable access to appropriate person-centred care (Larkin, 2017). Palliative care could start early at the point of diagnosis of dementia, however, there is controversy amongst palliative and dementia experts about whether this is too early (van der Steen et al., 2016). There are challenges with timing as cognitive decline across the disease trajectory can lead to reduced capacity and limited communication. Therefore, early advance care planning is recommended to include the person with dementia and their families in discussions about their future wishes (Eisenmann et al., 2020, Mogan et al., 2022).

Carers (both paid and family/unpaid carers) often lack the knowledge and skills of palliative care and yet are expected to be primary providers of palliative and end of life care. Co-ordinating complex physical and psychological care of a person with dementia and be responsible for making end of life decisions with little support can result in carers being burdened and a decline in their own physical and mental health (Fetherston et al., 2018, Jones et al., 2019).

Another biggest challenge is identifying when someone with dementia is approaching the end of their life (Handley et al., 2022, Sampson et al., 2018, Nishimura et al., 2022). Multiple complex factors such as physical co-morbidity, family and carers knowledge and care commonly provided by a generalist practitioner result in reactive emergency care at end of life (Sampson et al., 2018). People with dementia are often transferred to a hospital or long-term care facility for inappropriate lifesaving treatment as a result of poor acknowledgement of end-of-life care needs. Most people would prefer to die at home and yet people often die in nursing homes especially in the Netherlands (93%) and Wales (49%) (Eisenmann et al., 2020). Access to specialist palliative and end of life home care is lacking and although there is a willingness to increase specialist provision, the effectiveness on care and costs will need to be proved if this is to change (Miranda et al., 2021a). The growing ageing population and predicted rises in prevalence of people with dementia in future years brings a risk of substantial unmet needs for people with dementia and their families in Europe.

Palliative dementia care in Africa and other low- and middle-income countries

Dementia is a highly prevalent mental health condition in older persons (Alzheimer's Disease International, 2017), although early dementia is also common in patients with underlying conditions such as HIV, which is highly prevalent in Africa. This is because HIV has been found to affect the nervous system and is associated with cognitive impairments (Clifford and Ances, 2013), explaining the high prevalence of early dementia and other mental health illnesses among people living with HIV in sub-Saharan Africa (Nakasujja et al., 2010). A systematic review which aimed to determine the prevalence of neural degenerative disorders (HAND) among people living with HIV in Ethiopia reported a prevalence of 39% (Zenebe et al., 2021). A cross-sectional study conducted among ambulatory adults living with HIV reported a prevalence of probable dementia of 65% (Nakku et al., 2013). In sub-Saharan Africa the HIV burden is high, necessitating palliative psychiatry for people living with HIV despite the advent of antiretroviral therapy. Besides HIV, dementia is also common among older persons in Africa and this increasing trend in the prevalence is largely explained by the increasing life expectancy and incidence and prevalence of other non-communicable diseases. The lack of quality epidemiological data makes it difficult to estimate the true prevalence of dementia but a regional prevalence of 2.4% has been reported from a systematic review (George-Carey et al., 2012). Another review conducted in Nigeria reported a prevalence of 4.9% and the prevalence is expected to rise to about 7.62 million by 2050 (Adeloye et al., 2019).

In Africa, early stages of dementia may not be recognised due to the lack of awareness. At times it may be interpreted as a normal part of ageing and the affected may not seek care (George-Carey et al., 2012). As dementia progresses into the middle and late stages, people with dementia need support in terms of care and treatment for their complex symptoms and concerns (World Health Organization, 2006). Dementia is progressive and terminal and its progression comes with increased dependence on caregivers for care needs, complex symptoms and concerns (Reisberg et al., 1982). These include loss of capacity for autonomy and competent intellectual, emotional, and cognitive self-efficacy and hence self-actualisation. It brings on the need for one to depend on others for their day-to-day activities. The cognitive decline and physical dysfunction of people with Alzheimer's disease are accelerated by the behavioural and psychological symptoms of dementia, which also place a heavy load and stress on the carers of those with dementia (Kim et al., 2021). Primary palliative care is fundamental to quality care for people with advanced dementia and their family. Despite this need, the level of development and accessibility of palliative care remains limited in most African countries (Rhee et al., 2018) and it is even far less developed at primary health care level.

Mental health wellbeing is well embodied in the WHO definition of health as a state of complete physical, mental, and social well-being and not merely the absence of disease/infirmity (World Health Organization, 2022b). Mental well-being itself includes a subjective perceived self-efficacy, autonomy, competence to handle life's challenges, intergenerational dependence, and self-actualisation of one's intellectual and emotional potential; and not merely the absence of mental disorders (Garre-Olmo et al., 2010). Therefore, the WHO continues to urge member states to develop plans of action on dementia but by 2017 no action plans for the public health response on dementia had been developed (Alzheimer's Disease International, 2017). This gap continues to expose people with dementia and their families to avoidable health related suffering as well as family out of pocket costs. In 2015, dementia costed health systems in sub-Saharan Africa an estimate of USD 6.2 billion and two thirds to three quarters of the expenses went towards informal care (Alzheimer's Disease International, 2017).

In most African countries, patient care has been predominantly family based, although with the rising rate of labour and migration of the youth, some urban families are increasingly considering formal or paid models of care. A few families bring in paid caregivers at home to support the person with dementia while others may institutionalise people living with dementia due to their increasing care demands. To support people with dementia and families, effective communication, disclosure about the diagnosis, counselling and support to the person and family are important interventions with referrals to hospice or palliative psychiatry services where appropriate. Families are supported when navigating any risks or problems that people with dementia frequently encounter, such as falls, fractures, and activities of daily living (Garre-Olmo et al., 2010). The activities of daily living include feeding, sleeping, shopping, moving around, driving, finances and self-care (e.g., personal hygiene, bathing, toileting, and dressing).

Frailty in dementia occurs usually in advanced cases and often calls for 24-hour care. People with dementia commonly experience complex symptoms ranging from psychotic symptoms (hallucinations, delusions), affective symptoms (depression, mania, euphoria, dis-inhibition, anxiety, irritability, agitation), to behavioural symptoms (apathy, aberrant motor behaviour, aggression, sleep problems, eating problems, wandering) (Garre-Olmo et al., 2010). Those that wander may face violence in communities where awareness about dementia is low, some may be mistaken for witches who move around with an intention of causing harm. Care for people with advanced dementia is stressful to caregivers, who may also have to fend for the family. Families commonly seek pharmacological interventions where possible (Canevelli et al., 2013), while those who associate the condition with witchcraft may seek alternative traditional treatment options. Some people with dementia may be moved into nursing homes or into institutionalised care due to the overwhelming care needs which the family may not be able to meet.

Palliative psychiatry is an important component of care for people with severe and persistent mental illness, which aims to systematically manage biological, psychological, social, and existential factors of care, but not cure or remissions (Musisi, 2022, Stoll et al., 2022). The need to address caregiver burden is integral to the care action plan. The decision of where to care for people with dementia often arises. Some families need to be supported to make the decision. Options include home-based care, hospice care, respite care, long-term care such as nursing homes, outreach hospital visitations. Palliative psychiatry in dementia offers a support system to help people to live as actively as possible until death. The support focuses on giving the family support to cope with the person's progressive dementing illness. It calls for a multi-professional/multidisciplinary team approach to address the needs of people with dementia and their families to enhance their quality of life and positively influencing the course of illness (Zucchella et al., 2018).

Because dementia is incurable and is progressive, patients and their families should be empowered to make informed decisions to avoid heroics and unnecessary often expensive procedures and time-wasting medications. That said, the breaking of bad news should be done with compassion to minimise the risk of psychological distress which emerges from getting the news about the incurable nature of the disease, and controlled disclosures in family therapy sessions may be more appropriate when compared with insensitive breaking of the bad news (Briggs et al., 2017, Frank et al., 2018). Patients should be supported through advance care planning as well at an early stage possibly when they can make some decisions, with some degree of autonomy (Bryant et al., 2022). Treatments, medications, procedures, and advance directives including Do Not Resuscitate orders need to be discussed with the family (Piers et al., 2018). Individual and family support including spiritual care, traditional, complementary and alternative treatments need to be discussed with the family members and respected if they follow ethical standards (Azizi et al., 2022).

Conclusion

Common challenges have been identified to integrate palliative care into dementia practice in Asia, Europe, and Africa. Exploring and evaluating the appropriate approaches or models to manage complex symptoms such as the behavioural and psychological symptoms of dementia and address unmet needs of people with dementia and families has a long way to go. The socio-cultural context surrounding individuals influences the formation of care preferences, communication patterns, interpretation of different meanings of suffering, and decision-making processes about care, therefore, should be taken into consideration to ensure the provision of person-centred care. Improving palliative care for people with dementia and their families with cultural perspectives need to be further investigated. We conclude with recommendations of emphasising the need to work in partnerships with people living with dementia, their family members, communities, clinicians, and academic colleagues across the globe to identify and negotiate culturally meaningful care, reduce pain and improve quality of life, and ensure the highest quality palliative care for all affected by dementia, both domestically and internationally.

References

adeloye, D., Auta, A., Ezejimofor, M., Oyedokun, A., Harhay, M. O., Rudan, I. & Chan, K. Y. 2019. Prevalence of dementia in Nigeria: a systematic review of the evidence. *Journal of Global Health Reports,* 3, e2019014.

Alzheimer's Disease International. 2017. *Dementia in sub-Saharan Africa, Challenges and Opportunities* [Online]. Available: https://www.alzint.org/resource/dementia-in-sub-saharan-africa/ [Accessed 27 February 2023].

Alzheimer Europe. 2019. *Dementia in Europe yearbook 2019: Estimating the prevalence of dementia in Europe* [Online]. Available: https://www.alzheimer-europe.org/sites/default/files/alzheimer_europe_dementia_in_europe_yearbook_2019.pdf [Accessed 14 Febraury 2023].

Azizi, B., Tilburgs, B., Van Hout, H. P. J., Van Der Heide, I., Verheij, R. A., Achterberg, W. P., Van Der Steen, J. T. & Joling, K. J. 2022. Occurrence and Timing of Advance Care Planning in Persons With Dementia in General Practice: Analysis of Linked Electronic Health Records and Administrative Data. *Frontiers in Public Health,* 10.

Brazil, K., Galway, K., Carter, G. & Van Der Steen, J. T. 2017. Providing Optimal Palliative Care for Persons Living with Dementia: A Comparison of Physician Perceptions in the Netherlands and the United Kingdom. *Journal of Palliative Medicine,* 20**,** 473-477.

Briggs, R., Mchale, C., Fitzhenry, D., O'neill, D. & Kennelly, S. P. 2017. Dementia, disclosing the diagnosis. *QJM: An International Journal of Medicine,* 111**,** 215-216.

Bryant, J., Sellars, M., Waller, A., Detering, K., Sinclair, C., Ruseckaite, R., White, B. & Nolte, L. 2022. Advance care planning participation by people with dementia: a cross-sectional survey and medical record audit. *BMJ Supportive & Palliative Care,* 12**,** e464-e468.

Canevelli, M., Adali, N., Cantet, C., Andrieu, S., Bruno, G., Cesari, M. & Vellas, B. 2013. Impact of behavioral subsyndromes on cognitive decline in Alzheimer's disease: data from the ICTUS study. *Journal of Neurology,* 260**,** 1859-65.

Chen et al. 2022. Temporal trends of palliative care utilization in people with dementia: a nationwide study in Taiwan during 2007-2017. *2022 Alzheimer's Disease International (ADI) Asia Pacific Regional Conference.* Taipei, Taiwan.

Chen, P.-J., Ho, C.-H., Liao, J.-Y., Smits, L., Hsiung, C. A., Yu, S.-J., Zhang, K.-P., Petersen, I. & Sampson, E. L. 2020. The Association between Home Healthcare and Burdensome Transitions at the End-of-Life in People with Dementia: A 12-Year Nationwide Population-Based Cohort Study. *International Journal of Environmental Research and Public Health,* 17**,** 9255.

Chen, P. J. 2016. *Guidebook of palliative care for patients with dementia,* Tainan, Taiwan, Chi Mei Medical Center.

Chen, P. J., Liang, F. W., Ho, C. H., Cheng, S. Y., Chen, Y. C., Chen, Y. H. & Chen, Y. C. 2018. Association between palliative care and life-sustaining treatments for patients with dementia: A nationwide 5-year cohort study. *Palliat Med,* 32**,** 622-630.

Chen, Y.-H., Ho, C. H., Huang, C. C., Hsu, Y. W., Chen, Y. C., Chen, P. J., Chen, G. T. & Wang, J. J. 2017. Comparison of healthcare utilization and life-sustaining interventions between elderly patients with dementia and those with cancer near the end of life: A nationwide, population-based study in Taiwan. *Geriatrics Gerontology International,* 17, 2545-2551.

Clarfield, A. M., Monette, J., Bergman, H., Monette, M., Ben-Israel, Y., Caine, Y., Charles, J., Gordon, M. & Gore, B. 2006. Enteral feeding in end-stage dementia: a comparison of religious, ethnic, and national differences in Canada and Israel. *The Journals of Gerontology: Series A, Biological Sciences and Medical Sciences,* 61, 621-7.

Clifford, D. B. & Ances, B. M. 2013. HIV-associated neurocognitive disorder. *The Lancet Infectious Diseases,* 13, 976-986.

Dening, K. H., Sampson, E. L. & De Vries, K. 2019. Advance care planning in dementia: recommendations for healthcare professionals. *Palliative Care: Research and Treatment,* 12, 1178224219826579.

Eisenmann, Y., Golla, H., Schmidt, H., Voltz, R. & Perrar, K. M. 2020. Palliative Care in Advanced Dementia. *Frontiers in Psychiatry,* 11.

Fetherston, A. A., Rowley, G. & Allan, C. L. 2018. Challenges in end-of-life dementia care. *Evidence-Based Mental Health,* 21, 107-111.

Finkelstein, E. A., Bhadelia, A., Goh, C., Baid, D., Singh, R., Bhatnagar, S. & Connor, S. R. 2022. Cross Country Comparison of Expert Assessments of the Quality of Death and Dying 2021. *Journal of Pain and Symptom Management,* 63, e419-e429.

Fox, S., Fitzgerald, C., Harrison Dening, K., Irving, K., Kernohan, W. G., Treloar, A., Oliver, D., Guerin, S. & Timmons, S. 2017. Better palliative care for people with a dementia: summary of interdisciplinary workshop highlighting current gaps and recommendations for future research. *BMC Palliative Care,* 17, 9.

Frank, C. C., Lee, L. & Molnar, F. 2018. Disclosing a diagnosis of dementia. *Canadian Family Physician Medecin De Famille Canadien,* 64, 518-518.

Garre-Olmo, J., López-Pousa, S., Vilalta-Franch, J., De Gracia Blanco, M. & Vilarrasa, A. B. 2010. Grouping and trajectories of the neuropsychiatric symptoms in patients with Alzheimer's disease, part I: symptom clusters. *Journal of Alzheimer's Disease,* 22, 1157-67.

Gauthier, S., Webster, C., Servaes, S., Morais, J. & Rosa-Neto, P. 2022. World Alzheimer Report 2022: Life after diagnosis: Navigating treatment, care and support. London, England.

George-Carey, R., Adeloye, D., Chan, K. Y., Paul, A., Kolčić, I., Campbell, H. & Rudan, I. 2012. An estimate of the prevalence of dementia in Africa: A systematic analysis. *Journal of Global Health,* 2, 020401.

Handley, M., Parker, D., Bunn, F. & Goodman, C. 2022. A qualitative comparison of care home staff and palliative care specialists' experiences of providing end of life care to people living and dying with dementia in care homes in two countries: A focus group study. *Palliative Medicine,* 36, 114-123.

Houttekier, D., Vandervoort, A., Van Den Block, L., Van Der Steen, J. T., Vander Stichele, R. & Deliens, L. 2014. Hospitalizations of nursing home residents with dementia in the last month of life: Results from a nationwide survey. *Palliative Medicine,* 28, 1110-1117.

Hum, A., Tay, R. Y., Wong, Y. K. Y., Ali, N. B., Leong, I. Y. O., Wu, H. Y., Chin, J. J., Lee, A. O. K. & Koh, M. Y. H. 2020. Advanced dementia: an integrated homecare programme. *BMJ Supportive & Palliative Care,* 10, e40.

Hum, A. Y. M., Wu, H. Y., Ali, N. B., Leong, I. Y. O., Chin, J. J., Lee, A. O. K., Tay, R. Y. & Koh, M. Y. H. 2018. The dignity in advanced dementia (diadem) study: Developing an integrated geriatric palliative homecare program. *Progress in Palliative Care,* 26, 65-72.

Jones, K., Birchley, G., Huxtable, R., Clare, L., Walter, T. & Dixon, J. 2019. End of Life Care: A Scoping Review of Experiences of Advance Care Planning for People with Dementia. *Dementia (London),* 18, 825-845.

Kim, B., Noh, G. O. & Kim, K. 2021. Behavioural and psychological symptoms of dementia in patients with Alzheimer's disease and family caregiver burden: a path analysis. *BMC Geriatrics,* 21, 160.

Kupeli, N. 2020. More research is needed to understand how to provide optimal palliative dementia care to people living at home. *Evidence Based Nursing,* 23, 111-111.

Kwok, T., Twinn, S. & Yan, E. 2007. The attitudes of Chinese family caregivers of older people with dementia towards life sustaining treatments. *Journal of Advanced Nursing,* 58, 256-62.

Larkin, P. J. 2017. Palliative dementia care: lessons from a European perspective. *Annals of Palliative Medicine,* 6, 393-395.

Leniz, J., Gulliford, M., Higginson, I. J., Bajwah, S., Yi, D., Gao, W. & Sleeman, K. E. 2022. Primary care contacts, continuity, identification of palliative care needs, and hospital use: a population-based cohort study in people dying with dementia. *British Journal of General Practice,* 72, e684-e692.

MARTINSSON, L., LUNDSTRÖM, S. & SUNDELÖF, J. 2020. Better quality of end-of-life care for persons with advanced dementia in nursing homes compared to hospitals: a Swedish national register study. *BMC Palliative Care,* 19, 135.

MIRANDA, R., BUNN, F., LYNCH, J., VAN DEN BLOCK, L. & GOODMAN, C. 2019. Palliative care for people with dementia living at home: A systematic review of interventions. *Palliative Medicine,* 33, 726-742.

Miranda, R., Smets, T., De Schreye, R., Faes, K., Van Den Noortgate, N., Cohen, J. & Van Den Block, L. 2021a. Improved quality of care and reduced healthcare costs at the end-of-life among older people with dementia who received palliative home care: A nationwide propensity score-matched decedent cohort study. *Palliative Medicine,* 35, 1701-1712.

Miranda, R., Smets, T., Van Den Noortgate, N., Van Der Steen, J. T., Deliens, L., Payne, S., Szczerbińska, K., Pautex, S., Van Humbeeck, L., Gambassi, G., Kylänen, M., Van Den Block, L., Gatsolaeva, Y., Pivodic, L., Honinx, E., Tanghe, M., Van Hout, H., Froggatt, K., Onwuteaka-Philipsen, B., Pasman, H. R. W., Piers, R., Baranska, I., Oosterveld-Vlug, M., Wichmann, A. B., Engels, Y., Vernooij-Dassen, M., Hockley, J., Leppäaho, S., Bassal, C., Mammarella, F., Mercuri, M., Rossi, P., Segat, I., Stodolska, A., Adang, E., Andreasen, P., Kuitunen-Kaija, O., Hammar, T., Heikkilä, R., Moore, D. C., Kijowska, V., Ten Koppel, M., De Paula, E. M. & On Behalf Of, P. 2021b. No difference in effects of 'PACE steps to success' palliative care program for nursing home residents with and without dementia: a pre-planned subgroup analysis of the seven-country PACE trial. *BMC Palliative Care,* 20, 39.

Mogan, C., Harrison Dening, K., Dowrick, C. & Lloyd-Williams, M. 2022. Health and social care services for people with dementia at home at the end of life: A qualitative study of bereaved informal caregivers' experiences. *Palliative Medicine,* 36, 976-985.

Mura, T., Dartigues, J. F. & Berr, C. 2010. How many dementia cases in France and Europe? Alternative projections and scenarios 2010-2050. *European Journal of Neurology,* 17, 252-9.

Murray, S. A., Kendall, M., Boyd, K. & Sheikh, A. 2005. Illness trajectories and palliative care. *British Medical Journal,* 330, 1007-11.

Musisi, S. 2022. Integrating Mental Health In Palliative Care And Other Conditions. *7th African Palliative Care conference* Kampala African Palliative Care and Worldwide Hospice Palliative Care Alliance Conference.

Nakanishi, M., Endo, K., Hirooka, K., Granvik, E., Minthon, L., Nägga, K. & Nishida, A. 2018. Psychosocial behaviour management programme for home-dwelling people with dementia: A cluster-randomized controlled trial. *International Journal of Geriatric Psychiatry,* 33, 495-503.

Nakanishi, M., Ogawa, A. & Nishida, A. 2020. Availability of home palliative care services and dying at home in conditions needing palliative care: A population-based death certificate study. *Palliative Medicine,* 34, 504-512.

Nakanishi, M. & Van Der Steen, J. T. 2020. National dementia plans to address escalating global palliative care needs. *Palliative Medicine,* 34, 966-967.

Nakasujja, N., L Skolasky, R., Musisi, S., Allebeck, P., Robertson, K., Ronald, A., Katabira, E., Clifford, D. B. & Sacktor, N. 2010. Depression symptoms and cognitive function among individuals with advanced HIV infection initiating HAART in Uganda. *BMC Psychiatry,* 10, 44.

Nakku, J., Kinyanda, E. & Hoskins, S. 2013. Prevalence and factors associated with probable HIV dementia in an African population: A cross-sectional study of an HIV/AIDS clinic population. *BMC Psychiatry,* 13, 126.

Nishimura, M., Dening, K. H., Sampson, E. L., De Oliveira Vidal, E. I., De Abreu, W. C., Kaasalainen, S., Eisenmann, Y., Dempsey, L., Moore, K. J., Davies, N., Bolt, S. R., Meijers, J. M. M., Dekker, N. L., Miyashita, M., Nakanishi, M., Nakayama, T. & Van Der Steen, J. T. 2022. Cross-cultural conceptualization of a good end of life with dementia: a qualitative study. *BMC Palliative Care,* 21, 106.

Piers, R., Albers, G., Gilissen, J., De Lepeleire, J., Steyaert, J., Van Mechelen, W., Steeman, E., Dillen, L., Vanden Berghe, P. & Van Den Block, L. 2018. Advance care planning in dementia: recommendations for healthcare professionals. *BMC Palliative Care,* 17, 88.

Reisberg, B., Ferris, S. H., De Leon, M. J. & Crook, T. 1982. The Global Deterioration Scale for assessment of primary degenerative dementia. *American Journal of Psychiatry,* 139, 1136-9.

Rhee, J. Y., Garralda, E., Namisango, E., Luyirika, E., De Lima, L., Powell, R. A., López-Fidalgo, J. & Centeno, C. 2018. An Analysis of Palliative Care Development in Africa: A Ranking Based on Region-Specific Macroindicators. *Journal of Pain and Symptom Management,* 56, 230-238.

Sampson, E. L., Candy, B., Davis, S., Gola, A. B., Harrington, J., King, M., Kupeli, N., Leavey, G., Moore, K., Nazareth, I., Omar, R. Z., Vickerstaff, V. & Jones, L. 2018. Living and dying with advanced dementia: A prospective cohort study of symptoms, service use and care at the end of life. *Palliative Medicine,* 32, 668-681.

Sharp, B., Henderson, J., Brown, M., Jack-Waugh, A. & Macrae, R. 2020. Palliative and end of life care for people with advanced dementia. *Nursing Older People*.

Sleeman, K. E., De Brito, M., Etkind, S., Nkhoma, K., Guo, P., Higginson, I. J., Gomes, B. & Harding, R. 2019. The escalating global burden of serious health-related suffering: projections to 2060 by world regions, age groups, and health conditions. *The Lancet Global Health,* 7, e883-e892.

Smets, T., Onwuteaka-Philipsen, B. B. D., Miranda, R., Pivodic, L., Tanghe, M., Van Hout, H., Pasman, R., Oosterveld-Vlug, M., Piers, R., Van Den Noortgate, N., Wichmann, A. B., Engels, Y., Vernooij-Dassen, M., Hockley, J., Froggatt, K., Payne, S., Szczerbińska, K., Kylänen, M., Leppäaho, S., Barańska, I., Gambassi, G., Pautex, S., Bassal, C., Deliens, L. & Van Den Block, L. 2018. Integrating palliative care in long-term care facilities across Europe (PACE): protocol of a cluster randomized controlled trial of the 'PACE Steps to Success' intervention in seven countries. *BMC Palliative Care,* 17, 47.

Stoll, J., Mathew, A., Venkateswaran, C., Prabhakaran, A., Westermair, A. L. & Trachsel, M. 2022. Palliative Psychiatry for Patients With Severe and Persistent Mental Illness: A Survey on the Attitudes of Psychiatrists in India Compared to Psychiatrists in Switzerland. *Frontiers in Psychiatry,* 13.

Ten Koppel, M., Onwuteaka-Philipsen, B. D., Van Den Block, L., Deliens, L., Gambassi, G., Heymans, M. W., Kylänen, M., Oosterveld-Vlug, M. G., Pasman, H. R. W., Payne, S., Smets, T., Szczerbińska, K., Twisk, J. W., Van Der Steen, J. T., Groote, Z. D., Mammarella, F., Mercuri, M., Pivodic, L., Pac, A., Rossi, P., Segat, I., Sowerby, E., Stodolska, A., Van Hout, H., Wichmann, A., Adang, E., Andreasen, P., Finne-Soveri, H., Collingridge Moore, D., Froggatt, K., Kijowska, V., Van Den Noortgate, N. & Vernooij-Dassen, M. 2019. Palliative care provision in long-term care facilities differs across Europe: Results of a cross-sectional study in six European countries (PACE). *Palliative Medicine,* 33, 1176-1188.

The Economist Intelligence Unit 2010. The quality of death: Ranking end-of-life care across the world. Singapore: Lien Foundation.

The Economist Intelligence Unit 2015. The 2015 Quality of Death Index: Ranking palliative care across the world. Singapore: Lien Foundation.

Tilburgs, B., Vernooij-Dassen, M., Koopmans, R., Van Gennip, H., Engels, Y. & Perry, M. 2018. Barriers and facilitators for GPs in dementia advance care planning: A systematic integrative review. *PLoS One,* 13, e0198535.

Timmons, S., Fox, S., Drennan, J., Guerin, S. & Kernohan, W. G. 2022. Palliative care for older people with dementia—we need a paradigm shift in our approach. *Age and Ageing,* 51.

UK Legislation. 2005. *Mental Capacity Act* [Online]. Available: https://www.legislation.gov.uk/ukpga/2005/9/contents [Accessed 14 March 2023].

Van Der Steen, J. T., Radbruch, L., De Boer, M. E., Jünger, S., Hughes, J. C., Larkin, P., Gove, D., Francke, A. L., Koopmans, R. T. C. M., Firth, P., Volicer, L. & Hertogh, C. M. P. M. 2016. Achieving consensus and controversy around applicability of palliative care to dementia. *International Psychogeriatrics,* 28**,** 133-145.

Van Der Steen, J. T., Radbruch, L., Hertogh, C. M., De Boer, M. E., Hughes, J. C., Larkin, P., Francke, A. L., Jünger, S., Gove, D., Firth, P., Koopmans, R. T. & Volicer, L. 2014. White paper defining optimal palliative care in older people with dementia: A Delphi study and recommendations from the European Association for Palliative Care. *Palliative Medicine,* 28**,** 197-209.

Walsh, S. C., Murphy, E., Devane, D., Sampson, E. L., Connolly, S., Carney, P. & O'shea, E. 2021. Palliative care interventions in advanced dementia. *Cochrane Database of Systematic Reviews,* 9**,** Cd011513.

World Health Organization. 2006. *Neurological disorders: public health challenges* [Online]. Available: https://www.who.int/publications/i/item/9789241563369 [Accessed 14 March 2023].

World Health Organization. 2015. *The growing need for home health care for the elderly* [Online]. Geneva, Switzerland. Available: https://applications.emro.who.int/dsaf/EMROPUB_2015_EN_1901.pdf?ua=1 [Accessed 8 May 2020].

World Health Organization. 2020. *Palliative care* [Online]. Available: https://www.who.int/news-room/fact-sheets/detail/palliative-care [Accessed 17 February 2023].

World Health Organization. 2022a. *Ageing and Health* [Online]. Geneva, Switzerland: World Health Organization,. Available: https://www.who.int/news-room/fact-sheets/detail/ageing-and-health [Accessed 22 February 2023].

World Health Organization. 2022b. *Health and well-being* [Online]. Available: https://www.who.int/data/gho/data/major-themes/health-and-well-being#:~:text=The%20WHO%20constitution%20states%3A%20%22Health,of%20mental%20disorders%20or%20disabilities. [Accessed 15 March 2023].

Yamaguchi, T., Kuriya, M., Morita, T., Agar, M., Choi, Y. S., Goh, C., Lingegowda, K. B., Lim, R., Liu, R. K., Macleod, R., Ocampo, R., Cheng, S. Y., Phungrassami, T., Nguyen, Y. P. & Tsuneto, S. 2017. Palliative care development in the Asia-Pacific region: an international survey from the Asia Pacific Hospice Palliative Care Network (APHN). *BMJ Supportive & Palliative Care,* 7**,** 23-31.

Zenebe, Y., Akele, B., W/Selassie, M. & Necho, M. 2021. A systematic review and meta-analysis of HIV associated neurocognitive disorders (HAND) among people with HIV in Ethiopia. *AIDS Research and Therapy,* 18, 99.

Zucchella, C., Sinforiani, E., Tamburin, S., Federico, A., Mantovani, E., Bernini, S., Casale, R. & Bartolo, M. 2018. The Multidisciplinary Approach to Alzheimer's Disease and Dementia. A Narrative Review of Non-Pharmacological Treatment. *Frontiers in Neurology,* 9.

19

AN OVERVIEW OF CLINICAL CARE OF ENDSTAGE DEMENTIA

JONATHAN T. STEWART[1]

The author has no actual or potential financial, personal or other conflict of interest pertinent to this work. There was no sponsorship of this work, and no source of funding. This material has not been published or submitted for publication elsewhere.

Dementia may be the last frontier of hospice and palliative medicine. Dementia is common, affecting about 10% of individuals over 65 and almost half of those over 85, and is rarely reversible or arrestable[1]. The various dementias exhibit considerable heterogeneity initially, but at endstage all are similar and share common characteristics of other terminal illnesses: functional decline, weight loss, frailty, cachexia, and ultimately recurrent medical complications and a cascade of organ failures[2,3]. Median survival is about five years after diagnosis[4]. Nevertheless, dementia has been a latecomer for our discipline, the last major terminal condition to receive our full attention. As recently as 1995, less than 1% of hospice enrollments were for dementia[5] and there were few publications characterizing endstage dementia and its management. This has improved considerably only over the past two decades; in 2018, 15.6% of hospice enrollees in the United States had a primary diagnosis of dementia[6].

It is well established that the greatest barrier to palliative care for individuals with dementia is difficulty with prognostication[7-9]; while accuracy has improved over the years, dementia remains the most unpredictable of the major terminal conditions[3,10]. A more fundamental

[1] MD, DLFAPA, AGSF. Staff Geropsychiatrist (WOC), James A Haley VA Hospital, Collaborative Professor in Psychiatry and Geriatric Medicine, University of South Florida College of Medicine, Tampa FL, USA

barrier, though, may be the lack of perception of dementia as a terminal condition at all. Families and even professionals generally view dementia somewhat euphemistically as a "memory disorder," or perhaps more broadly as a cognitive disorder, and it is difficult to envision how forgetfulness or cognitive impairment could lead to death[2,3]. This conceptualization may logically lead to inappropriately aggressive treatment. For example, if a patient simply "forgets" when or how to eat, tube feeding is the logical solution; similarly, if there is no obvious causal relationship between pneumonia and memory impairment, aggressive treatment of the apparently unrelated recurrent pneumonia seems warranted.

Dementia is better conceived of as "brain failure," i.e., as a major end organ failure analogous to heart failure or respiratory failure, both ultimately terminal illnesses clearly within our purview[2,3,11]. The overall picture of functional decline, frailty and recurrent health crises, and the wisdom of withholding otherwise futile and burdensome treatment, becomes much clearer when dementia is so conceptualized.

There is abundant evidence of unrelieved suffering in individuals with advanced dementia[9,12,13]. Fearfulness and agitation are common, and pain, dyspnea and other discomfort often go unrecognized and untreated. Caring for a loved one with dementia is highly burdensome, and this burden only increases with progression to endstage; of all major terminal conditions, dementia is felt to be the most labor-intensive for families, both physically and emotionally[14]. Families are confronted with a gradual but fundamental loss of the parent, partner or loved one who once was, along with the burden of profound role changes, difficult behavioral problems, safety concerns, ambiguous medical information and possibly family conflicts[2]. Perhaps most difficult, though, is witnessing the unrelieved suffering of a loved one. The rigorous study of that suffering is relatively new, only evolving over the past two or three decades, and the gaps in our knowledge are numerous. This chapter will provide an overview of the difficulties encountered in advanced dementia and what is known about their management.

Prognostication

Prognostication is an essential skill in caring for patients with advanced dementia and their loved ones. As noted above, families are often unaware of the terminal nature of dementia, and stories of being blindsided by the unexpected death of their loved one are often heard. Of course, a general estimate of the time remaining will enter into many care decisions as well. Dementia remains the most difficult common terminal condition for prognostication[3,10]. Prognostic skill has improved over the past few decades; for example, a 1998 study by Aguero-Torres et al reported that fully 30% of hospice enrollees with a primary diagnosis of dementia were still alive three years after enrollment[15]. To this day, a primary diagnosis of dementia is a common cause of live discharge from hospice[16,17] and may occur in up to 25% of patients[18]; this is usually highly distressing to families.

One source of uncertainty in prognostication (and of confusion for families) is the typical course of advanced dementia. This had classically been described as one of slow but steady and inexorable decline, but some authors have suggested that the reality is more of slow decline punctuated by increasingly frequent health crises (often aspiration pneumonia, dehydration or an injurious fall)[2,3,19]. This pattern, and its attendant unpredictability and false hope of return to baseline, is akin to that seen in endstage COPD or heart failure.

A six month prognosis is most commonly established in accordance with the guidelines published by the National Hospice and Palliative Care Organization (NHPCO) in 1997[20]. These include a severity of stage 7 on Reisberg's Functional Assessment Staging Tool (FAST)[21] and one or more medical or nutritional comorbidities. Briefly, patients at stage 7 will be dependent in all activities of daily living (ADLs), doubly incontinent and will have speech characterized by no more than six words. Comorbidities may include recurrent aspiration pneumonia, recurrent sepsis, pyelonephritis, a fever that recurs immediately after cessation of antibiotics, a stage III or IV pressure ulcer, serum albumin less than 2.5g/dl or loss of greater than 10% of body weight over the previous six months. It should be borne in mind that these criteria are most applicable to Alzheimer's disease; other dementias may have a different trajectory.

In 2010, Mitchell et al developed the Advanced Dementia Prognostic Tool (ADEPT), which calculates prognosis based on items from the Minimum Data Set (MDS), a database collected on most patients admitted to skilled nursing facilities (SNFs) in the United States[8]. The ADEPT has been shown to have better predictive value than the NHPCO criteria but has only been validated in SNF populations to date.

Additionally, hip fracture[22] and the triad of dysphagia, anorexia and weight loss[23] are felt to portend an especially poor prognosis.

Advance planning

Advance care planning should begin soon after the initial shock of diagnosis, and should be an ongoing process revisited as the dementia progresses and as new problems arise or appear on the horizon[2,3]. Dementia by definition soon progresses to incapacity to engage in these decisions, although many individuals will have long-held ideas about their care; the capacity to communicate these wishes is generally not lost until the later stages of illness. Nevertheless, it is best to engage the patient in discussions early on when capacity is full, and to encourage consensus between the patient and surrogate(s) as capacity is gradually lost. It will be vital to ensure that patient and family understand that dementia is ultimately a terminal condition; we have found that gently framing the illness as "brain failure," as discussed above, sets the groundwork for productive discussion.

It will be found that many families have had discussions about dementia care, sometimes in response to an older relative's experiences[2]. These discussions will usually be somewhat uninformed, and promises may have been made that are impossible to keep. For example, a spouse may have promised many decades ago to never institutionalize the patient, but adequate care at home may now be impossible. Another concern, especially in jurisdictions that allow physician-assisted death, is that a patient may have indicated a preference for death over severe cognitive impairment ("when I can't recognize my loved ones" is a common threshold), but will likely be unaware of and possibly undisturbed by those deficits when that threshold is reached.

Unfortunately, the reality is that discussion of prognosis and of advance directives is often omitted. This is gradually improving; a 2009 study indicated that only 18% of families had heard any prognostic information at all[24], but this had improved to only 45% in a similar 2018 study[25]. Formal advance directive documents are also often neglected; in the United States, only about 37% of adults have an advance directive[26] and there is evidence that this is not improving[27]. It is also important to note that most standardized, boilerplate advance directives do not address typical decisions in endstage dementia, including artificial feeding and hydration, foregoing antibiotics and foregoing Emergency Department

(ED) visits or hospitalizations[2,3]. It is critical to discuss these issues in depth, emphasizing their minimal benefits and high burdens at the end of life. It is well established that provision of prognostic information leads to less aggressive and futile care and greater family confidence in decisions[24,28,29].

Behavior

Behavioral and psychological problems occur at some point in at least 90% of individuals with dementia[30] and are the major source of caregiver burden and institutionalization[31]. Behavior problems tend to become more prominent as the dementia progresses; more importantly, they tend to change qualitatively with progression[2,3,32]. For example, depression is more common in the earliest stages of dementia, delusions and hallucinations in the moderate stages and resistiveness to care in the later stages. Agitation of some sort is seen at some point in most patients, and its differential diagnosis is broad; to ask about the best medication or treatment for agitation is analogous to asking about the best medication or treatment for chest pain or fever. Unfortunately, a great deal of research over the past decades has treated "behavioral and psychological symptoms of dementia," or "BPSD," as a monolithic construct. The situation is especially challenging at the end of life, when almost any source of distress can manifest as nonspecific agitation and almost all patients are non-verbal and unable to contribute to the investigation[2,3]. Family members and nursing staff will often have insight into the source of distress but may still misattribute[2]. Signs of distress are manifold, and may include any sort of agitation, combativeness, screaming, crying, refusal of care or of feeding, or distressed facial expression. The most common sources of agitation and distress in endstage dementia are delirium, discomfort, fearfulness and resistiveness to care.

Delirium is very common near the end of life, in all terminal conditions[33,34]. Fortunately, lethargic delirium is much more common in the last days to weeks of life than the far more distressing and urgent hyperactive, agitated delirium[33,35]. The most robust risk factor for development of delirium is in fact pre-existing dementia[36]. Delirium can be quite difficult to identify in advanced dementia, though. Possibly the best-known framework for characterizing delirium is Inouye's Confusion Assessment Method (CAM): delirium is present if there are deficits in attention, disorganized thought, and either altered level of consciousness or an acute, fluctuating course[37]. In a non-verbal patient with advanced dementia, it will be difficult or impossible to detect a new problem with attention or disorganized thought, and many patients at this stage are mostly lethargic. This only leaves an acute (but often subtle) change in condition as a clue[3]. To further complicate matters, delirium in older patients may persist for weeks to even months after the precipitating condition resolves[3,38]. The differential diagnosis of delirium is broad, and an extensive workup will rarely be consistent with a patient's or family's goals of care. Any workup will be dependent on the intrusiveness of the evaluation, the intrusiveness and likely success (as defined by improved comfort and quality of life) of treatment if an etiology is found, anticipated life expectancy, and above all, patient and family preference.

Pain or discomfort, even seemingly trivial, is an important cause of agitation and distress in this population[2,3,39,40]. Many patients will have known sources of chronic pain (osteoarthritis, back pain, etc.) and this is often worsened by immobility. Acutely painful conditions, including unwitnessed falls or injuries, urinary retention or constipation, must be considered, as well as more serious sources of pain (acute coronary syndrome, for example). Detection and management of pain is discussed further below.

Agitation related to resistiveness to care is common late in the course of dementia[2,3,41], although this seems to abate in the last weeks to months of life, giving way to passivity and lethargy[2,3,7]. Resistiveness may be related to lack of understanding and fearfulness of carers, or to abulia (a general inertia and drive toward inactivity)[2,41]. The approach to resistiveness is nonpharmacologic and will involve limiting care to the minimum necessary to maintain comfort, a slow, gentle approach (care is sometimes tolerated better when approached from the side), pleasant distraction during care, and generally trying to personalize and optimize the approach. Some patients may also be fearful of being left alone, this is best managed by allowing them to spend time in common areas and by mobilizing the assistance of family and friends.

Sleep disturbance is nearly universal in most dementias, mostly as a result of disintegration of the normal circadian cycle[42]. Sleep problems are associated with wandering, falls and other hazards, and are a major source of distress to caregivers[2]. Often, though, they become less urgent in the last months of life as patients become bedridden and more lethargic. The first step in management will be to determine if the patient's safety and the environment can tolerate the disturbed sleep/wake cycle; the answer is often yes. Nonpharmacologic measures such as providing exposure to sunlight or bright lights during the day, keeping the patient awake and engaged during the day, ensuring adequate control of pain and nocturia and keeping the bedroom cool and quiet may be all that is needed[2,42]. If necessary for the wellbeing of the patient and family, an hypnotic may be prescribed[2,42]. Melatonin is very safe and has shown some efficacy for sleep disturbance in dementia[42]. Benzodiazepines and other sedative/hypnotics may be reasonable, but may increase risk of falls (if the patient is still at risk of getting out of bed unassisted) and aspiration.

The cornerstone of management of distress and problematic behavior is detective work, trying to identify and rectify the problem or problems that are driving the behavior. As noted above, evaluation of a presumptive delirium may or may not be warranted. Nevertheless, a limited evaluation for easily-remedied conditions may be reasonable. These may include drug toxicity (including anticholinergics, sedatives and opioid-induced neurotoxicity [OIN]; the latter is often characterized by agitation and myoclonus[43]), sedative withdrawal, electrolyte disturbances, hypo- or hyperglycemia, or dehydration. Empirical treatment for presumptive pain and evaluation for other potentially uncomfortable conditions (constipation, for example) is often reasonable[2,3,39,44], as is empirical opioid rotation (methadone is rarely associated with OIN and is often the best choice)[45-47]. It is also very safe and reasonable to try to increase meaningful activities and social contact; music therapy and aromatherapy can be used in this population, and there are a number of proprietary programs available for individuals with advanced dementia, including Snoezelen and Namaste Care[48,49]. Concurrently, it is essential to ensure safety by minimizing fall risk and the use of invasive devices that can be pulled out[2]. Overall, it is best to aim for a calm, somewhat understimulating but not sensory or socially depriving environment. Acetylcholinesterase inhibitors are clearly ineffective for delirium or behavioral problems[50].

Despite best efforts, medications will often be necessary to maintain patient comfort and safety. Neuroleptics are treatment of choice for hyperactive delirium and for fearfulness in dementia. While there are no high quality studies to date (most knowledge is extrapolated from studies of delirium in general hospital populations or sometimes hospice populations), most evidence and expert opinion supports this view[2,3,51-56]. All agents seem effective; haloperidol is the most commonly used agent due to its multiple routes of administration (intravenous, subcutaneous, oral, sublingual, rectal) and relative lack of autonomic effects[57]. The most common concerns are pseudoparkinsonism and other extrapyramidal effects (especially problematic in patients with Lewy body dementia), but these are likely less common with intravenous use[58]. Other concerns (QTc prolongation and torsades de pointes, tardive dyskinesia, metabolic syndrome, increased stroke risk and all-cause mortality in dementia) are usually irrelevant in endstage dementia. Second-generation neuroleptics also seem effective; many can be given sublingually and olanzapine can be given subcutaneously[59]. There are also a few reports of the utility of chlorpromazine in refractory terminal delirium[60]; it is highly sedating and can cause severe hypotension. Chlorpromazine is also quite irritating when given parenterally and should be given via a central line. The use of neuroleptics for agitation and distress in this population is somewhat analogous to the use of opioids for pain: they should be titrated so that the patient is at peace, but hopefully not excessively sedated[2]. Neuroleptics should not be used for hypoactive, lethargic delirium, but only for true distress.

Because of their potential adverse effects, neuroleptic use is often highly regulated. For example, in the United States the 2012 Center for Medicare and Medicaid Services' (CMS) National Partnership to Improve Dementia Care in Nursing Homes has designated neuroleptic use in skilled nursing facilities (other than for schizophrenia, Huntington's disease and Tourette syndrome) a negative quality measure, open to public scrutiny; hospice enrollment is not an exclusionary criterion. It has been noted that neuroleptic use in hospice populations has been declining over the past decade[61], and there is increasing interest in alternatives to manage hyperactive delirium and agitation. Most studies of delirium in general populations have demonstrated worse outcomes in patients treated with benzodiazepines[62,63], but again, these concerns are generally irrelevant in patients with endstage dementia and limited life expectancy. Worsening dysphagia and fall risk (in patients who are likely to try to stand or walk unassisted) may sometimes be concerns, however. Benzodiazepines may be used as an augmentation strategy in patients who do not respond adequately to neuroleptics[64], or as monotherapy[65]. Lorazepam is the most frequently used agent, it can be used intravenously and has a relatively short halflife with no active metabolites. Some authors have also documented the utility of diazepam, which has a much longer halflife and multiple active metabolites but is quite lipophilic and therefore rapidly acting[66]. There are also a few older anecdotal reports of the use of phenobarbital for refractory hyperactive delirium[67,68]. More recently, there have been reports of the utility of dexmedetomidine, an alpha-2 agonist, for hyperactive delirium at the end of life[69,70]. Dexmedetomidine is an appealing choice and is commonly used in intensive care units as it is not deliriogenic and does not cause respiratory suppression; limiting factors include hypotension, bradycardia and expense. Finally, palliative sedation may be necessary for a very select few patients with severe and refractory agitation[71,72]. In the United States, hyperactive terminal delirium is the most common indication for palliative sedation, the most commonly used agents are propofol and midazolam, and survival is generally under 24 hours[71].

Pain

Significant pain is seen in as many as 75% of hospice enrollees with advanced dementia[39], and it is well established that treatment of pain in this population improves both behavioral problems and quality of life[2,3,39,40]. Unfortunately, there is ample evidence that pain is frequently unrecognized or inadequately treated. Monroe et al reported that 40% of demented individuals with advanced malignancies had never received opioids[73], and Morrison and Siu reported that only 24% of patients with advanced dementia and acute hip fracture had received routine analgesics, ultimately receiving only 1/3 as much opioid as cognitively intact hip fracture patients[74]. The experience of pain is different in individuals with severe dementia, and detection can be challenging. Patients are usually non-verbal and unable to describe or localize pain, nor to reposition or make other efforts to relieve discomfort[2,3,75-77]. They are also unable to understand the context of pain; for example, they may be unable to recognize longstanding pain as benign and expected, or to interpret venipuncture as a transient discomfort with greater benefits[2,3,75-77]. The net result is that pain will often manifest as nonspecific agitation, even in reaction to apparently trivial discomfort.

It has sometimes been cynically stated that haloperidol is the most commonly used medication for pain in advanced dementia; pain in this population is clearly associated with increased use of psychotropic medications[40,74,77]. Detection of pain is indeed difficult in this population, and the most important step is to maintain a high index of suspicion. Families should be asked about pre-existing chronic pain[44] and a concerted effort should be made to detect any potentially painful or uncomfortable (however trivial) conditions. Families and experienced nursing staff will often be aware of subtle clues, but again, misattribution can occur[2]. There are also a number of validated pain assessment scales for non-verbal patients, including the PAINAD, the PACSLAC and the Doloplus-2 instruments[78]. If there is doubt, an empirical trial of an analgesic, either routine acetaminophen or an opioid, is warranted[2,3,39,44]. In treating pain, it is almost always best to prescribe routine analgesics, as non-verbal patients will usually not receive prn doses[2,3]. A routine laxative should almost always be prescribed when treating patients with opioids.

Anorexia

Decreased nutritional intake and weight loss are inevitable in dementia, may actually antedate any cognitive decline[79,80], and as noted above are important indicators of poor prognosis. Anorexia and weight loss likely contribute to poor quality of life (weakness, pressure ulcers, etc.)[81,82], and are also highly distressing to families given the strong symbolic significance of food[2]. The etiology of weight loss is multifactorial and incompletely understood. A number of factors contribute to anorexia, many of them remediable: visual agnosia (inability to recognize food), restlessness and distractibility at mealtimes, anosmia, unnecessarily restrictive diets, failure to honor longstanding food preferences, fear of being fed, inadequate time or resources for feeding, impersistent swallow, dysphagia, dental problems, drug-induced anorexia (about 20% of patients lose weight on acetylcholinesterase inhibitors, for example)[2,3].

Advanced dementia is also associated with chronic systemic inflammation and increased proinflammatory cytokine levels[80,82-85]. It is not clear when in the course of dementia this begins, but it is associated with cachexia, frailty and medical complications. Importantly, cachexia is clearly associated with a loss of appetite and patients rarely feel hunger[2,3,80,82]; it is probably correct to say that cachexia causes anorexia but that anorexia in and of itself does not cause cachexia[2,3]. As in the case of advanced malignancy, it is important to discuss the nature and inevitability of cachexia with families, who will often have concerns about their loved one "starving." At this stage, patients probably do not experience hunger and do not benefit physiologically from nutrition; this is the primary rationale for foregoing artificial nutrition.

Unfortunately, the futility of artificial nutrition and hydration is rarely discussed with families[86,87]. Percutaneous endoscopic gastrostomy (PEG) tubes are usually placed emergently during a health crisis, and discussion with families is usually limited to risks associated with the placement procedure itself[86,87]. It is well established that tube feeding does not improve health, strength or function, does not decrease the risk of pneumonia, does not promote wound healing, and neither improves quality nor quantity of life[80,86,88-91]. Tube feeding is also not ethically equivalent to natural feeding, nor is withholding tube feeding equivalent to "starving" the patient. It is essential to prepare families for the possibility that a PEG tube will be suggested. Fortunately, there is evidence that the prevalence of tube feeding in advanced dementia has been waning recently[92].

There are a number of options for feeding that may meet with limited success[2,3]. More importantly, they serve as an alternative for families and reassure that something is being done. As noted above, the first steps will always be family education about the inevitability of cachexia and weight loss and the futility of tube feeding. Many of the contributors to anorexia noted above will be modifiable. Families should be encouraged to bring in familiar and preferred foods from home and to assist with feeding. Patients with advanced dementia will sometimes prefer relatively monotonous and bland foods, softer textures or room temperature food, and will often prefer sweetened foods, including entrees. Preferred nutrient-dense meals and snacks should be provided on a 24 hour basis, in a pleasant and non-distracting environment. It may be appropriate for some patients to maintain modest dysphagia precautions, such as giving small bites of food, avoiding crumbly textures and encouraging upright posture and a chin tuck; patients will rarely tolerate thickened liquids[2,3]. Finally, there is a very limited role for appetite stimulants. Dronabinol and mirtazapine are probably best tolerated and may modestly improve intake and family satisfaction, although weight and lean body mass gain is rare[93,94].

Medical management

Intercurrent illness is a constant threat in advanced dementia, and the best care will be highly individualized. For every illness or health crisis, evaluation and treatment will be dependent on the tolerability of the evaluation, the likelihood that the evaluation will yield a treatment that will improve comfort and quality of life, the tolerability of that treatment, and above all, patient and family preference. As such, standing "comfort measures only" order sets are rarely adequate to meet the patient's and family's needs. It should be remembered that ED visits and hospitalizations are frightening to patients and rarely improve overall comfort[2,19,74]. Hospitalizations are still quite common, though; a 2022 study found that patients with dementia spent on average 19.6% of their last six months of life in a hospital[95].

Medication administration is often difficult in the resistive or lethargic patient. All medications should be continually reviewed, and those not likely to provide comfort in the estimated time remaining should be discontinued (acetylcholinesterase inhibitors and memantine are almost certainly unhelpful at this point). A compounding pharmacist can be quite helpful in formulating alternative routes of administration. Hypodermoclysis (subcutaneous infusion) is often an attractive option[2,96,97]; it is much simpler to implement than an intravenous line, often better tolerated (it can be placed in relatively inaccessible areas, such as medial to the scapula, to discourage dislodgement), is not associated with sepsis or thrombosis, and can be used to administer many medications, including morphine, haloperidol, lorazepam and furosemide. Hypodermoclysis can also be used for hydration, although this is rarely warranted.

As in most terminal conditions, poor fluid intake and dehydration are almost inevitable. Enteral or parenteral hydration may occasionally help with alertness and ability to interact with family and may decrease the risk of OIN, but can also cause edema and dyspnea and may be perceived as merely prolonging the dying process[98,99]. As such, it is rarely justified and if attempted should be done as a time-limited trial.

Advanced dementia is associated with both macro- and microaspiration[100]; about 70% of patients die from pneumonia[74,101-103], and when treated it generally recurs quickly. Again, family education about its inevitability as a consequence of "brain failure" is of paramount importance. Dyspnea is likely common in advanced dementia, both as a result of pneumonia and of generalized weakness[104]. Treatment of choice will be opioids[2,105]; supplemental oxygen generally only improves comfort in the presence of desaturation. Other measures, such as directing a gentle fan toward the face and avoidance of strong fragrances, may be helpful. Most studies show no survival or comfort benefit with antibiotics[102,106], although there is a single study suggesting a modest comfort benefit only[107].

Seizures will occasionally occur in advanced Alzheimer's disease, mostly in younger patients[108]. These generally respond well to most anticonvulsants; choice is often based on available routes of administration.

Pressure ulcers are also common in endstage dementia and are a poor prognostic indicator. Prevention is difficult, as patients are generally cachectic, immobile and often resistive to turning. Goals will generally be limited to managing pain and preventing infection; healing is rare[2].

Constipation is best managed with a combination of osmotic agents and stimulants, but is often difficult to manage in patients who are resistive to taking oral medications; suppositories and enemas are usually not tolerated well[2]. It is important to avoid constipating medications if possible; opioid-induced (only) constipation can be managed with subcutaneous methylnaltrexone[109]. Oral or enteral hydration can also be helpful if feasible; it is not clear whether parenteral hydration is useful for constipation, but it probably is not.

Bereavement

At the end of a long and difficult road, death is often anticlimactic[2,4,10,19,110,111], much more so in dementia where so much of the individual's identity and roles had been lost well before physical death. Bereavement always starts well before death[2,10,19,111], and in dementia there have been many smaller "deaths" along the way: the first time getting lost, the first time not recognizing a partner or child, the first episode of incontinence[2]. Role changes are difficult but inevitable transitions for loved ones[2,19,110]. Sometimes, there are family conflicts about the patient's affairs or medical care; thorough advance planning and documentation will be essential but frequently insufficient. When death ensues, it is not unusual for most of the grieving to have already been done, and some survivors will feel guilty about the lack of intense grief and feelings of relief that they may have[2,110,111].

There is much that we can do to ease the grief of loved ones left behind. This begins with a skilled palliative approach to the patient, thorough and continual advance planning, honest prognostication, and education about the broad range of normal bereavement reactions and behavior (including the usually anticlimactic and unburdening nature of death). This will generally involve much more listening than talking.

Most survivors cope well, but up to 10% may develop depression or pathological grief[2,110-112]. Warning signs of depression may include persistent guilt, anhedonia, sleep or appetite disturbances, or suicidal ideation. These depressive symptoms may overlap with those of pathological grief, which may also include persistent nightmares, persistent guilt or anger, reluctance to attend the funeral, to dispose of possessions or to speak of the deceased in the past tense[2,110]. Some authors have suggested that pathological grief is actually a form of post-traumatic stress disorder (PTSD)[112]. Survivors with such symptoms may do well with referral for individual or group bereavement counseling, and/or for treatment of depression[2,111,112].

Most predictors of pathological grief are not modifiable, including a poor relationship with the deceased, social isolation, a history of substance abuse or sometimes other psychiatric illness[2]. There is, however, one very modifiable predictor: bearing witness to the unrelieved suffering and struggling death of a loved one[2]. This is a traumatic memory that will never be forgotten, but one that is well within our power as clinicians to prevent. Equipped with knowledge and compassion, we can do much to ensure that our patients live and die with peace and dignity, leaving a positive legacy for those whom they leave behind.

References

1. 2021 Alzheimer's disease facts and figures. Alzheimers Dement 2021; 17:327-406.
2. Sekerak RJ, Stewart JT. Caring for the patient with end-stage dementia. Ann Long Term Care 2014; 22(12):36-43.
3. Hashimie J, Schultz SK, Stewart JT. Palliative care for dementia: 2020 Update. Clin Geriatr Med 2020; 36:329-339.
4. Wolf-Klein G, Pekmezaris R, Chin L, Weiner J. Conceptualizing Alzheimer's disease as a terminal medical illness. Am J Hosp Palliat Care 2007; 24:77-82.
5. Hanrahan P, Luchins DJ. Access to hospice programs in end-stage dementia: a national survey of hospice programs. J Am Geriatr Soc 1995; 43:56-59.
6. National Hospice and Palliative Care Organization. NCHPO Facts and Figures, 2020 Edition. www.nhpco.org/hospice-facts-figures, accessed 28 Jul 2022.
7. Shuster JL. Palliative care for advanced dementia. Clin Geriatr Med 2000; 16:373-386.
8. Mitchell SL, Miller SC, Teno JM, Kiely DK, Davis RB, Shaffer ML. Prediction of 6-month survival of nursing home residents with advanced dementia using ADEPT vs hospice eligibility guidelines. JAMA 2010; 304:1929-1935.

9. Harrison KL, Hunt LJ, Ritchie CS, Yaffe K. Dying with dementia: underrecognized and stigmatized. J Am Geriatr Soc 2019; 67:1548-1551.
10. Sampson EL. Palliative care for people with dementia. Br Med Bull 2010; 96:159-174.
11. Lee EE, Chang B, Huege S, Hirst J. Complex clinical intersection: palliative care in patients with dementia. Am J Geriatr Psychiatry 2018; 26:224-234.
12. Aminoff BZ, Adunsky A. Their last 6 months: suffering and survival of end-stage dementia patients. Age Ageing 2006; 35:597-601.
13. Soares LGL, Japiassu AM, Gomes LC, Pereira R, Peçanha C, Goldgaber T. Prevalence and intensity of dyspnea, pain, and agitation among people dying with late stage dementia compared with people dying with advanced cancer: a single-center preliminary study in Brazil. Ann Palliat Med 2018; 7:437-443.
14. Kumar V, Ankuda CK, Aldridge MD, Husain M, Ornstein KA. Family caregiving at the end of life and hospice use: a national study of Medicare beneficiaries. J Am Geriatr Soc 2020; 68:2288-2296.
15. Agüero-Torres H, Fratiglioni L, Winblad B. Natural history of Alzheimer's disease and other dementias: review of the literature in the light of the findings from the Kungsholmen Project. Int J Geriatr Psychiatry 1998; 13:755-766.
16. Rothenberg LR, Doberman D, Simon LE, Gryczynski J, Cordts G. Patients surviving six months in hospice care: who are they? J Palliat Med 2014; 17:899-905.
17. Hunt LJ, Gan S, Boscardin WJ, Yaffe K, Ritchie CS, Aldridge MD, Smith AK. A national study of disenrollment from hospice among people with dementia. J Am Geriatr Soc 2022 Jun 7. doi: 10.1111/jgs.17912. Epub ahead of print.
18. Luth EA, Russell DJ, Xu JC, Lauder B, Ryvicker MB, Dignam RR, Baughn R, Bowles KH, Prigerson HG. Survival in hospice patients with dementia: the effect of home hospice and nurse visits. J Am Geriatr Soc 2021; 69:1529-1538.
19. Sachs GA, Shega JW, Cox-Hayley D. Barriers to excellent end-of-life care for patients with dementia. J Gen Intern Med 2004; 19:1057-1063.
20. Luchins DJ, Hanrahan P, Murphy K. Criteria for enrolling dementia patients in hospice. J Am Geriatr Soc 1997; 45:1054-1059.
21. Reisberg B. Functional assessment staging (FAST). Psychopharmacol Bull 1988; 24:653-659.
22. Tarazona-Santabalbina FJ, Belenguer-Varea Á, Rovira Daudi E, Salcedo Mahiques E, Cuesta Peredó D, Doménech-Pascual JR, Gac

Espínola H, Avellana Zaragoza JA. Severity of cognitive impairment as a prognostic factor for mortality and functional recovery of geriatric patients with hip fracture. Geriatr Gerontol Int 2015; 15:289-295.

23. Chouinard J, Lavigne E, Villeneuve C. Weight loss, dysphagia, and outcome in advanced dementia. Dysphagia 1998; 13:151-155.
24. Mitchell SL, Teno JM, Kiely DK, Shaffer ML, Jones RN, Prigerson HG, Volicer L, Givens JL, Hamel MB. The clinical course of advanced dementia. N Engl J Med 2009; 361:1529-1538.
25. Gabbard J, Johnson D, Russell G, Spencer S, Williamson JD, McLouth LE, Ferris KG, Sink K, Brenes G, Yang M. Prognostic awareness, disease and palliative understanding among caregivers of patients with dementia. Am J Hosp Palliat Care 2020; 37:683-691.
26. Yadav KN, Gabler NB, Cooney E, Kent S, Kim J, Herbst N, Mante A, Halpern SD, Courtright KR. Approximately one in three US adults completes any type of advance directive for end-of-life care. Health Aff (Millwood) 2017; 36:1244-1251.
27. Gotanda H, Walling AM, Reuben DB, Lauzon M, Tsugawa Y. Trends in advance care planning and end-of-life care among persons living with dementia requiring surrogate decision-making. J Am Geriatr Soc 2022; 70:1394-1404.
28. Hanson LC, Kistler CE, Lavin K, Gabriel SL, Ernecoff NC, Lin FC, Sachs GA, Mitchell SL. Triggered palliative care for late-stage dementia: a pilot randomized trial. J Pain Symptom Manage 2019; 57:10-19.
29. Hochwald IH, Yakov G, Radomyslsky Z, Danon Y, Nissanholtz-Gannot R. Ethical challenges in end-stage dementia: perspectives of professionals and family care-givers. Nurs Ethics 2021; 28:1228-1243.
30. Steinberg M, Hess K, Corcoran C, Mielke MM, Norton M, Breitner J, Green R, Leoutsakos J, Welsh-Bohmer K, Lyketsos C, Tschanz J. Vascular risk factors and neuropsychiatric symptoms in Alzheimer's disease: the Cache County Study. Int J Geriatr Psychiatry 2014; 29:153-159.
31. Yang Y, Kandiah N, Kim S, Kwak YT. Clinical aspects of neurobehavioral symptoms of dementia. Dement Neurocogn Disord 2020; 19:54-64.
32. Teri L, Larson EB, Reifler BV. Behavioral disturbance in dementia of the Alzheimer's type. J Am Geriatr Soc 1988; 36:1-6.
33. Breitbart W, Alici Y. Agitation and delirium at the end of life: "We couldn't manage him". JAMA 2008; 300:2898-2910.

34. Knoepfel S, Bode L, Gehrke S, Spiller T, Fuchs S, Ernst J, von Känel R, Boettger S. Delirium at the end of life. Palliat Support Care 2021; 19:268-273.
35. Watt CL, Momoli F, Ansari MT, Sikora L, Bush SH, Hosie A, Kabir M, Rosenberg E, Kanji S, Lawlor PG. The incidence and prevalence of delirium across palliative care settings: a systematic review. Palliat Med 2019; 33:865-877.
36. Boettger S, Jenewein J, Breitbart W. Delirium in advanced age and dementia: a prolonged refractory course of delirium and lower functional status. Palliat Support Care 2015; 13:1113-1121.
37. Inouye SK, van Dyck CH, Alessi CA, Balkin S, Siegal AP, Horwitz RI. Clarifying confusion: the confusion assessment method. A new method for detection of delirium. Ann Intern Med 1990; 113:941-948.
38. Kiely DK, Marcantonio ER, Inouye SK, Shaffer ML, Bergmann MA, Yang FM, Fearing MA, Jones RN. Persistent delirium predicts greater mortality. J Am Geriatr Soc 2009; 57:55-61.
39. Romem A, Tom SE, Beauchene M, Babington L, Scharf SM, Romem A. Pain management at the end of life: a comparative study of cancer, dementia, and chronic obstructive pulmonary disease patients. Palliat Med 2015; 29:464-469.
40. Graham F, Beattie E, Fielding E. Hospital nurses' management of agitation in older cognitively impaired patients: do they recognise pain-related agitation? Age Ageing 2022; 51:afac140.
41. Stewart JT, Gonzalez-Perez E, Zhu Y, Robinson BE. Cognitive predictors of resistiveness in dementia patients. Am J Geriatr Psychiatry 1999; 7:259-263.
42. Salami O, Lyketsos C, Rao V. Treatment of sleep disturbance in Alzheimer's dementia. Int J Geriatr Psychiatry 2011; 26:771-782.
43. Bush SH, Bruera E. The assessment and management of delirium in cancer patients. Oncologist 2009; 14:1039-1049.
44. Snow AL, O'malley KJ, Cody M, Kunik ME, Ashton CM, Beck C, Bruera E, Novy D. A conceptual model of pain assessment for noncommunicative persons with dementia. Gerontologist 2004; 44:807-817.
45. Moryl N, Kogan M, Comfort C, Obbens E. Methadone in the treatment of pain and terminal delirum in advanced cancer patients. Palliat Support Care 2005; 3:311-317.
46. Mercadante S, Bruera E. Opioid switching: a systematic and critical review. Cancer Treat Rev 2006; 32:304-315.

47. Swart LM, van der Zanden V, Spies PE, de Rooij SE, van Munster BC. The comparative risk of delirium with different opioids: a systematic review. Drugs Aging 2017; 34:437-443.
48. Ernecoff NC, Lin FC, Wessell KL, Hanson LC. Quality of life with late-stage dementia: exploring opportunities to intervene. J Am Geriatr Soc 2019; 67:1189-1196.
49. Volicer L. Review of programs for persons facing death with dementia. Healthcare (Basel) 2019; 7:62.
50. Yu A, Wu S, Zhang Z, Dening T, Zhao S, Pinner G, Xia J, Yang D. Cholinesterase inhibitors for the treatment of delirium in non-ICU settings. Cochrane Database Syst Rev 2018; 6:CD012494.
51. Breitbart W, Marotta R, Platt MM, Weisman H, Derevenco M, Grau C, Corbera K, Raymond S, Lund S, Jacobson P. A double-blind trial of haloperidol, chlorpromazine, and lorazepam in the treatment of delirium in hospitalized AIDS patients. Am J Psychiatry 1996; 153:231-237.
52. Tahir TA. A review for usefulness of atypical antipsychotics and cholinesterase inhibitors in delirium. Pharmacopsychiatry 2012; 45:163.
53. Grassi L, Caraceni A, Mitchell AJ, Nanni MG, Berardi MA, Caruso R, Riba M. Management of delirium in palliative care: a review. Curr Psychiatry Rep 2015; 17:550.
54. Hui D, Dev R, Bruera E. Neuroleptics in the management of delirium in patients with advanced cancer. Curr Opin Support Palliat Care 2016; 10:316-323.
55. Hui D, De La Rosa A, Wilson A, Nguyen T, Wu J, Delgado-Guay M, Azhar A, Arthur J, Epner D, Haider A, De La Cruz M, Heung Y, Tanco K, Dalal S, Reddy A, Williams J, Amin S, Armstrong TS, Breitbart W, Bruera E. Neuroleptic strategies for terminal agitation in patients with cancer and delirium at an acute palliative care unit: a single-centre, double-blind, parallel-group, randomised trial. Lancet Oncol 2020; 21:989-998.
56. Maeda I, Ogawa A, Yoshiuchi K, Akechi T, Morita T, Oyamada S, Yamaguchi T, Imai K, Sakashita A, Matsumoto Y, Uemura K, Nakahara R, Iwase S; Phase-R Delirium Study Group. Safety and effectiveness of antipsychotic medication for delirium in patients with advanced cancer: a large-scale multicenter prospective observational study in real-world palliative care settings. Gen Hosp Psychiatry 2020; 67:35-41.

57. Sera L, McPherson ML, Holmes HM. Commonly prescribed medications in a population of hospice patients. Am J Hosp Palliat Care 2014; 31:126-131.
58. Beach SR, Gross AF, Hartney KE, Taylor JB, Rundell JR. Intravenous haloperidol: A systematic review of side effects and recommendations for clinical use. Gen Hosp Psychiatry 2020; 67:42-50.
59. Elsayem A, Bush SH, Munsell MF, Curry E 3rd, Calderon BB, Paraskevopoulos T, Fadul N, Bruera E. Subcutaneous olanzapine for hyperactive or mixed delirium in patients with advanced cancer: a preliminary study. J Pain Symptom Manage 2010; 40:774-782.
60. McIver B, Walsh D, Nelson K. The use of chlorpromazine for symptom control in dying cancer patients. J Pain Symptom Manage 1994: 9:341-345.
61. Gerlach LB, Fashaw S, Strominger J, Ogarek J, Zullo AR, Daiello LA, Teno J, Shireman TI, Bynum JPW. Trends in antipsychotic prescribing among long-term care residents receiving hospice care. J Am Geriatr Soc 2021; 69:2152-2162.
62. Clegg A, Young JB. Which medications to avoid in people at risk of delirium: a systematic review. Age Ageing 2011; 40:23-29.
63. Masopust J, Protopopová D, Vališ M, Pavelek Z, Klímová B. Treatment of behavioral and psychological symptoms of dementias with psychopharmaceuticals: a review. Neuropsychiatr Dis Treat 2018; 14:1211-1220.
64. Hui D, Frisbee-Hume S, Wilson A, Dibaj SS, Nguyen T, De La Cruz M, Walker P, Zhukovsky DS, Delgado-Guay M, Vidal M, Epner D, Reddy A, Tanco K, Williams J, Hall S, Liu D, Hess K, Amin S, Breitbart W, Bruera E. Effect of lorazepam with haloperidol vs haloperidol alone on agitated delirium in patients with advanced cancer receiving palliative care: a randomized clinical trial. JAMA 2017; 318:1047-1056.
65. Hui D. Benzodiazepines for agitation in patients with delirium: selecting the right patient, right time, and right indication. Curr Opin Support Palliat Care 2018; 12:489-494.
66. Howard P, Twycross R, Shuster J, Mihalyo M, Wilcock A. Benzodiazepines. J Pain Symptom Manage 2014; 47:955-964.
67. Stirling LC, Kurowska A, Tookman A. The use of phenobarbitone in the management of agitation and seizures at the end of life. J Pain Symptom Manage 1999; 17:363-368.
68. Hosgood JR, Kimbrel JM, McCrate Protus B, Grauer PA. Evaluation of subcutaneous phenobarbital administration in hospice patients. Am J Hosp Palliat Care 2016; 33:209-213.

69. Prommer E. Review article: dexmedetomidine: does it have potential in palliative medicine? Am J Hosp Palliat Care 2011; 28:276-283.
70. Thomas B, Lo WA, Nangati Z, Barclay G. Dexmedetomidine for hyperactive delirium at the end of life: an open-label single arm pilot study with dose escalation in adult patients admitted to an inpatient palliative care unit. Palliat Med 2021; 35:729-737.
71. Maltoni M, Scarpi E, Rosati M, Derni S, Fabbri L, Martini F, Amadori D, Nanni O. Palliative sedation in end-of-life care and survival: a systematic review. J Clin Oncol 2012; 30:1378-1383.
72. Arantzamendi M, Belar A, Payne S, Rijpstra M, Preston N, Menten J, Van der Elst M, Radbruch L, Hasselaar J, Centeno C. Clinical aspects of palliative sedation in prospective studies. A systematic review. J Pain Symptom Manage 2021; 61:831-844.
73. Monroe TB, Carter MA, Feldt KS, Dietrich MS, Cowan RL. Pain and hospice care in nursing home residents with dementia and terminal cancer. Geriatr Gerontol Int 2013; 13:1018-1025.
74. Morrison RS, Siu AL. A comparison of pain and its treatment in advanced dementia and cognitively intact patients with hip fracture. J Pain Symptom Manage 2000; 19:240-248.
75. Farrell MJ, Katz B, Helme RD. The impact of dementia on the pain experience. Pain 1996; 67:7-15.
76. Scherder E, Oosterman J, Swaab D, Herr K, Ooms M, Ribbe M, Sergeant J, Pickering G, Benedetti F. Recent developments in pain in dementia. BMJ 2005; 330:461-464.
77. Haasum Y, Fastbom J, Fratiglioni L, Kåreholt I, Johnell K. Pain treatment in elderly persons with and without dementia: a population-based study of institutionalized and home-dwelling elderly. Drugs Aging 2011; 28:283-293.
78. Zwakhalen SM, Hamers JP, Abu-Saad HH, Berger MP. Pain in elderly people with severe dementia: a systematic review of behavioural pain assessment tools. BMC Geriatr 2006; 6:3.
79. Johnson DK, Wilkins CH, Morris JC. Accelerated weight loss may precede diagnosis in Alzheimer disease. Arch Neurol 2006; 63:1312-1317.
80. Minaglia C, Giannotti C, Boccardi V, Mecocci P, Serafini G, Odetti P, Monacelli F. Cachexia and advanced dementia. J Cachexia Sarcopenia Muscle 2019; 10:263-277.
81. Smith KL, Greenwood CE. Weight loss and nutritional considerations in Alzheimer disease. J Nutr Elder 2008; 27:381-403.

82. von Haehling S, Anker SD. Cachexia as a major underestimated and unmet medical need: facts and numbers. J Cachexia Sarcopenia Muscle 2010; 1:1-5.
83. Perry RT, Collins JS, Wiener H, Acton R, Go RC. The role of TNF and its receptors in Alzheimer's disease. Neurobiol Aging 2001; 22:873-883.
84. Michaud M, Balardy L, Moulis G, Gaudin C, Peyrot C, Vellas B, Cesari M, Nourhashemi F. Proinflammatory cytokines, aging, and age-related diseases. J Am Med Dir Assoc 2013; 14:877-882.
85. Miwa K, Okazaki S, Sakaguchi M, Mochizuki H, Kitagawa K. Interleukin-6, interleukin-6 receptor gene variant, small-vessel disease and incident dementia. Eur J Neurol 2016; 23:656-663.
86. Palecek EJ, Teno JM, Casarett DJ, Hanson LC, Rhodes RL, Mitchell SL. Comfort feeding only: a proposal to bring clarity to decision-making regarding difficulty with eating for persons with advanced dementia. J Am Geriatr Soc 2010; 58:580-584.
87. Teno JM, Mitchell SL, Kuo SK, Gozalo PL, Rhodes RL, Lima JC, Mor V. Decision-making and outcomes of feeding tube insertion: a five-state study. J Am Geriatr Soc 2011; 59:881-886.
88. Mitchell SL, Kiely DK, Lipsitz LA. The risk factors and impact on survival of feeding tube placement in nursing home residents with severe cognitive impairment. Arch Intern Med 1997; 157:327-332.
89. Finucane TE, Christmas C, Travis K. Tube feeding in patients with advanced dementia: a review of the evidence. JAMA 1999; 282:1365-1370.
90. Ayman AR, Khoury T, Cohen J, Chen S, Yaari S, Daher S, Benson AA, Mizrahi M. PEG insertion in patients with dementia does not improve nutritional status and has worse outcomes as compared with PEG insertion for other indications. J Clin Gastroenterol 2017; 51:417-420.
91. Yuen JK, Luk JKH, Chan TC, Shea YF, Chu ST, Bernacki R, Chow DTY, Chan FHW. Reduced pneumonia risk in advanced dementia patients on careful hand feeding compared with nasogastric tube feeding. J Am Med Dir Assoc 2022 Apr 27:S1525-8610(22)00255-9. Epub ahead of print.
92. Mitchell SL, Mor V, Gozalo PL, Servadio JL, Teno JM. Tube feeding in US nursing home residents with advanced dementia, 2000-2014. JAMA 2016; 316:769-770.
93. Fox CB, Treadway AK, Blaszczyk AT, Sleeper RB. Megestrol acetate and mirtazapine for the treatment of unplanned weight loss in the elderly. Pharmacotherapy 2009; 29:383-397.

94. Howard ML, Hossaini R, Tolar C, Gaviola ML. Efficacy and safety of appetite-stimulating medications in the inpatient setting. Ann Pharmacother 2019; 53:261-267.
95. Yorganci E, Stewart R, Sampson EL, Sleeman KE. Patterns of unplanned hospital admissions among people with dementia: from diagnosis to the end of life. Age Ageing 2022; 51:afac098.
96. Rochon PA, Gill SS, Litner J, Fischbach M, Goodison AJ, Gordon M. A systematic review of the evidence for hypodermoclysis to treat dehydration in older people. J Gerontol A Biol Sci Med Sci 1997; 52:M169-176.
97. Fonzo-Christe C, Vukasovic C, Wasilewski-Rasca AF, Bonnabry P. Subcutaneous administration of drugs in the elderly: survey of practice and systematic literature review. Palliat Med 2005; 19:208-219.
98. Nakajima N, Hata Y, Kusumuto K. A clinical study on the influence of hydration volume on the signs of terminally ill cancer patients with abdominal malignancies. J Palliat Med 2013; 16:185-189.
99. Wu CY, Chen PJ, Ho TL, Lin WY, Cheng SY. To hydrate or not to hydrate? The effect of hydration on survival, symptoms and quality of dying among terminally ill cancer patients. BMC Palliat Care 2021; 20:13.
100. Matsuse T, Oka T, Kida K, Fukuchi Y. Importance of diffuse aspiration bronchiolitis caused by chronic occult aspiration in the elderly. Chest 1996; 110:1289-1293.
101. Keene J, Hope T, Fairburn CG, Jacoby R. Death and dementia. Int J Geriatr Psychiatry 2001; 16:969-974.
102. Givens JL, Jones RN, Shaffer ML, Kiely DK, Mitchell SL. Survival and comfort after treatment of pneumonia in advanced dementia. Arch Intern Med 2010; 170:1102-1107.
103. Manabe T, Mizukami K, Akatsu H, Hashizume Y, Ohkubo T, Kudo K, Hizawa N. Factors associated with pneumonia-caused death in older adults with autopsy-confirmed dementia. Intern Med 2017; 56:907-914.
104. Hendriks SA, Smalbrugge M, Galindo-Garre F, Hertogh CM, van der Steen JT. From admission to death: prevalence and course of pain, agitation, and shortness of breath, and treatment of these symptoms in nursing home residents with dementia. J Am Med Dir Assoc 2015; 16:475-481.
105. Elia G, Thomas J. The symptomatic relief of dyspnea. Curr Oncol Rep 2008; 10:319-325.
106. van der Maaden T, van der Steen JT, de Vet HC, Hertogh CM, Koopmans RT. Prospective observations of discomfort, pain, and

dyspnea in nursing home residents with dementia and pneumonia. J Am Med Dir Assoc 2016; 17:128-135.

107. Van Der Steen JT, Pasman HR, Ribbe MW, Van Der Wal G, Onwuteaka-Philipsen BD. Discomfort in dementia patients dying from pneumonia and its relief by antibiotics. Scand J Infect Dis 2009; 41:143-151.
108. Xu Y, Lavrencic L, Radford K, Booth A, Yoshimura S, Anstey KJ, Anderson CS, Peters R. Systematic review of coexistent epileptic seizures and Alzheimer's disease: incidence and prevalence. J Am Geriatr Soc 2021; 69:2011-2020.
109. Mozaffari S, Nikfar S, Abdollahi M. Methylnaltrexone bromide for the treatment of opioid-induced constipation. Expert Opin Pharmacother 2018; 19:1127-1135.
110. Noyes BB, Hill RD, Hicken BL, Luptak M, Rupper R, Dailey NK, Bair BD. The role of grief in dementia caregiving. Am J Alzheimers Dis Other Demen 2010; 25:9-17.
111. Hovland C. Welcoming death: exploring pre-death grief experiences of caregivers of older adults with dementia. J Soc Work End Life Palliat Care 2018; 14:274-290.
112. Maercker A, Lalor J. Diagnostic and clinical considerations in prolonged grief disorder. Dialogues Clin Neurosci 2012; 14:167-176.

20

PALLIATIVE CARE FOR PATIENTS WITH ADVANCED DEMENTIA IN LOW- AND MIDDLE-INCOME COUNTRIES: STATUS AND A FUTURE AGENDA

RICHARD A. POWELL[1], DR EVE NAMISANGO[2], DR SEGGANE MUSISI[3], DR SHEETAL RAJ[4], DR ALBERTO PÉREZ-MEDINA[5] AND DR TANIA PASTRANA[6]

Introduction

Increasing life expectancy has contributed to an aging world population (Sander et al., 2015), with those aged 65+ accounting for nearly a fifth of 'more developed' country populations in 2020 (Population Reference Bureau, 2020). By 2050 the worldwide population of older persons is projected to more than double its size from 2015, reaching nearly 2.1 billion, with the 'oldest old' numbering 434 million, tripling since 2015 (United Nations, Department of Economic and Social Affairs, Population Division

[1] Evaluation and Project Manager, Ethnicity and Health Unit, Department of Primary Care and Public Health, Imperial College London, London, England
[2] Research Manager, African Palliative Care Association, Kampala, Uganda
[3] Professor of Psychiatry, Department of Psychiatry, School of Medicine, Makerere University College of Health Sciences, Kampala, Uganda
[4] Associate Professor, Department of Medicine, Kasturba Medical College, Manipal Academy of Higher Education, Mangalore, India
[5] Consultant Psychiatrist and retired professor, Universidad del Quindío, Colombia
[6] Department of Palliative Medicine, Medical Faculty, RWTH Aachen University, Aachen, Germany

[UN], 2015). This demographic shift will be a significant driver of economic and social transformation, potentially affecting family structures, intergenerational connections and models of health care provision (UN, 2015), and mark an epidemiological transition to increased morbidity and mortality from non-communicable and age-related diagnoses (Phillips, 1994), including dementia.

Dementia is a syndrome comprised of an incurable deterioration in an individual's memory, thinking, behaviour and physical functioning (Mattap et al., 2022), with an illness trajectory characterised by progressive decline. Advanced dementia follows a more ambiguous disease trajectory, with transitions from mild-to-moderate advanced dementia to advanced dementia lacking in predictability. The prevalence, impact and financial cost of dementia has been overwhelmingly studied in high-income countries (HICs), despite more than two-thirds of the nearly 50 million people with dementia globally living in low- and middle-income countries (LMICs) (Prince, 2015; Wimo et al., 2017), where rapid demographic aging is occurring. The global cost of dementia—US$818 billion in 2015, projected to reach US$2 trillion by 2030 (Prince, 2015; Wimo et al., 2017)—is overwhelmingly accounted for by HICs, with the much lower financial estimates in LMICs compromised by limited economic studies (Mattap et al., 2022).

Growing evidence indicates that, given its incurability and symptomatology similar to other progressive, life-threatening illnesses, palliation and supportive care could positively manage advanced dementia for patients and affected families. In this way, palliative care—the active holistic care of individuals across all ages with serious health-related suffering (SHS) due to severe illness and especially of those near the end of life (Radbruch et al., 2020)—would potentially have applicability in reducing SHS and symptom burden, minimising overtreatment with unnecessary interventions, improving patients' and families' quality of life, and reducing caregiver burden on the latter.

However, minimal work has been undertaken exploring existing, and the potential for future, palliative care provision to alleviate suffering among this vulnerable group in LMICs. In many of these countries, residency in nursing home facilities and access to specialist palliative and hospice care that characterise advanced dementia care in some HICs (Sternberg et al., 2021) are non-existent. In these LMICs, availability of effective pain analgesics is typically much less common, familial support networks vary across cultures, palliative care services are less prevalent and developed, and have focused care provision on communicable (e.g., HIV/AIDS) and non-communicable diseases (NCDs) to the relative neglect of age-related progressive illnesses.

This chapter therefore first outlines existing palliative care service provision in three LMIC settings—Africa, South Asia (especially India), and Latin America (especially Colombia)—before highlighting generic challenges to potential palliative care responses to advanced dementia and localised challenges.

Palliative care services in LMICs

Globally the burden of SHS is projected to almost double by 2060, to 48 million people (47 percent of all deaths) (Sleeman et al., 2019). Over four-fifths of these deaths will occur in LMICs, with the largest proportional rise in SHS occurring in low-income countries (i.e., a 155 percent increase between 2016 and 2060) (Sleeman et al., 2019). Despite calls for global action to address this projected illness burden as an ethical and economic imperative, the development and integration of palliative care into health systems remains a divisive "access abyss" (Knaul et al., 2018), especially evident in LMICs.

In the latest global review of palliative care service provision, supporting policies, education and funding (Clark et al., 2020), the "patchy" palliative care development described by the authors is echoed across this chapter's target settings. Colombia is classified as having generalised palliative care provision (category 3b), and India is grouped under isolated palliative care provision (category 3a). While nine African countries are classified as either generalised provision (Gambia, Kenya and Zambia), a preliminary stage of integration with health systems (category 4a; Côte d'Ivoire, South Africa, Uganda and Zimbabwe) or as at an advanced integration stage (category 4b; countries being Malawi and Swaziland), the overwhelming majority have either isolated provision, capacity-building activities or no known activity. These contrasting developmental stages of palliative care provision inevitably have implications for the ability—in terms of technical skills, capacity and coverage—to address life-limiting illnesses generally, and advanced dementia specifically.

Sub-Saharan Africa

Prevalence

While the vast majority of Africa's population is young—almost 80 percent are below 30 years old (National Research Council, 2006)—the fastest growing portion is those aged 60 years and above (Prince et al., 2016; Apt, 2009). Studies in Uganda among older persons visiting hospital report depression and dementia are the most encountered neuropsychiatric problems, with prevalence rates of 13.2 (dementia), 24.4 (depression), and 28.4 percent (dementia) (Atim et al., 2021; Nakasujja et al., 2007). In a study conducted in a Nigerian nursing home, 48 percent of the population were diagnosed as having dementia (Baiyewu, Adeyemi and Ogunniyi, 1997), while in a South African community-based survey among people aged 65 and over, a prevalence of 11 percent was reported (de Jager et al., 2017). In contrast, much lower prevalence rates have been found in North and other West African countries; prevalence in Egypt among those aged 50 and above was found to be 2.3 percent (El Tallawy et al., 2012), and only 2.6 percent in a study conducted in rural Benin (Guerchet et al., 2009). This variation in prevalence estimates is in part explained by the criteria and screening methods employed (Cao et al., 2020) but does not negate the growing concern for dementia's incidence and prevalence on the continent.

Policies and frameworks

The World Health Organisation (WHO) (2017) notes that dementia requires a multi-sectoral response from all key stakeholders, including the health and social care system—public and private—and other government sectors. Such a response helps governments coordinate and respond to the complex symptoms and concerns faced by affected patients. The WHO developed a global action plan for the public health response to dementia, with the setting up of policies, guidelines, and strategy frameworks—be they stand-alone or integrated in existing documents—one of the necessary actions. Seventy five percent of countries globally were meant to have developed or updated their national policies, strategies or frameworks accordingly. As of 2020, slow progress in making these changes was reported, with only a few African countries (i.e., Ethiopia, Ghana, Kenya and South Africa) having strategies that are, however, not yet operationalized, while other sub-Saharan African countries have no known policies or strategies (Ddumba, 2020).

Service provision and staff capacity

The level of palliative care service development in Africa has been on the increase (Rhee et al., 2018). Models of service delivery include hospices, home-based care, and hospital-based palliative care. Notable challenges include a lack of access to essential medicines commonly used in palliative care, lack of a critical mass for staff to deliver care, lack of policies to support the integration of palliative care into health systems, and the lack of awareness about palliative care *per se*.

Palliative psychiatry aims at reducing symptoms, misery and suffering rather than seeking cure or remission (Musisi, 2022). Psychiatric and palliative care are both grounded in the biopsychosocial model, operating within multi-professional and multidisciplinary teams, that involve families in the care giving process (Prince et al., 2016; Musisi, 2022). Most African palliative care services have not yet, however, integrated mental health services into their service models; consequently, most patients rely on referrals to tertiary mental health care centres (e.g., Butabika referral hospital in Uganda). This results in fragmented rather than comprehensive care for patients and their affected families. In Zimbabwe, however, innovative models using lay workers have been found to be effective in detecting mental health disorders in people living with HIV (Chibanda et al., 2015), and these models are potentially scalable to palliative care settings for people with dementia.

Indeed, it is the impact of the progressive, degenerative and terminal impact of dementia, and patients increased dependency upon informal caregivers for their complex symptomatic care needs and concerns (Reisberg et al., 1982; Moens, Higginson and Harding, 2014), that necessitates an additional focus on caregivers themselves. Palliative psychiatry not only offers a support system to help patients live as actively as possible until death, but also offers a support system to family members to cope with the patients' illness (Stewart and Schultz, 2018; Musisi, 2022). This entails providing support to families and patients in coping with and accepting the distressing mental and physical symptoms of dementia by affirming life but acknowledging that the illness is progressive and terminal.

Challenges to care provision

Lack of understanding

One of the significant challenges to dementia care provision is the lack of understanding of the diagnosis, with ignorance of the condition, its causes and manifestations resulting in stigmatisation and persecution. For example, in Kenya reports exist of dementia patients being burned as witches, their condition not seen as a part of the aging process but rather as a form of demonic madness threatening others. This lack of awareness is not necessarily limited to general public members. In rural Kenya, Musyimi et al. (2021) reported negative stereotypes of dementia, limited knowledge of the condition, and neglect and abuse of dementia patients, who were seen as a risk to others and described in derogatory terms among dementia carers and healthcare providers, as well as the public.

Familial and financial support systems

In previous generations, the extended family that characterised many African cultures helped ensure the welfare of elderly members, with strong inter-generational familial networks (Guerchet et al., 2009; Stewart and Schultz, 2018). However, many African societies are undergoing rapid demographic and socio-economic transitions, with younger, more economically active populations migrating from villages to towns or migrating overseas as part of the continent's "brain drain" in search of employment.

Across Africa there are often no official social security systems, pensions or universal health insurance. Juxtaposed with what is seen as an alien practice in many African cultures of placing the elderly, with or without dementia, in nursing homes or in hospice care (Stewart and Schultz, 2018), caring for the elderly is left with immediate families, with the caretaker burden primarily being borne by women, younger wives or daughters (Stewart and Schultz, 2018). It has been argued that facing the new African family realities necessitates revisiting the traditional family support system and modifying it to suit the changed lifestyles and realities faced by many Africans today. One example is merging African traditions of caring for the old, as the wise elders who bind society together (Guerchet et al., 2009), with adjustments to domestic settings by building "granny apartments" to ensure dignified and respectful care at the end of their lives (Stewart and Schultz, 2018).

Impact of epidemics

Epidemics and pandemics have taken a significant toll on care for the elderly, especially those with dementia (Musisi, 2022). HIV/AIDS left many elderly people looking after the needs of orphaned grandchildren following the death of their parents, the generation that would have been expected to care for the old. This became more obvious in the COVID-19 pandemic, which exposed gaps in health care. Access to palliative care and mental health services were grossly affected, with this impact compounded for those with complex needs, including those living with advanced dementia and in need of palliative psychiatry.

Training gaps

The limited capacity of existing palliative care services to address the specific needs of advanced dementia patients are compounded by the lack of specific training in the needs of these patients. Palliative care calls for quality communication, disclosure of and sharing the diagnosis, counselling and support to patients and families throughout the progression of the illness, and referral to hospice care when appropriate.

Mental health services should be integrated with palliative care services to help address these needs (Musisi, 2015). However, while a systematic review to identify training interventions for African healthcare workers on mental health reported several education and training courses, the efficacy of the training techniques is inadequate and potentially insufficient to support the integration of mental health into existing health systems generally (Liu et al., 2016), including palliative care services. More positively, best practices exist in HIV programmes where mental health services are provided by lay workers and integrated into HIV services (Chibanda et al., 2015). Palliative care services must endeavour to learn from such success stories. Reciprocally training mental health workers in palliative care approaches and palliative care teams in mental health care is a pressing need to provide more comprehensive services for those with advanced dementia.

South Asia and India

Prevalence

The crude estimated prevalence rate of dementia for South Asia is 3.7 percent (Alzheimer's and Related Disorders Society of India, 2010). An estimated 5.3 million people in India alone above the age of 60 have dementia, equating to one in 27 people (Kumar et al., 2019), with the states of Maharashtra, West Bengal, Andhra Pradesh and Tamil Nadu having the greatest prevalence rates. It is predicted that by 2030, country prevalence will increase to 7.61 million, and to 14.32 million by 2050 (Kumar et al., 2019; Alzheimer's and Related Disorders Society of India, 2010).

Policies and frameworks

The National Program for Palliative Care, launched in 2012, provides operational and financial guidelines for the implementation of palliative care services across the nation through the National Health Mission (NHM), the flagship program for strengthening Indian health services. Established in 2012, the NHM initially focussed on reproductive and child health services. In the past decade it has shifted and upgraded its focus to be more comprehensive and include NCDs, under which elder care and palliative services are listed. Upgraded services have provision for conceptualisation, and the infrastructure, funding and human resource development necessary for the implementation of an advanced dementia care program. However, despite that potential and the possibility of its future seamless inclusion, currently dementia care is not specifically mentioned within the program (National Health Mission, no date).

There are a number of legislative enactments and policies that, while not specifically dedicated to palliative care, impact upon care for people with advanced dementia. For example, the 2017 Mental Health Care Act has provisions for psychiatric advance directives for a person to appoint a nominated representative, consent for treatment and the right to access mental health care. In 2016 India ratified the Rights of Persons with Disabilities Act, which has provisions for: a) guardianship; b) disability welfare and social benefits provision, and; c) the right to access justice. Moreover, the Maintenance and Welfare of Parents and Senior Citizens Act of 2007 makes it obligatory for children / heirs to provide sufficient maintenance to senior citizens. Similarly, the 2011 National Policy for Senior Citizens, and the National Policy on Older Persons from 1999, are comprehensive in their coverage of older adult issues of welfare schemes, financial security, healthcare and nutrition. With the establishment of the Health and Wellness Centre, under the Ayushman Bharat Scheme, the policy environment has never been better placed for the introduction of a care program specifically for dementia care, especially for patients with advanced dementia. However, unless incorporated as a separate care module, dementia care could be left on the peripheries at best, and neglected at worse.

Service provision and staff capacity

In India palliative care has developed as a specialty in the last two decades, and less than 1 percent of its population has access to its approach to care provision (Bag et al., 2020). Most Indian states provide palliative care, but more than two thirds of services are located in the state of Kerala, which constitutes only 3 percent of the country's population (Philip et al., 2018). The NHM has upgraded its primary health centres through the establishment of 150,000 Health and Wellness Centres, which aim to provide an expanded spectrum of services that include elderly and palliative care services. Through this mission, there is provision to train grassroot-level workers—called ASHA workers (i.e., Accredited Social Health Activist)—on all aspects of basic elder care and palliative care. While the coverage is comprehensive and is designed to include all cases eligible for palliative care, it does not specify dementia care as one aspect of service provision. The NHM is working, in tandem with the Indian Association of Palliative Care, to create training modules for palliative care at the community health centre level (Directorate General of Health Services, no date). However, while the staffing infrastructure and training is extensive in its reach and comprehensive in its nature, extending from neonatal care to reproductive health and palliative care, it might not be specifically focussed on dementia care.

Outside of the palliative care field, the Alzheimer's and Related Disorders Society of India is dedicated to developing care and support services for dementia patients and advancing necessary research into the illness. The society's fourteen chapters spread out across the country, along with organizations like HelpAge India, Dignity Foundation, Nightingales Trust, the Dementia Society of Goa, Sangath, Silver Innings Foundation, Christian Medical College Vellore, St. John's Medical College Bangalore and Voluntary Health Services Chennai, are providing care services either alone or in collaboration with others (Alzheimer's and Related Disorders Society of India, 2010).

Only six fully residential facilities exist for dementia care in India (Alzheimer's and Related Disorders Society of India, 2010), all of which are registered as not-for-profit services reliant on financial donations, public contributions and service charges collected from those utilising the facilities. These agencies reflect the efforts of individuals and private bodies working separately within small domains. They lack a single, centralised organisation to coordinate dementia care generally, identify advanced dementia specifically as a priority, and provide the necessary substantive financial support. These organisations, however, which provide specialist experience in dementia care, could be utilised by the Indian government to help in the development of nationwide services for advanced dementia care.

Consequently, a greater proportion of advanced dementia patients' care needs in India is provided by informal carers, most of whom are family members and women. However, as is evident in other parts of the world, there is a gradual eroding of the multi-generational families that provided support networks and their replacement by nuclear families, where women are often employed and increasingly unavailable as caregivers (Kumar et al., 2019). Moreover, the financial dimension to care provision can be prohibitive. The estimated household cost of caring for a person with dementia is Rs29,272 – 95,208 (equivalent to USD$354 – USD$1,152) per household annually in rural areas, and Rs65,755 – 291,933 (USD$795 to USD$3,531) in urban areas (Kumar et al., 2019). Putting these monetary figures in context, the average annual household income of a rural household is Rs167,833 (USD$2,030), while that of an urban household is Rs267,656 (USD$3,237) (Shukla, 2021).

Challenges

Data limitations

Most of the insights into dementia prevalence rates for India has been derived from sparse data (Kumar et al., 2019). There is a significant need for methodologically rigorous epidemiological studies to determine the overall and comparative urban and rural prevalence of dementia and advanced dementia. There are no data available specifically for advanced dementia or regarding utilisation of palliative services by advanced dementia patients and their families, which documents their needs, their variation over the trajectory of the illness, the costs of and satisfaction with service provision, and the cultural and attitudinal factors that potentially manifest in community and facility settings.

Staff training gaps

There is a huge dearth of trained health care professionals needed to care for advanced dementia patients (Kumar et al., 2019). Also, structured dementia care facilities are scarce in India, with the cost of care in such facilities being prohibitively high (Ravindranath and Sundarakumar, 2021). Training programs for doctors and nurses in palliative and geriatric care started in the last decade (Salins, 2015). Due to the lack of financial incentives, these topic subjects are not widely pursued by healthcare workers. However, there has been a burgeoning of training programs for geriatric and palliative care during the last ten years.

Awareness and community mobilisation

There is a need to improve awareness of dementia generally among all stakeholders, from care providers to the communities within which patients and their families live. Dementia is still not recognised as a disease but is instead considered a natural consequence of ageing, with the behavioural and psychological symptoms of the illness often viewed with stigma that can delay seeking needed care (Kumar et al., 2019).

South America and Colombia

Prevalence

The prevalence of dementia across Latin America and the Caribbean (LAC) is growing rapidly. Among people aged 60 and above, it is estimated to grow more than three-fold over the next thirty years, from 6.86 million in 2020 to 9.94 million in 2030, and 19.33 million in 2050 (Xiang et al., 2021), contrasting with stable or declining rates in Europe and North America (GBD 2019 Dementia Forecasting Collaborators, 2022). This implies a disproportionate clinical, social, and economic burden for patients and caregivers, especially women, lower-educated and rural residents, exacerbated by the negative social determinants of health, fragile and fragmented healthcare systems, unstable economies, and multiple inequalities (Baez and Ibáñez, 2016; Ibáñez et al., 2021a; Ibáñez et al., 2021b; Ribeiro et al., 2022).

With more than 50 million people, Colombia is the third most populous country in Latin America, with the number of persons aged >65 years old more than four million (8.2 percent of the total population) (World Bank, 2023). In 2019 the number of people living with dementia in the country was 369,422, and between 2019 and 2050 this number is expected to increase at a rate of 272% (GBD 2019 Dementia Forecasting Collaborators, 2022), contrasted with a minor increase in the age-standardized prevalence of 3.1 percent (GBD 2019 Diseases and Injuries Collaborators, 2020). For the past five years (GBD 2019 Diseases and Injuries Collaborators, 2020; IHME, 2023), dementia has been the fifth leading cause of death in Colombia, accounting for 13,672 deaths (GBD 2019 Collaborators, 2021). In 2019, dementia caused 188 thousand Disability-Adjusted Life Years (DALYs) among all ages, representing an age-standardized rate of DALYs of 336 per 100,000 (GBD 2019 Diseases and Injuries Collaborators, 2020). Using the methodology of the Lancet Commission on Palliative Care and Pain Relief, it is calculated that of the number of persons with dementia in the country, almost 44,000 are experiencing SHS, of which women are 1.4 more times affected than men (Knaul et al., 2018), which may be alleviated with palliative care interventions.

Policies and frameworks

The Pan American Health Organization (PAHO) declared dementia in the elderly as one of the eight key health issues in Latin America, agreeing on an action plan with long-term investments that emphasize improved treatment and comprehensive care and research into the needs of affected people (PAHO, 2015). Colombia has a robust legal framework for the care of persons with dementia through the law for promoting mental health as an integral element of guaranteeing the right to health (Congreso de la República de Colombia, 2013), the signature and ratification of the Inter-American Convention on protecting the human rights of older persons (A-70) through law 2055 10th September 2020 (Congreso de la República de Colombia, 2020) and also the law for palliative care, which includes the provision of palliative care to persons experiencing SHS due to dementia in advanced stages (Congreso de la República de Colombia, 2014). However, dementia is mentioned once in the National Mental Health Program (Ministerio de Salud y Protección Social, 2018) and there is no national plan specifically for dementia. Additionally, the limited allocation of 2 percent of the public health budget to mental health, and the poor implementation of the laws mentioned above, suggest dementia lacks priority in the national policy and program agenda (Buraye and Quijano-Martínez, 2019). This contrasts with other countries in Latin America: Chile (Ministerio de Salud, 2017, Costa Rica (Consejo Nacional de la persona adulta mayor, 2014), Cuba (Bosch et al., 2019), Dominican Republic (Ministerio de Salud Pública, 2020), Mexico (Gutiérrez and Arrieta, 2014) and Peru (Presidente de la República, 2018) have national plans on dementia, while those from Dominica Republic and Mexico include palliative care. There are, however, gaps between public policy and implementation.

The legalization of assisted dying by The Constitutional Court of Colombia, opened the question of the availability of medical assistance in dying for patients with dementia, given that dementia can be viewed as intolerable, and causing SHS, especially when leading to physical, emotional, and financial dependency on others.

Challenges

Delayed detection

The actual prevalence of missed and/or delayed diagnoses of dementia is unknown. Buraye and Quijano-Martínez (2019) estimate that in Colombia less than 10 percent of dementia cases are detected and treated. Initial symptoms are often ignored or normalized by the family and by the healthcare provider. If detected, no classification studies are performed and, as such, often the time to use effective pharmacological and non-pharmacological therapies is missed. Consequently, there is a progression of the disease to advance stages, with intensification in the amount of care needed due to increasing functional dependence. Even then the referral of patients with dementia to palliative care for a multidisciplinary approach is sporadic, impeding the discussion of legal issues and legal representation for decision-making or advance care planning, provision of end-of-life care and bereavement care.

Social impact

Public awareness and knowledge about dementia and palliative care is low in the region. Dementia is not recognised as a disease; rather, ageing is conceived as a negative process associated with physical and mental decline. Commonly, persons with dementia are mainly cared for by families, and sometimes friends and neighbors. Care is time-intensive and emotionally and physically exhausting, people have no prior training and are not reimbursed for it. This is the case in Colombia, partly due to cultural reasons, but also because caregivers are legally responsible for the care of their relatives (Corte Constitucional de Colombia. Sentencia T, 2013).

This challenging situation has relevant and frequently underestimated negative effects on patient and family quality of life, health, and income due to direct and indirect costs, as studies in Chile (Slachevsky et al., 2013) and Brazil (Ferretti et al., 2018) have shown, in the absence of data from Colombia. Sometimes, when the dementia is advanced or severe, the family hires a professional or informal caregiver, but the family must also bear these costs, increasing the already high cost of advanced and end-of-life care.

Dementia and COVID-19

The fragility of health systems and structural inequalities in the region hindered the control of the COVID-19 pandemic (Ibanez and Kosik, 2020). The lack of integration of palliative care, informed consent and advance directives to the protocols for action and hospital admissions of older adults led to an ethical catastrophe regarding the distribution of healthcare resources: a predominance of utilitarian criteria determining patients' chances of survival (Tudela et al., 2022).

In 2021, the region had approximately a fifth of the confirmed cases of COVID-19 and about 30 percent of deaths worldwide, despite having only 8.4 percent of the world's population (Pan American Health Organization, 2021). Although no data in Latin America are available, it is possibly similar to other countries, such as Canada, where a significant portion of those aged 85 years or more who died of COVID-19 in 2020 had dementia (Beauchet and Allali, 2022). Additionally, even if the elderly did not contract COVID-19, they had a high risk of having neuropsychiatric symptoms aggravated by social isolation, psychosocial stressors and disruption in the health system (Beauchet and Allali, 2022; Slomski, 2022).

Future agenda

LMICs are not homogenous blocks but highly heterogenous in nature, with differing stages of economic development, health systems and palliative care services with differing requirements for their further advance. A reasonable future, cross-cutting agenda for the management of advanced dementia patients by palliative care services in LMICs is, however, multi-dimensional in nature and includes: research; awareness raising; service development and staff training; and supportive policies and frameworks.

Research

There is a need to develop screening tools to help identify people with dementia in communities (Fam, Mahendran and Kua, 2019). While audit measures exist (e.g., the APCA African Palliative Outcome Scale [Harding et al., 2010; Powell et al., 2007]) that can monitor patient symptomatology and quality of life domains over time, there is a need to explore dementia-specific measures and their development in LMIC settings.

More generally, there is a need for good quality research that originates within LMICs themselves that can form the reliable evidence base to inform service and policy development. For example, several global and regional initiatives (Ibañez et al., 2021a; Ibañez et al., 2021b; Sexton et al., 2021; Crivelli, 2020; Washington University School of Medicine, 2023; Chan et al., 2019; Parra et al., 2021; Duran-Aniotz et al., 2022; Eyre et al., 2022) offer a promising conceptual and philosophical framework for research in prevention, diagnosis and intersectoral treatment of dementias in Latin America, which should include palliative care (World Health Organization, 2017). While this evidence base must be observational (e.g., mapping and comparing dementia interventions shown to be effective locally [Salcher-Konrad et al.,, 2019]) and epidemiological in nature, it must also be evaluative, testing interventions for their efficacy, effectiveness and cost implications.

Awareness raising

The ignorance and misunderstanding of dementia as an illness not only adds to delays in accessing health support systems but stigmatises both the affected patient and their family. Campaigns aimed at destigmatising dementia should be coupled with those aimed at increasing knowledge of, and sensitivity to, the illness from its earlier symptoms among the general public and health professionals (Fam, Mahendran and Kua, 2019).

Service provision and staff training

Investing in dedicated dementia services is unrealistic in many LMICs. Equally, expecting over-stretched and poorly funded palliative care services to meet existing and future need for advanced dementia patients is largely misplaced. A way forward for many of these providers is therefore to integrate and broaden palliative care services by including a dementia care component. This component could be developed by engaging in networked partnerships with those agencies that work specifically for and with dementia patients.

Existing community-orientated palliative care services should also be sensitised to, and trained in, the signs of advanced dementia, helping to identify those in need of home-based support and care for individual as well as familial clinical and social needs. This could entail training community volunteers and family members to ensure treatment intervention, continuity and quality of life. This mobilisation of social resources and community volunteers can draw lessons from the successful Kerala model of palliative care, an example of how society and community members can foster interdependence and provide supportive care (Azeez and Anbuselvi, 2021). Moreover, to compensate for the challenges to strained palliative care services, another option to consider for service provision is distance support using mobile apps. These can be highly affordable, as well as culturally and linguistically acceptable, such as the Demensia KITA app being developed in Malaysia (Rashid, et al., 2022).

More generally, while the involvement of people living with dementia in service design and planning is more common in HICs, there is a need for that approach to be adopted in LMICs following the four principles identified by Breuer et al. (2021): 1) respecting the rights of people with dementia to self-determination; 2) valuing people with dementia's unique understanding of the illness; 3) creating a culture of active inclusion that creates space for people with dementia to participate, and; 4) ensuring appropriate accommodations are in place to maximise participation.

Policies and frameworks

To face the burgeoning number of people diagnosed with dementia, and advanced dementia, and the profound impact on people living with the condition, their family and associated networks, and society at large, governments and legislators need to incorporate dementia into national mental health plans, and ensure palliative care is an integral component of all dementia programs and initiatives. It is imperative that the most vulnerable in society–including those with mental health problems who are facing the end of their lives–can access the care they need with palliative care provision.

Conclusions

People with advanced dementia have complex care needs that can benefit from palliative care interventions focussing on reducing symptom burden and SHS, and enhancing existing quality of life. Similarly, family carers of relatives with advanced dementia can gain emotionally, physically and practically from palliative support that addresses information needs at the end of life and support with proxy decision-making. There are, however, multiple challenges to providing effective palliative care service and community support in LMICs where palliative care services themselves are variably developed at best, and non-existent at worst, with limited and uncertain financial models supporting their work.

References

Alzheimer's and Related Disorders Society of India. 2010. *The Dementia India Report: prevalence, impact, costs and services for dementia*. New Delhi: ARDSI.

Apt NA. *Ageing in Africa: Revisiting Traditional Safety Nets*. 2009. University of Ghana, Legon: Center for Social Policy Studies.

Atim LM, Kaggwa MM, Mamun MA, Ashaba S, Maling S. 2021. "Prevalence of Severe Neurocognitive Impairment and its Association with Socio-Demographics and Functionality Among Ugandan Older Persons: A Hospital-Based Study." *Clin Interv Aging* 16: 1415-1425.

Azeez EPA, Anbuselvi G. 2021. "Is the Kerala Model of Community-Based Palliative Care Operations Sustainable? Evidence from the Field." *Indian J Palliat Care* 27 (1): 18-22.

Baez S, Ibáñez A. 2016. "Dementia in Latin America: An Emergent Silent Tsunami." *Front Aging Neurosci* 8: 253.

Bag S, Mohanty S, Deep N, Salins N, Bag S. 2020. "Palliative and End of Life Care in India: Current Scenario and the Way Forward." *Journal of the Association of Physicians of India* 68: 11.

Baiyewu O, Adeyemi JD, Ogunniyi A. 1997. "Psychiatric Disorders in Nigerian Nursing Home Residents." *Int J Geriatr Psychiatry* 12 (12): 1146-50.

Beauchet O, Allali G. 2022. "The Prevention of Major Neurocognitive Disorders in the Next Phase of COVID-19 Pandemic: On Being Proactive." *Maturitas* 162:67-8.

Bosch Bayard RI, Fernández Seco AE, Llibre Rodríguez JdJ, Zayas Llerena T, Hernández Ulloa E, Rodríguez Blanco AL. 2019. Cuba implementa el Plan global de acción para la demencia aprobado por la Organización Mundial de la Salud 2017. Revista Habanera de Ciencias Médicas [Internet] 18: 529-38. Available from: https://revhabanera.sld.cu/index.php/rhab/article/view/2120.

Breuer E, Freeman E, Alladi S, Breedt M, Govia I, López-Ortega M, Musyimi C, Oliveira D, Pattabiraman M, Sani TP, Schneider M, Swaffer K, Taylor D, Taylor E, Comas-Herrera A. 2022. "Active Inclusion of People Living with Dementia in Planning for Dementia Care and Services in Low- and Middle-Income Countries." *Dementia* 21 (2): 380-395.

Buraye JA, Quijano-Martínez MC. 2019. Colombia. In *Dementia Care: International Perspectives*, edited by A. Burns and P. Robert, 337-43. Oxford: Oxford University Press.

Cao Q, Tan CC, Xu W, Hu H, Cao XP, Dong Q, Tan L, Yu JT. 2020. "The Prevalence of Dementia: A Systematic Review and Meta-Analysis." *J Alzheimers Dis* 73 (3): 1157-66.

Chan KY, Adeloye D, Asante KP, Calia C, Campbell H, Danso SO, Juvekar S, Luz S, Mohan D, Muniz-Terrera G, Nitrini R, Noroozian M, Nulkar A, Nyame S, Paralikar V, Rodriguez MAP, Poon AN, Reidpath DD, Rudan I, Stephan BCM, Su T, Wang H, Watermeyer T, Wilkinson H, Yassuda MS, Yu X, Ritchie C, and on behalf of the Global Dementia Prevention Program (GloDePP). 2019. "Tackling Dementia Globally: The Global Dementia Prevention Program (GloDePP) collaboration." *J Glob Health* 9 (2): 020103.

Chibanda D, Bowers T, Verhey R, Rusakaniko S, Abas M, Weiss HA, Araya R. 2015. "The Friendship Bench Programme: A Cluster Randomised Controlled Trial of a Brief Psychological Intervention for Common Mental Disorders Delivered by Lay Health Workers in Zimbabwe." *International Journal of Mental Health Systems* 9: 21.

Clark D, Baur N, Clelland D, Garralda E, López-Fidalgo J, Connor S, Centeno C. 2020. "Mapping Levels of Palliative Care Development in 198 Countries: The Situation in 2017." *J Pain Symptom Manage* 59 (4): 794-807.

Congreso de la República de Colombia. Ley 12055 (10 Sep 2020) Por medio de la cual se aprueba la Convención interamericana sobre la protección de los derechos humanos de las personas mayores https://www.funcionpublica.gov.co/eva/gestornormativo/norma.php?i=141981. 2020.

Congreso de la República de Colombia. Ley 1616 (21 Ene 2013) por medio de la cual se expide la ley de salud mental y se dictan otras disposiciones https://www.minsalud.gov.co/sites/rid/Lists/BibliotecaDigital/RIDE/DE/DIJ/ley-1616-del-21-de-enero-2013.pdf. 2013.

Congreso de la República de Colombia. Ley 1733 (8 Sep 2014) Ley Consuelo Devis Saavedra, mediante la cual se regulan los servicios de cuidados paliativos para el manejo integral de pacientes con enfermedades terminales, crónicas degenerativas e irreversibles en cualquier fase de la enfermedad de alto impacto en la calidad de vida http://wsp.presidencia.gov.co/Normativa/Leyes/Documents/LEY%201733%20DEL%2008%20DE%20SEPTIEMBRE%20DE%202014.pdf. 2014.

Consejo Nacional de la persona adulta mayor. Plan Nacional para la Enfermedad de Alzheimer y Demencias Relacionadas 2014-2024 (National Plan for Alzheimer's Disease and Related Diseases 2014-2024) https://www.binasss.sa.cr/opac-ms/media/digitales/Plan%20nacional%20para%20la%20enfermedad%20de%20Alzheimer%20y%20demencias%20relacionadas.%20Esfuerzos%20compartidos%202014-2024.pdf. 2014.

Corte Constitucional de Colombia. Sentencia T - 782 https://www.corteconstitucional.gov.co/relatoria/2013/T-782-13.htm. 2013.

Crivelli L. LatAm-FINGERS (Latin America). 2020. *Alzheimer's and Dementia* 16 (S10): e046953.

Ddumba I. 2020. "Implementation of Global Action Plan on the Public Health Response to Dementia (GAPD) in Sub-Saharan Africa: Comprehensive Reviews." *Alzheimer's and Dementia* 16 (S8): e043363.

de Jager CA, Msemburi W, Pepper K, Combrincka MI. 2017. "Dementia Prevalence in a Rural Region of South Africa: A Cross-Sectional Community Study." *J Alzheimer's Disease* 60 (3): 1087-96.

Directorate General of Health Services. Ministry of Health and Family Welfare, Government of India; [cited 2023Feb28]. Available from: https://dghs.gov.in/content/1351_3_NationalProgramforPalliativeCare.aspx].

Duran-Aniotz C, Sanhueza J, Grinberg LT, Slachevsky A, Valcour V, Robertson I, Lawlor B, Miller B, Ibáñez A. 2022. "The Latin American

Brain Health Institute, a Regional Initiative to Reduce the Scale and Impact of Dementia." *Alzheimers Dement* 18 (9): 1696-98.

El Tallawy HN, Farghly WMA, Shehata GA, Rageh TA, Hakeem NA, Abo-Elfetoh N, Hegazy AM, Rayan I, El-Moselhy EA. 2012. "Prevalence of Dementia in Al Kharga District, New Valley Governorate, Egypt." *Neuroepidemiology* 38 (3): 130-37.

Eyre HA, Smith E, Ibanez A, Berk M. 2023. "Toward a Brain Capital Living Lab Model: Multi-Scale Opportunities." *Braz J Psychiatry* 45 (1): 1–2.

Fam J, Mahendran R, Kua EH. 2019. "Dementia Care in Low and Middle-Income Countries." *Curr Opin Psychiatry* 32 (5): 461-64.

Ferretti C, Sarti FM, Nitrini R, Ferreira FF, Brucki SMD. 2018. "An Assessment of Direct and Indirect Costs of Dementia in Brazil." *Plos One* 13: e0193209.

GBD 2019 Collaborators. 2021. "Global Mortality from Dementia: Application of a New Method and Results from the Global Burden of Disease Study 2019." *Alzheimer's and Dementia* 7 (1): e12200.

GBD 2019 Dementia Forecasting Collaborators. 2022. "Estimation of the Global Prevalence of Dementia in 2019 and Forecasted Prevalence in 2050: An Analysis for the Global Burden of Disease Study 2019. The *Lancet Public Health* 7 (2): e105-e25.

GBD 2019 Diseases and Injuries Collaborators. 2020. "Global Burden of 369 Diseases and Injuries in 204 Countries and Territories, 1990–2019: A Systematic Analysis for the Global Burden of Disease Study 2019. *Lancet* 396 (10258): 1204-22.

Guerchet M, Houinato D, Paraiso MN, von Ahsen N, Nubukpo P, Otto M, Clément JP, Preux PM, Dartigues JF. 2009. "Cognitive Impairment and Dementia in Elderly People Living in Rural Benin, West Africa." *Dementia and Geriatric Cognitive Disorders* 27 (1): 34-41.

Gutiérrez Robledo L, Arrieta Cruz I. Plan de acción Alzheimer y otras demencias. México. 2014 http://diariote.mx/docs/plan_alzheimer_WEB.pdf. 2014.

Harding R, Selman L, Agupio G, Dinat N, Downing J, Gwyther L, Mashao T, Mmoledi K, Moll T, Sebuyira LM, Panjatovic B, Higginson IJ. 2010. "Validation of a Core Outcome Measure for Palliative Care in Africa: The APCA African Palliative Outcome Scale." *Health Qual Life Outcomes* 8: 10.

Ibañez A, Kosik KS, Latin America and the Caribbean Consortium on Dementia. 2020. "COVID-19 in Older People with Cognitive Impairment in Latin America." *Lancet Neurol* 19 (9): 719-21.

Ibañez A, Pina-Escudero SD, Possin KL, Quiroz YT, Peres FA, Slachevsky A, Sosa AL, Brucki SMD, Miller BL; Multi-Partner Consortium to

Expand Dementia Research in Latin America. 2021a. "Dementia Caregiving Across Latin America and the Caribbean and Brain Health Diplomacy." *Lancet Healthy Longev* 2 (4): e222-e31.

Ibañez A, Yokoyama JS, Possin KL, Matallana D, Lopera F, Nitrini R, Takada LT, Custodio N, Ortiz ALS, Avila-Funes JA, Behrens MI, Slachevsky A, Myers RM, Cochran JN, Brusco LI, Bruno MA, Brucki SMD, Pina-Escudero SD, de Oliveira MO, Kehoe PD, Garcia AM, Cardona JF, Santamaria-Garcia H, Moguilner S, Duran-Aniotz C, Tagliazucchi E, Maito M, Ibarrola EML, Pintado-Caipa M, Godoy ME, Bakman V, Javandel S, Kosik KS, Valcour V, Miller BL. 2021b. "The Multi-Partner Consortium to Expand Dementia Research in Latin America (ReDLat): Driving Multicentric Research and Implementation Science." *Front Neurol* 12: 631722.

Institute for Health Metrics and Evaluation (IHME). What causes the most deaths? https://www.healthdata.org/colombia.

Knaul FM, Farmer PE, Krakauer EL, De Lima L, Bhadelia A, Kwete XJ, Arreola-Ornelas H, Gómez-Dantés O, Rodriguez NM, Alleyne GAO, Connor SR, Hunter DJ, Lohman D, Radbruch L, Del Rocío Sáenz Madrigal M, Atun R, Foley KM, Frenk J, Jamison DT, Rajagopal MR; Lancet Commission on Palliative Care and Pain Relief Study Group. 2018. "Alleviating the Access Abyss in Palliative Care and Pain Relief - An Imperative of Universal Health Coverage: The Lancet Commission report." *Lancet* 391 (10128): 1391-1454.

Kumar CTS, Shaji KS, Varghese M, Nair MKC, eds. 2019. *Dementia in India 2020*. Cochin: Alzheimer's and Related Disorders Society of India (ARDSI).

Liu G, Jack H, Piette A, Mangezi W, Machando D, Rwafa C, Goldenberg M, Abas M. 2016. "Mental Health Training for Health Workers in Africa: A Systematic Review." *Lancet Psychiatry* 3 (1): 65-76.

Mattap SM, Mohan D, McGrattan AM, Allotey P, Stephan BCM, Reidpath DD, Siervo M, Robinson L, Chaiyakunapruk N. 2022. "The Economic Burden of Dementia in Low- and Middle-Income Countries (LMICs): A Systematic Review. *BMJ Glob Health* 7 (4): e007409.

Ministerio de Salud Pública. Plan de Respuesta a las Demencias en la República Dominicana 2020-2025. Santo Domingo: Ministerio de Salud Pública; 2020.

Ministerio de Salud y Protección Social. Política Nacional de Salud Mental https://www.minsalud.gov.co/sites/rid/Lists/BibliotecaDigital/RIDE/VS/PP/politica-nacional-salud-mental.pdf. 2018.

Ministerio de Salud. Plan Nacional de Demencia https://www.minsal.cl/wp-content/uploads/2017/11/PLAN-DE-DEMENCIA.pdf. 2017.

Moens K, Higginson IJ, Harding R; EURO IMPACT. 2014. "Are There Differences in the Prevalence of Palliative Care-Related Problems in People Living with Advanced Cancer and Eight Non-Cancer Conditions? A Systematic Review. *J Pain Symptom Manage* 48 (4): 660-77.

Musisi S. 2022. Integrating Mental Health in Palliative Care and Other Conditions. International African Palliative Care and Worldwide Hospice Palliative Care Alliance Conference, August 24-26th. Uganda: Kampala.

Musisi, S. 2015. "Caring for the Elderly with Dementia in Africa." In Brain Degeneration and Dementia in Sub-Saharan Africa, edited by S. Musisi and S. Jacobson, pp287-97. New York: Springer

Musyimi CW, Ndetei DM, Evans-Lacko S, Oliveira D, Mutunga E, Farina N. 2021. "Perceptions and Experiences of Dementia and its Care in Rural Kenya." *Dementia* (London) 20 (8): 2802-19.

Nakasujja N, Musisi S, Walugembe J, Wallace D. 2007. "Psychiatric Disorders Among the Elderly on Non-Psychiatric Wards in an African Setting." *International J. Psychogeriatrics* 19 (4): 691-704.

National Health Mission. Ministry of Health and Family Welfare, Government of India; [cited 2023Feb28]. Available from: https://nhm.gov.in/].

National Research Council (US) Committee on Population. *Aging in Sub-Saharan Africa: Recommendation for Furthering Research*, M.J. Cohen B, Editor. Washington (DC), 2006.

Pan American Health Organization (PAHO). Strategy and plan of action on dementias in older persons (CD54/8, Rev. 1). https://iris.paho.org/handle/10665.2/28348, 2015.

Pan American Health Organization (PAHO). The prolongation of the health crisis and its impact on health, the economy and social development https://iris.paho.org/handle/10665.2/54991. 2021.

Parra MA, Baez S, Sedeño L, Gonzalez Campo C, Santamaría-García H, Aprahamian I, et al. 2021. "Dementia in Latin America: Paving the Way Toward a Regional Action Plan." *Alzheimers Dement* 17 (2): 295-313.

Philip RR, Philip S, Tripathy JP, Manima A, Venables E. 2018. "Twenty Years of Home-Based Palliative Care in Malappuram, Kerala, India: A Descriptive Study of Patients and Their Caregivers." *BMC Palliat Care* 17: 26.

Phillips D. 1994. *Health and Development*. London: Routledge.

Population Reference Bureau. 2020. *2020 World Population Data Sheet*. Washington DC: Population Reference Bureau.

Powell RA, Downing J, Harding R, Mwangi-Powell F, Connor S, APCA. 2007. "Development of the APCA African Palliative Outcome Scale." *Journal of Pain and Symptom Management* 33 (2): 229-32.

Presidente de la República. Decreto Supremo que aprueba el Reglamento de la Ley N° 30795, Ley para la Prevención y Tratamiento de la Enfermedad de Alzheimer y Otras Demencias N° 030-2018-SA (Viernes 28 de diciembre 2018) https://busquedas.elperuano.pe/normaslegales/decreto-supremo-que-aprueba-el-reglamento-de-la-ley-n-30795-decreto-supremo-n-030-2018-sa-1727064-14/. 2018.

Prince M, Ali G-C, Guerchet M, Prina AM, Albanese E, Wu Y-T. 2016. "Recent Global Trends in the Prevalence and Incidence of Dementia, and Survival with Dementia." *Alzheimer's research and therapy* 8 (1): 23.

Prince MJ. 2015. *World Alzheimer's report 2015: the global impact of dementia – and analysis of prevalence, incidence, cost and trends*. London: Alzheimer's Disease International.

Radbruch L, De Lima L, Knaul F, Wenk R, Ali Z, Bhatnaghar S, Blanchard C, Bruera E, Buitrago R, Burla C, Callaway M, Munyoro EC, Centeno C, Cleary J, Connor S, Davaasuren O, Downing J, Foley K, Goh C, Gomez-Garcia W, Harding R, Khan QT, Larkin P, Leng M, Luyirika E, Marston J, Moine S, Osman H, Pettus K, Puchalski C, Rajagopal MR, Spence D, Spruijt O, Venkateswaran C, Wee B, Woodruff R, Yong J, Pastrana T. 2020. "Redefining palliative care—a new consensus-based definition." *J Pain Symptom Manage* 60 (4): 754-764.

Rashid NSA, Chen XW, Marzuki MFM, Takshe AA, Okasha A, Maarof F, Yunus RM. 2022. "Development and Usability Assessment of a Mobile App (Demensia KITA) to Support Dementia Caregivers in Malaysia: A Study Protocol." *Int J Environ Res Public Health* 19 (19): 11880.

Ravindranath V, Sundarakumar JS. 2021. "Changing Demography and the Challenge of Dementia in India." *Nat Rev Neurol* 17 (12): 747-58.

Reisberg B, Ferris SH, de Leon MJ, Crook T. 1982. "The Global Deterioration Scale for Assessment of Primary Degenerative Dementia." *Am J Psychiatry* 139 (9): 1136-9.

Rhee JY, Garralda E. Namisango E, Luyirika E, de Lima L, Powell RA, López-Fidalgo J, Centeno C. 2018. "An Analysis of Palliative Care Development in Africa: A Ranking Based on Region-Specific Macroindicators." *J Pain Symptom Manage* 56 (2): 230-38.

Ribeiro F, Teixeira-Santos AC, Caramelli P, Leist AK. 2022. "Prevalence of Dementia in Latin America and Caribbean Countries: Systematic

Review and Meta-Analyses Exploring Age, Sex, Rurality, and Education as Possible Determinants." *Ageing Res Rev* 81: 101703.

Salcher-Konrad M, Naci H, McDaid D, Alladi S, Oliveira D, Fry A, Hussein S, Knapp M, Musyimi CW, Ndetei DM, Lopez-Ortega M, Comas-Herrera A. 2019. "Effectiveness of Interventions for Dementia in Low- and Middle-Income Countries: Protocol for a Systematic Review, Pairwise and Network Meta-Analysis." *BMJ Open* 9 (6): e027851.

Salins N. 2015. "Specialist Palliative Medicine Training in India." *Indian J Palliat Care* 21 (3): 257.

Sander M, Oxlund B, Jespersen A, Krasnik A, Mortensen EL, Westendorp RGJ, Rasmussen LJ. 2015. "The Challenges of Human Population Ageing." *Age Ageing* 44 (2): 185-7.

Sexton C, Snyder HM, Chandrasekaran L, Worley S, Carrillo MC. 2021. "Expanding Representation of Low and Middle Income Countries in Global Dementia Research: Commentary from the Alzheimer's Association." *Front Neurol* 12: 633777.

Shukla S. 2021. Urban households powering up income, expenditure and saving. ICE 360 Insights. https://www.ice360.in/blog/urban-households-powering-up-income-expenditure-and-saving/.

Slachevsky A, Budinich M, Miranda-Castillo C, Núñez-Huasaf J, Silva JR, Muñoz-Neira C, Gloger S, Jimenez O, Martorell B, Delgado C. 2013. "The CUIDEME Study: Determinants of Burden in Chilean Primary Caregivers of Patients with Dementia. *J Alzheimers Dis* 35 (2): 297-306.

Sleeman KE, de Brito M, Etkind S, Nkhoma K, Guo P, Higginson IJ, Gomes B, Harding R. 2019. "The Escalating Global Burden of Serious Health-Related Suffering: Projections to 2060 by World Regions, Age Groups, and Health Conditions." *Lancet Glob Health* 7 (7): e883-e892.

Slomski A. 2022. "Greater Excess Mortality in 2020 for People with Dementia." *JAMA* 327 (17): 1641.

Sternberg SA, Shinan-Altman S, Volicer L, Casarett DJ, van der Steen JT. 2021. "Palliative Care in Advanced Dementia: Comparison of Strategies in Three Countries." *Geriatrics (Basel)* 6 (2): 44.

Stewart JT, Schultz SK. 2018. "Palliative Care for Dementia." *The Psychiatric Clinics of North America* 41 (1): 141-51.

Tudela Cuenca J, De los Ríos Uriarte ME, Hernández González JA. 2022. "Ethical distribution of resources, palliative care,and other bioethical aspects in times of pandemic in Mexico." *Medicina y Ética* 33: 473-504.

United Nations, Department of Economic and Social Affairs, Population Division. *World Population Ageing 2015* (ST/ESA/SER.A/390), 2015.

Washington University School of Medicine. The Dominantly Inherited Alzheimer Network Trials Unit (DIAN-TU). https://dian.wustl.edu/our-research/our-collaborators/. 2023.

Wimo A, Guerchet M, Ali G-C, Wu Y-T, Prina AM, Winblad B, Jönsson L, Liu Z, Prince M. 2017. "The Worldwide Costs of Dementia 2015 and Comparisons with 2010." *Alzheimers Dement* 13 (1): 1-7.

World Bank. Population estimates and projections https://databank.worldbank.org/source/population-estimates-and-projections#. 2023.

World Health Organization. 2017. *Global Action Plan on the Public Health Response to Dementia 2017-2025*. Geneva: World Health Organization.

Xiang Y, Vilmenay K, Poon AN, Ayanian S, Aitken CF, Chan KY. 2021. "Systematic Review Estimating the Burden of Dementia in the Latin America and Caribbean Region: A Bayesian Approach." *Frontiers in Neurology* 12: 628520.

21

Palliative Care for People with Dementia: An Islamic Perspective

Mohammad Al Qadire, PhD[1]
and Maen Aljezawi, RN, PhD[2]

Abstract

This book chapter discusses the challenges of providing palliative care for people with dementia as they approach the end of their lives. It highlights that people with dementia have complex physical, mental, and social needs that require attention, particularly in the period before hospitalization. The chapter stresses the importance of using a palliative approach to care that focuses on symptom management, identification of caregivers, and the best place for the person with dementia to die. The authors also examine the Islamic perspective on death, noting that it is considered a natural part of life and that reducing suffering and pain is encouraged. Additionally, the chapter emphasizes the importance of family care in the Islamic culture, as the Quran and Shariah mandate that families provide care for elderly and sick parents. It is important to note that palliative care for people with dementia is a complex and multidisciplinary task that needs to be addressed by a team of healthcare professionals and caretakers who appreciate patients cultural background and religious beliefs.

Keywords: Islam, Muslims, Dementia, end of life, Palliative.

---

[1] Professor of Oncology and Palliative Nursing, Adult Health Department, School of Nursing
[2] Professor of Gerontology, Community Health Department, School of Nursing

Palliative care for people living with dementia

Dementia is a progressive deterioration of an individual's mental status, resulting in decreased physical, cognitive, and psychological abilities over time, eventually leading to complete dependence on a caregiver (Shankardass, 2021). Risk factors include aging, family history, head trauma, hypertension, high cholesterol, and smoking. Palliative care can improve quality of life, manage symptoms, and reduce suffering in individuals with dementia, who experience burdensome conditions similar to those of patients with cancer (Hashimie et al., 2020). While the percentage of dementia patients benefiting from palliative care has increased to 20.9% in 2019, barriers to access remain due to challenges in diagnosis, perception of dementia as non-life-limiting, and lack of resources (National Hospice and Palliative Care Organization, 2021; Hanrahan & Luchins, 1995). Despite these barriers, palliative care should be incorporated at early stages to provide comfort, symptom management, communication, and advance care planning for persons with dementia.

Behavioral and psychiatric problems

Most people with dementia experience at least one or two behavioral and psychiatric symptoms. These symptoms include agitation, resistiveness to care, delirium, apathy, anxiety, and depression (Hashimie et al., 2020). They are correlated with poor quality of life and might indicate unmet needs such as pain relive. With presence of infection, use of various medications, and other risk factors, delirium might be experience. It comes suddenly and deteriorate patients' condition, however, it become less common with the advanced dementia (Eisenmann et al., 2020a; Mitchell, 2015). So, early recognition is paramount, four key characteristics of delirium need to be observed. That are decreased attentions span, sudden onset, disorganized thinking, and deteriorated level of consciousness (Matzo & Sherman, 2018). However, in the context of dementia, it is not always straight forward. Having already disorganized thought, difficulty in speaking, and frailty making the diagnosis difficult and complex (Matzo & Sherman, 2018; Schmidt et al., 2018). Most of the time, it is drug associated although other causes were documented like dehydration, infection, and hyponatremia. This might be combined with agitation and resistive behaviour complicating the case (Eisenmann et al., 2020a). The current practice suggests the use of haloperidol orally every four hours or the use of risperidone. However, the use and the effectiveness of antipsychotic drug is questionable because of it side effects profile that may deteriorate the health status of this fragile group of patients.

Healthcare providers and family caregivers can identify any changes in patients' health status or behaviors (Eisenmann et al., 2020a; Matzo & Sherman, 2018). Having family member present and interact with the patients may provide comfort. In addition, reducing the stimulants, distractors and unneeded procedures may help as well. In Islamic culture, caring for parents is often considered a mandatory duty, which presents an opportunity to promote human well-being and quality of life through religious teachings. This include respect of parent, feeding them, paying their costs, and being with them whenever they needed. Bearing in mind the goal of enhancing patients comfort and quality of life, this may avoid patients aggressive and intense treatment (Matzo & Sherman, 2018).

Communication

People with dementia gradually loss their ability to speak and communicate their needs or complains. This becomes obvious as they progress to the advanced stage. They may understand conversion but unable to respond or they may have global aphasia (Matzo & Sherman, 2018; Shankardass, 2021). Under the pressure of their unmet needs and inability to verbally deliver them, people with dementia become frustrated and depressed. Also, this contributes to their social isolation and withdraw from group activities (Kelley & Morrison, 2015). Assessment plan that is multi-disciplinary needed to assess individual communication abilities and needs. Also, some nonverbal behaviors in people with dementia may indicate unmet need such as pain relive, hunger, thirst etc. As results of assessment, care plan is set and implemented considering wishes and preference of the individual (Kelley & Morrison, 2015; Matzo & Sherman, 2018).

Several approaches can be used for better communications. For example, it is recommended to have consistent caregiver, so this aid in understanding speech and being sensitive to any change in individual behaviors. In addition, anticipating and attending needs lessen the frustration combined to inability to verbalize. Further, maintain eye to eye contact, touch and message could be used. Furthermore, having family member may give feeling of security and safeness. Finally, better communication might be achieved within a calm environment, using clear calm voice, and building a rapport with the individual with dementia (Matzo & Sherman, 2018).

Advanced care planning from Islamic perspective

Advanced care planning (ACP) is a process that involves discussing and documenting a person's preferences and goals for their future health care, especially in the context of a serious or life-limiting illness such as dementia. In Islamic tradition, it is believed that preserving life is a high priority, and that suffering is a test of faith and an opportunity for reward in the hereafter (Chamsi-Pasha & Albar, 2017). However, quality of life is also valued, and there are teachings that encourage the use of all available means to relieve pain and suffering.

In the context of dementia, ACP can be particularly important, as people with dementia may lose their capacity to make decisions and communicate their wishes. Islamic teachings emphasize the importance of family support and involvement in decision-making, as well as the value of respecting the autonomy and dignity of the individual(Alsolamy, 2014). This can involve discussing with the person and their family what types of medical interventions they would or would not want, and what types of supportive care would be most meaningful to them (Alsolamy, 2014; Chamsi-Pasha & Albar, 2017).

It is also important to consider the ethical and legal implications of ACP in Islamic tradition. Islamic law recognizes the concept of "wasiyah" or a will, which can be used to provide guidance on the distribution of one's assets after death. There are also teachings that encourage Muslims to leave behind a legacy of good deeds and charitable works, which can be incorporated into ACP discussions. In terms of specific recommendations for ACP in dementia from an Islamic perspective, there is limited literature available. However, general principles of respecting the dignity and autonomy of the person, involving family and loved ones, and using all available means to relieve suffering can be applied. It is also important to consider the legal and ethical implications of ACP, and to seek guidance from qualified Islamic scholars or healthcare professionals with expertise in Islamic bioethics.

Dying with dementia

People with dementia tend to have a shorter lifespan than those without the condition. Approximately one third of older people aged 65 years and above will die because of dementia or while having dementia. Persons living with dementia have a complex physical, mental, and social needs, that needs to be addressed especially as they reach their end of life (Bunn et al., 2018). Evidence for interventions that addresses an effective symptoms management is lacking, most studies in this area focus primarily on the last 24 hours of life, that is the period of hospitalization or residential nursing homes. Caretakers at home are an important element in the caring process, as the period of dying extends for much more time before hospitalization. Providing care in this period is a challenging task as in this stage there is not only deterioration in the cognitive abilities, but also more complex physical problems that start to appear, such as eating difficulties, fecal and urinary incontinence, and mobility problems that eventually make the person with dementia bedridden. Caring for the persons dying with dementia entails using a palliative approach of care that has three important components, namely: end of life symptom management, identification of the care taker, and the best place to die in peacefully (Bunn et al., 2018; Eisenmann et al., 2020b; Shankardass, 2021)

Best place to die

It is essential that people with dementia are supported at their end of life to die at preferred place. Although nursing homes are common places for end-of-life and many people with dementia die in nursing homes or hospitals, still their preferred place to die is their home. Enabling persons to die in their usual place of residence has been marked as a "good death". If given a hypothetical choice most people living with dementia prefer to die at home or a nursing home, with people whom they love and trust. Literature has shown that preferring to die at home is associated with higher socioeconomic status, being married, having higher level of activity, and referral to palliative care. Understanding these factors can encourage health care professionals to provide more care activates and personnel in people preferred place to death (Wiggins et al., 2019).

Islam perspective of death

According to Quran and Shariah (Islamic law) death is not to be resisted or hastened, as Islam consider the life as several terminals, death is the last one which marks the end of a Muslim journey in the current life. The life to come after death is the eternal abode (Sheikh, 1998).

Physical aspect during death has a place in Islam. Islamic Shariah is against undue suffering, so it is encouraged in Islam to give medication that can lessen suffering and minimize pain. Islam also delt with the psychosocial aspect during death. From an ideal point of view, death in a remote place rather than home is not preferred. Muslims prefer to die at home surrounded by family, relatives, and friends. Visiting sick and dying people is mandated in Islam (J., 1994). Visitors are encouraged to pray and recite Quran for the dying person for his\her welfares after death. Also, the death is a time to ask forgiveness from both the visitor and the dying person, for any excesses that may have been committed in previous time. Also doing the five prayers has an essential role in the Muslim daily life. The role of prayers is even greater when the person is dying, as so, family members encourage their beloved ones to continue praying as long as they are capable doing (Gatrad, 1994).

Family care within the Islamic culture

Family is the basic building block and the primary institution providing care among other societal institution in the Islamic society. About third of the Islamic laws mentioned in the Quran are related to family function and regulations (Ahmad, 1974). One of the most important functions of the family in Islam is to provide care for parents especially when they get old and sick.

Almighty Allah (God) said in the holy Quran about caring for parents when they get older: "Thy Lord hath decreed that ye worship none but Him, and that ye be kind to parents. Whether one or both of them attain old age in thy life, say not to them a word of contempt, nor repel them, but address them in terms of honor". (Quran, 17-23 Al Isra). This mean that God (Allah) commanded, that he is the solely to worship, and, that offspring must show, kindness to parents, by being dutiful to them, if they should reach old age one of them or both. Providing care to diseased or weak family members is not just a virtue in Islam, or a good deed to be rewarded upon, it is a command from God. Structuring the family care in Islam in a form of a mandate function, ensures its implementation (Franceschelli & O'Brien, 2014).

Providing care in the Islamic family is not just restricted to physical care it also extends to cover, social and spiritual care. In Islam family visits and socialization are encouraged. This is evident in the Holy Quran: "God commands justice, and good conduct, and giving to relatives, and forbids sexual immorality, and perversity, and sectarian zealotry. He admonishes you, that you might take heed" (Quran, 16-90 Nahl). This will enhance the social health of people and relieve will bring peace of mind to members of the family. Also, family members help each other to connect with God and seek help with patience and prayer, this will be reflected as spiritual wellness that has an important role in the caring process. Asking for atonement (Tuba) is also another mean of family care in Islam. Family can help its individuals in expressing a genuine remorse for transgressions and a removal of the unhealthy effects of that state by turning to God and seeking divine grace through prayer, charity, and reciting Quran (Schultz et al., 2012).

The role of the family in care also extends to providing care during death. According to Islamic rituals when a Muslim individual is dying, the family has a role in comforting this event, through the following: prayers of allegiance to God, recite Quran and help the dying person to recite if possible, encouraging visits by their beloved ones and relatives, lay the dying person on his right side with the bed arranged to face Mecca, and to recite Shahada at the very last moments of death (There is no God but God (Allah – i.e. there is none worthy of worship but Allah), and Muhammad is the Messenger of Allah). These Islamic rituals can help the dying to overcome his fears of death (Ott et al., 2003).

Home care for persons living with dementia

With a growing number of people having dementia and the increasing burden on health care systems, providing home care for dementia has become a public health priority in many countries. Family members for persons living with dementia are the primary caregivers. Providing home care for persons living with dementia caries a larger burden. Family members for persons living with dementia provide up to 75% more effort and time compared to persons without dementia (Breen et al., 2022). Interventions focusing on optimal symptom management, continuity of care and psychosocial support, were the most reported in high quality studies for persons living with dementia (Miranda et al., 2019). The best evidence suggests that caring out these interventions is best persons living with dementia is best at home, this evidence is combined with the rising cost of high quality institutional care (Saragosa et al., 2022).

Some ethnic groups consider dementia as a concealed dilemma. Islamic regulation through Quran and Hadith (prophet Mohammad piece be upon him talk), encourages the acceptance of dementia as a disease to deal with not as a stigma to hide. Muslim caregivers do not classify themselves as caregivers, they consider themselves as family members obligated to provide care for their loved ones. In the Islamic contextual, family has a major responsibility to take care of their week family members or sick. This also include caring for elderly people, and that younger people in the family should provide care for their elders and pay respect to them (Kiwi et al., 2018).

In the Islamic culture the role of caregiving is not usually assigned to a particular person, usually it starts as one family member requires a significant care with the onset of a debilitating illness (including dementia) (Hammad et al., 2022). Members of the Muslim family consider themselves as good Muslims, if they fear from Allah (God) displeasure for not providing the necessary care for their older family members living with dementia. The Islamic religious believes, are the source to derive norms and values and acts consistently r to increase interpersonal motives and obligations to provide care from their family members at home. It could be argued that providing care to family members in need is more important than receiving external support (Hossain & Mughal, 2021). Performing the activities of care is a way to fulfill religious duties in aiming for felicity in the afterlife. In a similar manner, the thought of sending a family member with dementia to a care home is deemed not only as a last alternative, but morally and culturally deplorable and not accepted by the general community (Ahmad, 1974; Franceschelli & O'Brien, 2014).

Role of Islamic commands in caring for people with dementia

Religion could have a profound effect on organizing how people deal and cope with illness. This implies also to neurodegenerative disease like dementia. Religious and spiritual views affect how care is approached and delivered (Sayegh & Knight, 2013).The Health Belief Model also considered religion as a factor that affects perception of illness and health, this implies how people will react to and manage different diseases (Rosenstock et al., 1988). In this context cognitive abilities which is the main thing affected in dementia is well recognized in Islam, for instance, a person should have intact cognitive abilities to be considered obligated to practice religious practices such as prayers (Daher-Nashif et al., 2021).

Islam has organized life through stringent laws (the Sharia) brought by four sources. The primary two source are the holy Quran and the Sunnah, as distilled from the traditions and customs of Muhammad" or "the words (Hadiths), actions and silent assertions of him. Muslim scholars covered matters that were not mentioned in these two sources were covered through consensus (Ijma) and analogical reasoning (Qiyas) by Islamic scholars (Coulson, 2017).

Caring for older adults especially those with mental illness is structured through these sources through obligations and rewards, this implies that offspring are obligated to take care of their parents, and in the same time they are rewarded in the hereafter. Previous studies concluded that this role is well-practiced by family members and extended family members based on their faith cementing this role. In fact, many studies conducted in the Muslim societies revealed that caregivers for persons living with dementia is considered a source of blessing, this increases the feeling of sympathy with these people from the caregivers perspective (Cipriani & Borin, 2015; TARNÓCZY, 1981). This is reflected as a stronger family support system for the people living with dementia and a more positive attitude (Abdelmoneium & Alharahsheh, 2016).

Muslim families based on the teachings of Islam find themselves blessed and in place to receive rewards from God as they obey the command regarding elderly care (Daher-Nashif et al., 2021). Islamic commands considered family as the primary caregiver for elderly especially those who are chronically ill, and home is the setting. It is now will established that ill people especially elderly are more comfortable receiving care at home because family can provide emotional and social support in addition to emotional. Studies that were conducted in the Muslim countries supported this conclusion. The teachings of Islam effects the caregiver's motivation and role as a caregiver, thus the quality of care. It produces a higher positive intrinsic motivation that eventually builds resilience among caregivers and reduces associated burnout (Zahed et al., 2019).

Summary

In the Islamic perspective, death is not something to be resisted or hastened, but rather accepted as the final stage of a person's journey in this life. Physical and emotional suffering should be minimized through medication and other interventions, and it is preferred for individuals to die at home surrounded by loved ones. Additionally, prayer and recitation of the Quran are important practices in providing spiritual support for the dying person.
In the Islamic culture, family plays a central role in providing care for loved ones during the end of life. This includes caring for older and sick parents, as well as providing emotional and spiritual support for the dying person. It is important for healthcare professionals to understand and respect these

cultural beliefs and practices when providing care for Muslim individuals and their families.

References

Abdelmoneium, A. O., & Alharahsheh, S. (2016). Family home caregivers for old persons in the Arab region: perceived challenges and policy implications. *Open Journal of Social Sciences*, *4*(1), 151-164.

Ahmad, K. (1974). *Family life in Islam*. Islamic Foundation.

Alsolamy, S. (2014). Islamic views on artificial nutrition and hydration in terminally ill patients. *Bioethics*, *28*(2), 96-99.

Breen, R., Savundranayagam, M. Y., Orange, J. B., & Kothari, A. (2022). Quality home care for persons living with dementia: Personal support workers' perspectives in Ontario, Canada. *Health & social care in the community*, *30*(5), e2497-e2506.

Bunn, F., Lynch, J., Goodman, C., Sharpe, R., Walshe, C., Preston, N., & Froggatt, K. (2018). Improving living and dying for people with advanced dementia living in care homes: a realist review of Namaste care and other multisensory interventions. *BMC Geriatric*, *18*(1), 1-15.

Chamsi-Pasha, H., & Albar, M. A. (2017). Ethical dilemmas at the end of life: Islamic perspective. *Journal of Religion and Health*, *56*, 400-410.

Cipriani, G., & Borin, G. (2015). Understanding dementia in the sociocultural context: A review. *International Journal of Social Psychiatry*, *61*(2), 198-204.

Coulson, N. J. (2017). *A history of Islamic law*. Routledge.

Daher-Nashif, S., Hammad, S. H., Kane, T., & Al-Wattary, N. (2021). Islam and mental disorders of the older adults: Religious text, belief system and caregiving practices. *Journal of religion and health*, *60*(3), 2051-2065.

Eisenmann, Y., Golla, H., Schmidt, H., Voltz, R., & Perrar, K. M. (2020a). Palliative care in advanced dementia. *Frontiers in Psychiatry*, *11*, 699.

Eisenmann, Y., Golla, H., Schmidt, H., Voltz, R., & Perrar, K. M. (2020b). Palliative care in advanced dementia. *Frontiers in Psychiatry*, *11*(1), 1-13.

Franceschelli, M., & O'Brien, M. (2014). 'Islamic capital'and family life: The role of Islam in parenting. *Sociology*, *48*(6), 1190-1206.

Gatrad, A. R. (1994). Muslim customs surrounding death, bereavement, postmortem examinations, and organ transplants. *BMJ*, *309*(6953), 521-523.

Hammad, S. H., Daher-Nashif, S., Kane, T., & Al-Wattary, N. (2022). Sociocultural insights on dementia care-giving in Arab and Muslim communities: the perspectives of family care-givers. *Ageing & Society*, 1-28.

Hashimie, J., Schultz, S. K., & Stewart, J. T. (2020). Palliative care for dementia: 2020 update. *Clinics in Geriatric Medicine*, *36*(2), 329-339.

Hossain, M. Z., & Mughal, F. (2021). Dementia and revivalist Islam: New perspectives to understanding dementia and tackling stigma. *Journal of Evaluation in Clinical Practice*, *27*(2), 213-217.

J., N. (1994). *Caring for Dying Patients of DjJerent Faiths* (2nd ed.). Mosby.

Kelley, A. S., & Morrison, R. S. (2015). Palliative care for the seriously ill. *New England Journal of Medicine*, *373*(8), 747-755.

Kiwi, M., Hydén, L.-C., & Antelius, E. (2018). Deciding upon transition to residential care for persons living with dementia: Why do Iranian family caregivers living in Sweden cease caregiving at home? *Journal of cross-cultural gerontology*, *33*(1), 21-42.

Matzo, M. L., & Sherman, D. W. (2018). *Palliative care nursing: Quality care to the end of life*. Springer Publishing Company.

Miranda, R., Bunn, F., Lynch, J., Van den Block, L., & Goodman, C. (2019). Palliative care for people with dementia living at home: a systematic review of interventions. *Palliative medicine*, *33*(7), 726-742.

Mitchell, S. L. (2015). Advanced dementia. *New England Journal of Medicine*, *372*(26), 2533-2540.

Ott, B. B., Al-Khadhuri, J., & Al-Junaibi. (2003). Preventing ethical dilemmas: understanding Islamic health care practices. *Pediatric Nursing*, *29*(3), 227.

Quran. (17-23 Al Isra). Holy Quran. In.

Quran. (16-90 Nahl). Holy Quran. In.

Rosenstock, I. M., Strecher, V. J., & Becker, M. H. (1988). Social learning theory and the health belief model. *Health education quarterly*, *15*(2), 175-183.

Saragosa, M., Jeffs, L., Okrainec, K., & Kuluski, K. (2022). Towards defining quality in home care for persons living with dementia. *Plos one*, *17*(9), e0274269.

Sayegh, P., & Knight, B. G. (2013). Cross-cultural differences in dementia: the Sociocultural Health Belief Model. *International psychogeriatrics*, *25*(4), 517-530.

Schmidt, H., Eisenmann, Y., Golla, H., Voltz, R., & Perrar, K. M. (2018). Needs of people with advanced dementia in their final phase of life: a multi-perspective qualitative study in nursing homes. *Palliative medicine*, *32*(3), 657-667.

Schultz, M., Baddarni, K., & Bar-Sela, G. (2012). Reflections on palliative care from the Jewish and Islamic tradition. *Evidence-Based Complementary Alternative Medicine, 2012*.

Shankardass, M. K. (2021). *Dementia Care: Issues, Responses and International Perspectives*. Springer Nature.

Sheikh, A. (1998). Death and dying—a Muslim perspective. *Journal of the Royal Society of Medicine*, *91*(3), 138-140.

TARNÓCZY, T. (1981). Mentek. *Acta Linguistica Academiae Scientiarum Hungaricae*, *31*(4), 291-297.

Wiggins, N., Droney, J., Mohammed, K., Riley, J., & Sleeman, K. (2019). Understanding the factors associated with patients with dementia achieving their preferred place of death: a retrospective cohort study. *Age and Aging*, *48*(3), 433-439.

Zahed, S., Emami, M., Bazargan-Hejazi, S., Eslami, A. A., Barekatain, M., & Zamani-Alavijeh, F. (2019). What motivates informal caregivers of people with dementia (PWD): a qualitative study. *BMC palliative care*, *18*(1), 1-7.

III

RELIGION, SPIRITUALITY AND CULTURAL ASPECTS IN DEMENTIA CARE

22

Palliative Care in Dementia Patients

Wilson Astudillo A[1],
Carmen Mendinueta A[1],
Antonio Salinas M[1], Folaju O. Oyebola[2],
Michael Silbermann, John Comba[1],
Carmen De la Fuente[1] and
Zemilson Bastos de Sousa[3]

> "Alzheimer's is really like an insidious fog, barely perceptible until everything around you disappears completely … Then the fog dissipates and the precipice appears beneath your feet".
>
> —John Bayley, *Elegy for Iris*

Keywords: dementias, types, symptoms, common problems, advanced planning stigmas, cultural aspects, support measures

Introduction

Dementias are a group of diseases known as "major neurocognitive disorders" that cause much suffering for those afflicted and their families. Is a major cause of disability and dependency among older adults. Their prevalence increases with age, ranging from 6.4 % at age 65 to 25%–47% by age 85, and they are a major burden on the healthcare system. It is estimated that 50 million people were affected worldwide in 2015, more than 60% in low- and middle-income countries (LMICs) and most new cases (71%) are expected to ocurr in those countries. With ten million new cases per year (WHO,2017) and one new case every three seconds, a projected 82 million will be affected in 2030 and 152 million in 2050 (5%–

[1] Paliativos Sin Fronteras Spain. [2] PSF Nigeria. [3]PSF Brasil

8% of the elderly population) (1-4). Pharmacological treatment is scarce, with new drugs in development and generally only for the early stages. Palliative care (PC) is the basis for achieving greater well-being through anticipating care needs, identifying and alleviating symptoms, reducing the burden of care for caregivers, and helping to ensure that the decisions that are made respect the values of the patients and their families (4). This paper reviews the most common dementias, behavioral problems, their treatment, and support for caregivers (5).

Characteristics of Dementias

Dementias may arise in the context of a systemic disease, be accompanied by other evidence of neurological involvement, or be the sole manifestation of the disease. They are one of the major causes of disability and dependence in the elderly, and present clinically as memory decline of an organic and multicausal nature that persists for more than 3–6 months, with progressive loss of acquired intellectual functions (learning, attention, concentration, verbal facility, numerical dexterity, visuospatial perception, emotional control, and behavior), without alteration of alertness (6). These signs should not be confused with major depression or schizophrenia or with reversible metabolic, structural, or endocrine disorders. The dementia scenario changes the personality of patients and their relationships with others, makes them socially and occupationally incapacitated, and creates a great need for care that exceeds 40 hours a week.

There are several types of dementia, the most common being Alzheimer's disease (AD), which accounts for more than 60%–80% of the total. The first thing to be noticed in this type of dementia is episodic memory, followed by difficulty in finding words and executive disorders, with difficulties in calculation and disorientation. It is progressive and ends in disability and death within four to ten years, while limiting the patient's possibility of living alone. Dementia with Lewy body (DLB) accounts for 15%–20% of dementia cases. It presents with vivid, complex visual hallucinations, fluctuations in consciousness, progressive extrapyramidal disturbances, and sensitivity to neuroleptics that may increase behavioral disturbances. Multi-infarct dementia (MID), which accounts for 10%–20% of dementia cases, is caused by ischemic or hemorrhagic cerebrovascular lesions. MID is manifested by global slowing, gait, speech problems, vision problems, sphincter disturbances, spasmodic laughing and crying with abrupt changes, and neurological signs. Memory loss and cognitive impairment can appear after a stroke, but does not always progress and even improves with appropriate preventive treatment.

Most dementia sufferers have a vascular element and AD components that are difficult to quantify. Frontotemporal dementia (FTD), also called Pick's disease (5%–10%), is a focal degeneration of the frontal and temporal lobes that affects people at a younger age relative to AD (45 to 65 years old). It manifests with language disorders such as anomia, aphasia, and echolalia of the reiterative type, and with personality, emotional, and behavioral changes. It is also associated with genetic mutations. Parkinson's dementia, present in 27 and 78 % of advanced cases, is accompanied by tremor, rigidity, bradykinesia and gait disorders. It is considered part of DLB. Major neurocognitive disorders are also seen in Huntington's disease, traumatic brain injury, HIV, and prion disease (4-9). While there is a definite correlation between anatomopathology and dementia, there are often people without dementia with significant levels of neuropathology and others with clinical dementia with little or no anatomopathological alterations. Additionally, non-modificable genetic risk factors exist that increase a person´s risk of developing dementia (1). Tau and amyloid β biomarkers indicate risk of progression to AD, but most people with normal cognition never develop AD (3).

Dementias are the ultimate consequence of diseases that must be identified at an early stage and that are up to 40% preventable with proactive management of modifiable risk factors, according to WHO (1-3). Thus, dementias can be reduced by 7% in early age groups if the effort is made to increase the cognitive reserve by providing primary and secondary education for all; in the middle age group, dementias can be reduced by up to 8% by attenuating hearing loss (with hearing aids and noise protection) and visual loss, better control of hypertension (2%), obesity (1%), alcohol consumption (1%), head injuries (3%), and pollution (2%). In older age groups, they can be reduced by smoking cessation (5%), treatment of depression (4%), physical inactivity (2%), reduction of social isolation (4%), and diabetes (1%). Non-communicable risk factors are genetic polymorphisms, age, gender, race/ethnicity, and family history. All patients with cognitive impairment should receive information from the WHO to prevent dementia (9). Dementia accounts for 11,9 % of the years lived with disability due to a noncommunicable disease (1).

Natural History

Differential diagnosis is essential, considering the difficulties in distinguishing dementia from normal aging, from depression or encephalopathy and from secondary dementias caused by or related to diseases such as HIV, head injury, multiple sclerosis, thyroid disorders or Vitamin B12 deficiency. There is a wide range of causes of cognitive loss among individuals with dementia, so it is essential to obtain a proper assessment of cognitive status using the Mini Mental State Examination (MMSE), and to conduct physical and neurological examinations in order to formulate treatment plans and assess the patients' concerns and functional deficits, particularly auditory and visual deficits, troublesome symptoms, infections, trigger impact on the patient and the caregiver. The quality of care should be assessed and the family should be informed and accompanied. It is important to obtain the patients' perspective, their values and those of the family, and to ask for support from other disciplines such as social workers. As the relationship with the patient becomes more difficult, efforts should be put in place to empower the patient's family or caregivers (10). One of the most essential goals at each level should be to maximize comfort and to help patients feel well, particularly in the final phase, when their suffering is greatest (7-9,11-13). Patients need to be provided with holistic post-diagnostic care that encompasses their physical, mental, and social health, and their carers must be supported with multidisciplinary team care interventions.

There are several scales for assessment of dementia such as the Clinical Dementia Rating (CDR), which provides descriptive domains that help clinicians make assessments based on interview data and clinical judgment. Ratings range from 0 (no impairment), to 0.5, (very mild), 1 (mild), 2 (moderate), and 3 (severe). A CDR of 3 is severe dementia. Reisberg's Global Deterioration Scale (GDS) allows to categorize the stage of severity, as Bouchard and Rossor's, The Functional Assessment Staging (FAST) scale ranges from 1 to 7, with higher levels according to greater severity and is widely used to measure cognitive impairment although many patients do not follow the stages sequentially (13-15). **Table 1.** For vital prognosis, Karnofsky Performance Status are more useful than FAST and the Advanced Dementia Prognostic Tool has an especificity of 89 % and a sensibility of 27 % .

Table 1. Summary of the stages of functional assessment of dementias (FAST)(15)

Stage	Skill
1	No subjective or objective difficulties
2	Complaints of missing objects, subjective difficulty with word finding
3	Difficulties in carrying out work with others. Difficulties with organization
4	Disturbances in instrumental life activities
5	Needs assistance with getting dressed according to time and occasion.
6	6 (a-2) Difficulty in getting dressed, bathing, toileting without assistance (stage 6 a-c), occasional or more frequent urinary incontinence (6-d), fecal incontinence (6-e)
7	(a-f) Language limited to less than six words/day (7a), to one or less (7b), inability to move by self (7c), sit up unaided (7d), smile (7e) and keep head on something (7f)

Reisberg, B (1988) Functional assessment staging (FAST) Psychopharmacol Bul. 23 (4),653-9

Cultural Aspects of Dementia

Dementia in the elderly is a universal phenomenon that is culturally determined and has not been well studied in non-Western settings. It relies upon biomedicine's ability to name and give form to a collection of changes, behaviors, and experiences (16,17). Cross-cultural research identifies how understandings of dementia as either a natural part of the aging process or a result of brain disease are culturally shaped. Concepts of dementia may also be shaped by social location. There is a growing recognition that social class has a significant role in the ways in which dementia is both experienced and conceptualized (17). Cohen's research (18) in India showed that cultural representations of dementia also become entwined with other social meanings, such as the social expectations of aging, the implications of these cultural representations for those living with the condition, and how these implications may differ according to a person's social location. More data is needed on the socio-cultural context or meaning of the disease for patients and their caregivers and the variation across cultures in definitions of normal aging, mild and severe dementia, and the thresholds that separate them (16). It is essential to harmonize the methods of studying cognitive functions with the culture and language of the population being studied and to know which activities of daily life are perceived as irrelevant or inappropriate.

Low and Purwaningrum (19) reviewed a total of 60 articles and found that dementia was often equated with Alzheimer's disease. It was almost always depicted in conjunction with aging in popular culture and associated with negative images and feelings, such as social distance between people with dementia and those without. These authors found several common frames for dementia, including a biomedical frame, in which dementia involves a deterioration of the brain for which there is no current cure; a natural disaster or epidemic frame, in which dementia is a force of nature which will overwhelm mankind; and a 'living-dead' frame, in which people with dementia lose their brains, memories, minds, and consequently their personhood and human rights. The stereotype was framed so that the person with dementia is not fully human and does not have a voice. Feelings commonly associated with dementia were fear, shame, compassion, and guilt, and depictions often resulted in a sense of social distance.

Dementia stigma is a key concern of dementia advocacy. Stigma is defined as negative stereotyped beliefs, feelings, behaviors, and attitudes. The prevailing stereotypes often depict the later stages of the disease, when a person is most impaired and fully dependent upon others for care (20). Cultural stigma is society's shared negative beliefs, prejudices, and discriminatory structures. Examples of this cultural stigma include public fear of dementia, therapeutic nihilism, and locked dementia care units. Dementia stigma contributes to delayed help-seeking and self-education about the disease, a reluctance by health professionals to give a dementia diagnosis, and human rights violations of people with dementia. This means that people with dementia frequently feel denied and ignored and experience discrimination in healthcare. For care partners, the stigma is associated with depression, anxiety, and lower self-esteem, lower personal control and activity participation, and depression. It can also lead to poor reactions by people, such as patronizing, isolating, and discriminating against a person with the disease. Decades ago in some African villages, anecdotal observations showed that undiagnosed dementia in otherwise healthy elderly individual, that hallucinate, confabulate and talking irrationally could be regarded as witch confessing her past wicked atrocities and are usually discriminated upon or punished. This is why, when talking about and depicting people with dementia, we need to be mindful about the social impact of the words, images, and messages that we use.

Understanding the composition of beliefs, attitudes, and expectations about AD dementia held by the general public could help inform specific strategies to mitigate stigma and its consequences. Reducing public stigma of AD is important for facilitating the success of AD prevention. It could help identify gaps in current policy protections, whereby concerns among the public are common, but policy protections are lacking or insufficient (19-20). Stites et al., (20) consider that the way in which advances in the science of AD therapies are communicated, such as offering improved longevity versus retaining functioning or preventing declines, could radically affect the social and psychological experience of the disease. Other counter-frames for dementia are that dementia is a natural part of aging, carpe diem, family reciprocity of care, and a moral duty to provide loving care. A diagnosis of AD dementia can mitigate against some forms of stigma, such as harsh judgments about a person's poor hygiene or esthetics (19,20).

There are many ways of unlocking and challenging the assumptions that underpin cultural understandings of dementia, as many of these depictions in film, literature, and art are beginning to do. Hillman and Latimer (17) discuss the example of the film *Iris* by Richard Eyre, based on the book by John Bayley (*Elegy for Iris*), as offering a nuanced message. This film shows how dementia challenges the complex social processes that produce, the appearance at least, of the discrete individual, including cooperation, or what sociologists may observe as a person's capacity to fit in, get along, and pass as a member of society. The film helps to trouble and challenge the discourse of waging war on dementia. Hillman (17) also considers that *Iris,* as well as the film *Still Alice* (2015), embody the contradictions that make up contemporary images of dementia:

> "On the one hand, they reflect our fears of obliteration, the tragedy of a gradual chipping away of our humanity; while on the other hand, we are met with characters who remain present as a moral force, who feel pleasure and pain, who have emotional responses and connections to their social and material worlds. Perhaps the effects of the disease are less of a tragedy than the torment of our own contradictions. At the end of Iris, we see her husband and her friends accepting that she is someone different, with Iris herself happy in a new environment where she is able to be the person that she has become rather than who she once was"

There are worldwide programs for destigmatizing dementia using new social formations that create possibilities for living with dementia differently, such as dementia-friendly communities across Europe, Japan, and the United States (17,19-20). These communities present a positive frame by showing people with dementia as friendly, an approach that has been shown to reduce stigma (16). In these ways, alongside biomedical and public health programs for addressing whether there are disease processes that underpin dementia and which can be remedied, finding alternative ways of being in the world that are more accepting and embracing the kinds of disruptions that dementia can produce.

Advanced Care Planning

A common symptom of cognitive impairment is anosognosia or lack of awareness of illness, and while it does not occur in all cases, it is essential to know the patient's wishes at the end of life and to obtain advance directives (AD), or living wills in the mild or moderate phases, and always act in his/her best interests about what to do in the future with possible common medical interventions, non-cardiopulmonary resuscitation, non-hospitalization, admission to a hospice, artificial nutrition by tube, hydration, comfort, quality of life, or other actions with long-term benefit, especially if his/her wishes are not clear. Patients should be encouraged to choose a representative who can make decisions on their behalf in case of possible incapacity and to ensure that both patients and family understand the diagnosis, prognosis, and possible trajectory, before a crisis occurs. Between 62% and 90% of patients prefer wellness care over aggressive options (11). Low MMSE scores (<16 de 30) indicate impaired decision-making capacity, so if AD is left too late, it might not be possible for sufferers to participate in decision-making about their health, personal care, and finances (4,21-27). A frequent reason for their non-participation in decision-making is that the family does not realize the importance of this discussion. It is helpful to consider dementia as a terminal illness. The presentation of a video or guide with dementia patients can improve communication and decision-making if it includes not only the goals of care, but also the beneficial and harmful effects of various medical interventions (6,8,12). Videos:
https://www.dementiacarecentral.com/wp-content/uploads/2009/02/what-is-dementia.mp4.

Common Health Problems in Dementia Patients

Two-thirds of dementia patients have a treatable, intercurrent pathology with more problems in communicating their symptoms than others of the same age, and since their wishes are not known and it is difficult for them to consent to their treatments and to organize their care, they often have more difficulty accessing health care systems. Many suffer malnutrition, weight loss, diabetes, urinary or respiratory infections, sensory defects, and avitaminosis; nonetheless, half of them improve their cognitive functions when these problems are treated correctly, if they are better hydrated, if their daily routine is simplified, or if they are kept in a familiar environment.

The care of a patient with dementia will focus on the search for their well-being because if they are physically and emotionally comfortable, they will tend to show and act better, with less confusion and behavioral problems. Such care comprises a wide approach of anticipating their needs, timely correction of conflicting situations that arise, detecting concomitant diseases, managing symptoms, avoiding anything that is aggressive, burdensome or futile, and supporting the patient and caregivers (27,28). Any sudden worsening of an elderly person's mental status should raise suspicion of a vascular event of cardiac origin, embolism, a new urinary or respiratory infection, depression, or a drug reaction. The physician should consider whether increased confusion or psychiatric symptoms indicate the progression of an underlying brain disease, metabolic disorders, depression, environmental modification, and other psychosocial factors (6,28).

Problems associated with increased mortality are infections, dysphagia, pain, dyspnea and agitation, pressure ulcers, verbal and physical agitation, falls, frailty, and epilepsy, while hip fracture and cardiac infarction are more occasional (5). Recognizing them early on can have positive effects in restoring balance, reducing irritability with a calmer environment, and using medication (4,8,27). Hypertension and diabetes should be treated more conservatively to avoid postural hypotension and hypoglycemia. Identification and control of risk factors for stroke and cerebrovascular disease is an important strategy in the early stages to slow the progression of cognitive decline, especially in AD and MID. The presence of associated intercurrent diseases deteriorates dementias in the late phase.

Teams should try to have more time to listen to patients and attend to their carers, who will be asked about behaviors of concern, hallucinations, whether they see things or hear voices, and how they sleep. When talking to patients, simple sentences and yes/no or closed questions should be used and ambiguous terms and giving instructions over the phone should be avoided. Teams should use long-term memory as a basis for conversation and should do so clearly and calmly, in an audible but non-aggressive tone. Teams will get more attention by using the patient's name, gestures, light touch, calm facial expressions, slower body and postural movements, and eye contact (10). The team must be particularly skilled at interpreting symptoms, communicating with the elderly, appreciating changes in the patient's condition, and acting on them. In symptom management, there are three basic rules: (1) believe what the patients say; (2) never abandon them, because care and support are always possible; and (3) ask "why can this be", to try to clarify the causes of their problem.

Confusional States

Confusional states are common in dementias as death approaches, particularly apathy, depression, agitation, and wandering. Less common but more problematic are frank psychosis with hallucinations and abnormal ideas and violent or aggressive behavior. Possible causes should be sought, including pain, organ failure, hypoxia, hypercapnia, effects of medication, CNS disease, urinary or respiratory infection, hunger, thirst, loneliness, isolation, lack of intimacy, and other concerns. Hearing loss or deafness cause difficulty in understanding and accelerates cognitive loss and auditory hallucinations, and doubles the risk of agitation (4,6, 27-29). Table 2 presents possible measures to address behavioral disorders.

Table 2. Actions to address behavioral disorders

- Identify types of behavioral disorders
- Rule out infection or dehydration
- Assess change in patients' environment and routines
- Consider potential adverse effects of medication and interactions
- Assess withdrawal or lower doses of anticholinergic drugs and benzodiazepines
- Closely supervise patients to avoid accidents and monitor their nutrition
- Assess possibility of vision and hearing correction
- Avoid overstimulation, excessive noise, and crowds
- Attempt behavior modification techniques

The psychological symptoms of adaptation—anxiety disorders, depression, lack of interest—may lead to outbursts of anger and restlessness in the early stages of dementia, but they should be differentiated from the psychiatric disorders that appear as the disease progresses. For the former, relationship interventions, accompaniment, and the use of coping strategies are useful. Biographical information, provided by the patient and family, allows to determine which behavioral patterns are transient responses and which are largely characteristic of the individual's personality (8, 27-30). Thus, if there is a history of past physical or psychological trauma, the person is likely to respond in the only way they know how: agitation and violence. If it is known that they have never demonstrated an ability to share, it will be understood why they have difficulty being in a shared room, or if they have been very dominant in relationships all their lives, why it is difficult for them to be under the control of others. Self-centeredness replaces altruism, as impaired awareness of others reduces the capacity for empathy.

Non-Pharmacological Measures

A proactive approach comprising early recognition and treatment of symptoms and behavioral disorders, together with training of caregivers, support from the healthcare team, and improvement of patients' physical environment, can provide many benefits and reduce the use of antipsychotics. Minimizing stress and preventing distress must be an inherent part of dementia care, as it is necessary to create an appropriate environment for the patients. Proper communication is especially important for minimizing stress and is essential to improve quality of life. Communication must be conducted in an emotionally engaged way, through sharing knowledge about the person and establishing a collaborative social relationship (29-33).

Patients' mild confusion and agitation can respond to interpersonal and environmental manipulations, such as reassurance, soft voice, tact, non-threatening postures, avoiding arguments, not responding verbally or physically to aggression, and asking for help. Counseling measures, behavioral treatments with differential reinforcement, stimulus control, structured activities, simple commands, sensory stimulation (music, massage, face-to-face social contact, family videos), use of hearing aids, and good pain management are helpful (see **Table 3**). Other therapies, such as occupational therapy, serve to stimulate self-identity and self-esteem, maintain or enhance preserved abilities, avoid disconnection with the environment, strengthen social relationships, provide security, promote autonomy in daily living activities, and minimize stress.

Table 3. Measures to prevent violent behavior

- The presence of familiar faces or friends often brings more peace
- Maintain routine or make changes gradually
- Reduce pain and use painkillers before painful treatments
- Encourage the patient to express what is going on (anxiety, anger, or fear)

- Provide emotional support, frequent reorientation
- Correcting dehydration, hearing loss, cognitive stimulation
- Remove unnecessary catheters and safety measures
- Reducing noise and other disturbing stimuli
- Write directions in large, legible print
- Use signs, words, or pictures on drawers and cupboards to identify contents
- Have visible clocks and calendars
- Ensure that they take their medication and have an adequate diet
- Encourage movement and exercise
- Aromatherapy, reflexology, multi-sensory stimulation, massages
- Animal-assisted therapy
- Various psychosocial interventions, psychomotor, labor therapy, reminiscence

Psychiatric Disorders in Dementias

Behavioral and psychological symptoms of dementia (agitation, psychosis, depression, anxiety, and disinhibition) are almost omnipresent in mild dementia and may influence the course of dementia more than memory impairment. They may determine prognosis, frequency of emergency department visits, hospitalizations, and nursing home admissions. Neurodegeneration may promote increased vulnerability to stressors in 60%–90% of people with dementia. Cognitive impairment is expressed in maladaptation, emotional symptoms, behavioral problems, difficulties in establishing positive relationships with others, in impulse control, and in taking responsibility and judging reality. Major personality disorders (apathy, disinhibition), mood changes (depression, euphoria), psychotic symptoms (hallucinations and delusions), and agitation (inappropriate vocal or motor) are more striking and common as dementia progresses and are associated with tau and amyloid neuropathology (4,6,11,24-29). They can be considered behavioral excesses, where the occurrence of a behavior is the problem (e.g., hitting, wandering, restlessness, screaming), or behavioral deficits, where the lack of behavioral occurrence is the reason (e.g., introversion, apathy). Their treatment is complex and individual.

Management of psychosis in dementia will start with non-pharmacological interventions and control of possible triggering causes such as infections, pain, severe constipation, thirst, cardiovascular disease, pulmonary disease, dehydration, hyponatraemia, acid-base disorders, hypoglycemia, thyroid dysfunction, hypercalcemia, sensory deprivation, and drug reactions

(4,6,12,27, 29-37). Neuroleptic therapy should be recommended: 1) if there is a justifiable risk of harm to the patient or others, (2) if symptom distress is significant, and (3) if non-pharmacological therapeutic interventions have been unsuccessful and symptomatic relief is important. Typical or atypical antipsychotics are not the first choice but may be used for a short time at low doses to treat behavioral or psychological symptoms of dementia if they are sufficiently severe to impact the patient's life in significant psychosis (with hallucinations or disturbed thinking). In these cases, haloperidol (0.5-1 mg/oral), lorazepam (0.5-1 mg), midazolam (7.5-15 mg), quetiapine (12.5 mg), or risperidone (0.25 mg/day oral to 0.75 mg/day) may be administered. In acute control of unacceptable behavior, olanzapine (2.5-5 mg/day) is useful (6,11-13).

Depression

Depression is present in 15%–90 % of patients. Its diagnosis is complicated because it may be combined with symptoms and signs of cognitive impairment, apathy, aphasia, sleep disturbance, and social withdrawal, or it may be an undesirable effect (e.g., of anticonvulsants, B-adrenergic antagonists, metoclopramide). Depression is a common initial symptom that is considered a risk factor for AD and that can exacerbate cognitive and functional impairment in dementia. A therapeutic trial with antidepressants such as sertraline (at an initial dose of 25 mg-medium dose) or citalopram (at less than 20 mg per day) may improve psychotic or behavioral symptoms and reduce the progression of AD. Tricyclics are not well tolerated (4,13).

Anxiety

Anxiety is manifested in excessive and unwarranted nervousness in the face of new or complex environmental demands. The patient is irritable, restless, tense with the difficulty of concentrating, sweating, palpitations, nausea, diarrhea, dyspnea, dizziness, dry mouth, tremors and motor restlessness, and tends to wander around the house, go out or get lost. It can lead to accidents and loss of sleep for caregivers. Benzodiazepines should be limited to agitation associated with procedures or crises for a short time; short-acting ones should be used such as lorazepam (0.5 mg c/4-6 hours). If agitation is nocturnal, haloperidol (0.5) or tiapride (50-100 mg c/8-12 h) can be used.

Apathy

Apathy is very frequent in up to 75% of cases. It consists of lack of motivation, of initiative, of interest with diminished behavior, and cognition with reduced activity (27). It can occur with or without depression, appear early and persist over time. It can be treated with non-pharmacological methods, such as a cholinesterase inhibitor (donepezil, amantadine), if the patient has not used them before. If no response, a trial with 5 to 10 mg/day of methylphenidate is tried. Apathy may be associated with citalopram in the elderly with major depression.

Agitation and aggression

Most dementia sufferers exhibit various forms of agitation, such as physical and verbal aggression, related to infection or drug toxicity, untreated pain, hunger, thirst, inappropriate temperature, noise, confusion due to lack of sleep, the disease itself, or being overwhelmed by provocation (8, 11-13,30). These reactions are more severe in FTD than in AD and can occur up to three years before diagnosis. Efforts should be made to assess and meet the needs of sufferers, improve communication, modify procedures, and educate caregivers (e.g., to use analgesics before painful treatments). Atypical antipsychotics or haloperidol can be used in AD. risperidone (0.25 mg/day), olanzapine (2.5 mg starting dose and titrated up to a maximum of 5 mg twice daily), and quetiapine as an alternative (with a starting dose of 25 mg/night up to 75 mg/2 times daily), together with lorazepam (0.25 mg/day) are useful. The use of restraints leads to many undesirable effects such as increased agitation. A group of individuals with impaired cognitive function found restraints to be the third most bothersome medical procedure. They do not decrease the incidence of falls or may increase their frequency and the occurrence of pressure ulcers (4,6,30-34).

Delusions and hallucinations

Delusions and hallucinations appear when the individual becomes unable to recognize the environment, and there is an overload of stimuli due to severe systemic illness such as infection, toxins, and adverse effects of medication. They arise as an acute confusional state with changes in attention and behavior that appear in a short time and fluctuate throughout the day. They may be hyperactive (characterized by agitation, restlessness, or emotional lability) or more often hypoactive (with flat affect, apathy, lethargy, or poor responsiveness). They tend to reverse with adequate pain control, urinary or respiratory infection, review of polypharmacy, hydration and nutrition, and the presence of a familiar person. DLB dementia has many behavioral disorders and psychotic symptoms (between 7% and 33%), especially visual hallucinations (these are less frequent in Parkinson's dementia), with a high risk of severe neuroleptic sensitivity. Therefore, many typical and atypical antipsychotics should be avoided, any psychoactive medication should be reduced, eliminating dopamine agonists, anticholinergics, and even carbidopa/levopa. Delusions and hallucinations are very distressing for the patient and caregivers and more intense in severe dementia. They respond well to low doses of antipsychotics such as risperidone (0.5-1.0 mg/day). Quetiapine (25 mg night) or olanzapine (2.5-10 mg/day) have a lower antidopaminergic profile and can be used (6,27). Benzodiazepines (BZD) are not recommended because they may worsen gait and should be limited for stressful episodes due to change of residence or an anxiety-provoking event (30).

Executive dysfunction syndrome

This is a combination of disinhibition and fixation to stimuli that produces disinhibited and inappropriate behaviors that make caregivers uncomfortable and distressed. It is an important symptom in FT dementias, as they are related to the disruption of frontal subcortical circuits. While executive dysfunction syndrome is less common than depression, psychosis, and apathy, it may present a safety risk, either through being injured by incessant walking or by a slap by the offended person. Treatment with amantadine, SSRIs, and sodium valproate is not always successful (4,6,29-31).

Paranoid delusions

These are misinterpretations of external stimuli. The patients may see objects larger or smaller than they are, as well as distorted objects. In 30% of cases, the paranoid delusions can be severe. Delusions include beliefs that the house has been invaded, theft of personal objects, replacement of family members by impostors, and infidelity of spouses. A low dose of risperidone is helpful.

Obsessive compulsive and repetitive symptoms

These include recurrent thought patterns and vocalizations. Repetitive acts without purpose are noticeable in Parkinsonian patients and FT dementia.

Hypersexuality

This sometimes occurs in Kluver Bucy syndrome due to temporal lobe involvement. Hypersexuality occurs in 15%–25% of patients with vascular dementia, AD, and other neurodegenerative dementias. This can be reduced or ameliorated by risperidone and antiandrogen therapy (e.g., flutamide).

Noisy behavior

May be seen in dementias as an undesirable reaction to medication, a partial seizure, or when the patient is delirious. The cause is usually not found and is treated with neuroleptics and low doses of carbamazepine and trazodone.

Wandering

The possibility of getting hurt, lost, or dying is a concern for family or caregivers and is more common when left alone in very hot or cold weather where there is a greater chance of death. Wandering may be due to distractibility and restlessness, memory loss, and spatial disorientation (5) and is often caused by a change of environment and sometimes resolves on return home. Wandering improves with risperidone. Compulsive wandering is an indication for placement in secure units to control this behavior.

Sleep disturbances

Sleep disturbances are common in up to two-thirds of patients and may be due to depression and anxiety, decreased physical activity, nocturia, undesirable drug effects, and changes in circadian rhythms. Some suffer from severe agitation associated with premature awakening in depressive illnesses, or become more confused and behaviorally impaired in the evening and at night (sundowners syndrome). They may improve with increased daytime exercise, natural light in the morning, limiting night-time drinks, withdrawing alcohol and coffee, reducing noise, not waking for vital signs or night-time medication, and bringing residents together according to their sleep patterns (6). Trazodone (25 mg initial dose/night) is well tolerated and is used in the onset of sleep disorders with dementia. It can be used in the first weeks until SSRIs take effect. Another possibility: melatonin (2 mg/1 h before bedtime, max. 13 weeks) or zolpidem (5 mg before bedtime, max. 4 weeks). Hypersomnia can be caused by use of hypnotics, antiepileptics, anticholinergics, infections, and various stimuli. If sleep apnea is suspected, refer to polysomnography or a sleep specialist. CPAP improves cognition and decreases the risk of dementia.

Resistance to attention

This comprises various behaviors whereby patients resist the efforts of caregivers. While it can occur in mild dementia, it is more common when impairment is very severe and the ability to understand spoken language is diminished. Resistance to attention may be accompanied by delusions, hallucinations, or depression, but the most important factor in managing it is the caregiver's approach, who should maintain a relaxed attitude and avoid making requests that create stress or go beyond the person's capacity. The caregiver should always try to be within the person's field of vision and express respect by allowing the person to maintain some control (4,8,21,27,29). Distraction methods can serve to shift patients' attention away from the stimulus that is causing them stress. Engaging them in conversation and reminiscing about happy times can help and will be better if there are two caregivers. The bathroom should be clean and regarded as private and personal, with relaxing music, soft lighting, and low noise levels. If shower baths are difficult, they should be replaced by bed hygiene, which may be less stressful. Encouraging patients' participation in their care and bathing may reduce confusion. If a painful treatment is to be given, painkillers should be administered first.

Drugs and Dementia

The brain is a vulnerable organ in dementia, as is the heart in heart disease. Current drugs do not effectively control many of the most annoying behaviors, so it is essential to train caregivers in non-pharmacological methods for better care on their part, because the best results are not produced by drug treatment. Alzheimer's disease is associated with reduced acetylcholine synthesis and altered cortical cholinergic function, which is why cholinesterase inhibitors are used: donepezil (5-10 mg/day), galantamine (16-24 mg/day), rivastigmine (6-12 mg/day), and memantine (with another mechanism; 10 mg/day in mild to moderate phases of AD) with a modest benefit to cognition without changing the underlying pathology or disease. There is more benefit in DLB and Parkinson's, with improvement in behavioral symptoms and hallucinations and small improvements in cognition (22). There is very limited evidence to support the use of cholinesterase inhibitors in severe dementia, so it is reasonable to discontinue them progressively (50% every 4 weeks) according to the patient's preferences, their previous wishes, and in collaboration with the family : if there has been a significant worsening in the previous six months, if there has been no improvement or significant changes, if the dementia is severe or terminal, or if intolerable undesirable effects (nausea, vomiting, and diarrhea) appear in one-third of patients. Other causes of suspension are anorexia, weight loss, risks of syncope, bradycardia, using a pacemaker and hip fracture but is posible to continue if there are positive effects on cognition, behavior and functional status (9). These medications are considered to offer little benefit and divert the clinician's attention from other interventions (1-3-7,11-13).

The very common polypharmacy in the elderly can affect the cognitive level and the relationship with the environment, even causing acute confusional symptoms. Sedatives, first-generation antihistamines, amitriptyline, chlorpropamide, oral meperidine, pentazocine, diuretics, digitalis, oral antacids, NSAIDs cimetidine, BZP, opioids, and antipsychotics are responsible, especially in patients with Parkinson's. The adverse effects of polypharmacy in dementia can add up and increase cognitive deterioration. Therefore, periodic reviews of the list of medications should be made, along with an attempt to use the minimum doses required to obtain clinical benefit and suspension of unnecessary ones. Before prescribing a new drug, adverse effects should be thought of as possible causes of a new symptom, and non-pharmacological measures should begin when possible. In dementia, there is a risk of a prescription cascade effect when giving a new drug for an unrecognized side effect of a pre-existing therapy (e.g. oxybutynin, which is an anticholinergic, for incontinence) (23-26).

Patient Support Measures

Caring for a person with mental disorders is more emotionally burdensome than caring for someone with physical problems and involves changes in the daily life of the carer, particularly if the patient is restless, talks too much, is upset at night, and causes problems for the neighbors (6). Patients are often confused, anxious, and irritable, with a loss of self-esteem and depression; therefore, they should be spoken to face-to-face, without startling them, with simple words, asking them only one thing at a time, with the help of gestures if it is possible and giving enough time to respond (6,27-42). It is necessary to encourage families to provide the patient with verbal instructions or simple visual cues, such as starting to perform the movement—with a toothbrush, for example—when they are unable to start on their own. The maxim: "*start slow and go slow*" is helpful in adjusting your pace. You will be asked to simplify the tasks you perform, with simpler guidelines, schedule predictable activities, limit options and decision making. They will need to wear glasses or hearing aids if needed and will have orientation stimuli, calendars and clocks in their environment It is helpful if they wear a name tag indicating than their address and phone number, and keep them active during the day so they sleep better at night.

Physical exercises and walks improve mood, strength, muscle tone, and sleep, help maintain good balance, and prevent pneumonia and urinary tract infection (4,8). With the progression of dementia, patients present unsteadiness, gait in small steps, inability to walk and avoid obstacles, with more falls. It is recognized that good periodic control, adequate nutrition, treatment of chronic ailments, good sleep, occupational therapy, and regular exercise, such as a walking, prevent memory symptoms from appearing worse than they really are. Memory conservation does not depend only on the patient but on their environment, so old friends should be invited, one or two at a time, and the family photo album should be reviewed. Developing simple interests can stimulate and give the patient satisfaction. Making it easier for patients to maintain some activity, even at the simplest levels, is important for maintaining dignified social relationships. Religious, artistic, movement, dance, and pet therapy practices are useful (6-10,29).
An occupational therapist can help patients exercise certain functions, and a music therapist may find a delicate way to provoke and renew motivation in life through music, using songs that the patient likes or old songs that are familiar to everyone. Music can stimulate preserved areas of the brain and creates emotional connections (6,29). Observing patients' response to music can be invaluable in illuminating a sad and hopeless life with a brief spark. Patients can be encouraged to sing or even play an instrument if they had a musical background (See: https://youtu.be/ NKDXuCE7LeQ.) Music can itself become a bridge between reality and the unreal world in which the patient isolates or seeks refuge. Getting up and singing for pleasure can give patients, even for a moment, a sense of dignity by participating in an activity that is neither material nor utilitarian.

Some families who provide the bulk of chronic care may think they will never feel normal again because the burden is too heavy, the information scanty, and the doubts too great. It is preferable to provide care within the family when possible, due to the strong ties that transcend cultural and racial differences, but inadequate, poor quality, or ineffective care can be much more expensive and less desirable for individuals. Patients, even when severely disturbed and unable to communicate, need and appreciate family affection. Holding their hands, hugging them, or just sitting next to them are important ways to maintain communication. Anxiety may be due to feeling confused in an apparently unfamiliar place (26-31). We must speak simply and softly to patients, with few words, allowing them to participate in decisions as much as possible. High pitch, even in those with hearing loss, can be perceived as a nonverbal signal of irritation. The delicate physical care given to them conveys the concern of their peers and increases their sense of security.

Personalized Attention

Maintaining the quality of life of patients with advanced dementia is very important. Volicer and Simard (8,12,26,42) developed a program called Namaste Care, a Hindu term that means '*honoring the inner spirit*', to treat residents with advanced dementia in an individualized and person-centered way in a welcoming environment with multiple visual, tactile, and aural stimuli. The criteria for enrollment into this program are MMSE ≤ 7, non-ambulatory, sleeping most of the time, limited vocalization, in need of total care, and unable to actively participate in activities (8,22,26-29,33-43). Caregivers in this program seek to work on patients' physical, psychosocial, and spiritual needs, with meaningful and caring activities that reduce their isolation and facilitate the intervention of family members who feel that they can continue doing something for their loved ones. The results are positive and the staff and family feel grateful for having an activity with meaning for the sick.

The Family and the Care of the Patient with Dementia

Dementia is usually unfamiliar territory that most families are unable to navigate, so we must point out that the active roles and rights of the patient should be respected, and various forms of communication with them should be promoted while paying attention to all the patients' signals. Caregivers usually have difficulties distinguishing between dementia symptoms and the patient's personality and may be either aware, partially aware, or unaware of the disease. Caregiver unawareness may be an attempt to maintain the integrity of the patient's identity. Family caregivers may experience an increased burden caused by anticipatory grief when confronted with a diagnosis of dementia. Sometimes, caregivers may deny the disease and loss of roles, increasing their emotional distance from the patient (44).

To improve awareness, it is very important to involve caregivers in psychoeducational interventions and provide information about the condition, its prognosis, and ways of coping with it. These interventions help caregivers understand that their role is not only associated with rehabilitation or retarding the course of the disease; they also provide belief clarifications, in which caregivers are stimulated to view their situation with some distance and to develop strategies to deal with immediate and recurrent caregiving situations (35-43). Thus, they become more aware of the emotional impact of their actions on the patients (44). In terms of the significance of the burden of giving care to a dementia patient, black family caregivers appear to experience less burden than white caregivers, similar to African Americans, Chinese Americans, Jewish Americans, and those of Latin origin. This demonstrates a relationship between cultural factors and disease history. Non-white caregivers demonstrate less stress, burden and depression, believe more in the support of their children, and tend to use more prayer, faith, or religion as coping mechanisms. The hegemony of the biomedical discourse has influence on the fact that the sensibilities, meanings, and concerns of family caregivers of persons with EA in different cultural contexts tend to be similar. Therefore, it is necessary to legitimize the knowledge of the family members because they are experienced caregivers (44).

The motivation to provide care is determined by both cultural and individual aspects and may influence disease awareness, depending on whether caregivers are able to identify negative or positive aspects related to activities of caring. Social representations of family and religion are additional cultural aspects that may influence awareness. Tradition and spirituality, which are secondary reasons for becoming a caregiver, are considered social norms, especially in Latin American countries. Faith often appears as a source of support in the face of difficulties and suffering, offering strength to overcome them. Caregivers' cultural background and the resulting attitudes toward the disease may also partially determine their investment in the care of their loved ones and thus increase or decrease the burden of care. The majority of caregivers tend to have difficulties coping with the behavioral and psychological symptoms of dementia (44-45). These symptoms may arouse negative feelings, such as entrapment, shame, or guilt, which may lead to higher levels of depression and physical symptoms. It is also essential to detect in time caregivers' mental health and possible overload in order to promote a self-care program for them, because they have a greater risk of losing their health, and suffering from depression, sadness, anger, resentment, and isolation. These data suggest that clinicians need to be more sensitive to the cultural aspects of dementia and should ask patients and their families about the meaning of aging and help them understand the meaning of dementia symptoms. This will also help them to understand whether or not they need care.

In the final phase, families prefer to care for the patients at home, especially if they have the support of a palliative team. Knowing how to ask for help from other relatives or to hire other caregivers, identifying and offering them the existing support resources in the community (6,22, 29,37-42). For these reasons, professionals should inform families of the following: (a) about human and physical resources available in the community to reduce the burden of care and what to do in each phase and how to deal with various circumstances; (b) the importance of having close emotional support; (c) forms of rest in their tasks and possibilities of entertaining themselves and continuing with their habitual customs; (d) the possibility of respite admission of the patient, and; (e) the need for admission to palliative care if there are other pathologies and difficulties.

Caregiver overload is the greatest determinant of hospitalization or admission and must be regularly evaluated with the Zarit Scale in the follow-up of patients. Various counseling and support measures can reduce the anxiety of the caregiver; day centers and respite programs are very useful. Care teams must provide the family with easier access to consultation, by telephone or at home, adapt schedules, and reduce waiting times with good coordination of all services and support resources. Aides must have significant social, financial and employment implications (38-41).

Prospects

The 2020 Lancet Commission report (3) considers that it is never too early or too late to reduce the risk and mitigate dementia. This can be accomplished by promoting a culture that reduces the poverty and inequality being suffered by ethnic groups such as Blacks, Asians, and vulnerable populations and by the creation of environments where physical activity is a more normal occurrence, hypertension, obesity, and hyperlipidemia are controlled, levels of exposure to excessive noise are reduced, and nutrition is improved. According to the WHO(2), it is essential to implement the global action plan 2017-2025 for a response to dementia because this disease affects all countries, especially the poor and medium-income countries.The impact of dementia is not only significant in financial terms,but also reresents substancial human costs to countries, societies, families and individuals. Priority interventions should be made to ensure that people with dementia and their carers can live well and receive the care and support they need with dignity, respect, autonomy, and equality. The WHO plan comprises seven action areas: dementia as a public health priority; awareness of insanity and kindness; dementia and risk reduction; dementia diagnosis, treatment and support; support for dementia carers; dementia information systems; and dementia and innovation. With this, it is expected that by 2025, at least 50% of people with dementia will be diagnosed in at least 50% of countries. Attention to social circumstances and support throughout life is recommended, including poverty reduction strategies and opportunities for social commitments such as volunteering and continuing education, which help people maintain stimulating activities.

One of the most active research topics at the moment is trying to answer the following question: by what mechanisms is a stored perception retrieved from memory and how can we influence the recall of that perception? Several investigations are underway for the development of new therapeutic means. Thus, in AD, efforts are being made to achieve effective treatments because it is considered that the formation of neurofibrillary tangles of the tau protein and the accumulation of plaques of beta-amyloid protein are responsible for neuronal isolation (46). According to studies by Lars Lannfelt, as a result of finding the arctic or APPE693G mutation in a Swedish family in which 11 members developed dementia before the age of 60, it is believed that the origin of AD may lie in a genetic defect. Based on this finding, a monoclonal antibody BAN2401 has been developed, called lecanemab, which slows down the progress of dementia by 27% compared to placebo in patients in the initial phase with slight deterioration. Although the majority of patients do not share this benefit, it can help in the case of families with several members with dementia. The two most recent, significant developments in this field are the progressive development of vaccines for Alzheimer's disease and monoclonal antibody (3-7).

Summary

Dementia is a progressive illness and a social problem with a well-characterized clinical course, requiring compassionate care measures based on evidence and shared decision-making to alleviate bothersome symptoms and the suffering of affected patients, especially in LMICS. Palliative care seeks to provide the greatest possible well-being to patients and help them adapt to progressive losses and create a new model in relationships. With a global effort and friendly dementia policies that reduce stigmatization, 40% of dementia sufferers can achieve a good quality of life.

Bibliography

1. Risk reduction of Cognitive decline and dementia. WHO Guidelines, 2019.
2. Global Action plan on the public health response to dementia 2017-2025, WHO, 2017.
3. Livingston G. Huntley J., Sommerlard A. et al. Dementia prevention, intervention and care,2020 Report of the Lancet Commission. Lancet 2020.396-413-46
4. Widera E., Talebreza S., Bernacki R. Dementia. In: Oxford Textbook of Palliative care, edited by Cherny N. Fallon M.T., Kaasa S., Russell K, Oxford University Press, 2021, 987-993
5. Press D. Management of the patient with dementia. UpTo Date, Last Updated Dec. 22,2021
6. Astudillo W., Arriola E y Mendinueta C. El paciente con demencia. Cuidado personal y apoyo a la familia. En: Medicina Paliativa: Cuidados del enfermo en el final de la vida y atención a su familia. Editado por W. Astudillo, C. Mendinueta y E. Astudillo. EUNSA, 6 Edición, 2018, 779-802.
7. Sabbag N. McCarthy M., Martin G. Determining and defining Advanced dementia. Palliative care for advanced Alzheimer´s and dementia. Springer Publishing co. Alzheimer Asociation. Desert Southwest chapter,3-9 2011
8. Volicer L. Simard J. Tratamiento de la demencia avanzada. En: Manual de Enfermedad de Alzheimer y otras demencias,editado por M.F. Weiner y A. Lipton. Editorial Médica Panamericana, 2010, 533-349,
9. Ismail, Z, Blanck, S., Camicioli R, et al, Recommendations of the 5 th Canadian Consensus Conference on the diagnosis and treatment of dementia. Alzheimer´s & Dementia, 2020;16:1182-1195
10. Adelman R. Greene M. Silva M. Communication challenges with the elderly. In: Oxford Textbook of Communication in Oncology and Palliative care. 2 ed. Oxford University Press, 2017, 334-343
11. Mitchel S- Care of patients with advanced dementia, UpToDate Nov. 2022
12. Volicer L. Palliative Medicine in dementia. In: Oxford Texbook of Palliative Medicine, edited by G. Hanks, N. I. Cherny, N. Christakis, M. Fallon, S. Kaasa, R. Portenoy, R. Oxford University Press. 4th Edition, 2010, 1376-1384.

13. Widera E. Bernacky R., Dementia, Oxford Textbook of Palliative Medicine, edited by N. Cherny, M.Y. Fallon, S. Kaasa, R. Portenoy and D. Currow, 2015, Oxford Univ.Press. 991-993
14. Mitchell SL., Miller SC., Teno JM, Kiely DK., etal. Prediction of 6 month survival of nursing home residents with advanced dementia using ADEPT vs hospice elegibility guidelines. JAMA 2010:304 (17):1929
15. Reisberg B. Functional assessment staging (FAST), Psychopharmacology Bulletin, Vol, 23, Issue, 4, pp. 653-9, 1988
16. Herbert C.P. Cultural aspects of Dementia. Can. J. Neurol. Sci. 2001,28; Suppl. 1- S77-S82
17. Hillman, A., Latimer, J. Cultural representations of Dementia. Cultural representations of Dementia. PLoS Med 14(3):e1002274. Doi: 10.1371/journal.pmed.1002274
18. Cohen, l. Toward an anthropology of senility: anger, weakness and Alzheimer´s in Banaras, India. Medical Anthropology Quartely,1995, 9(3):314-334-
19. Low, L.F. Purwaningrum F. Negative stereotypes, fear and social distance: a systematic review of depictions of dementia in popular culture in the context of stigma. BMC Geriatrics https://doi.org/10.1186/s12877-020-01754x
20. Stites, D.S., Rubright J., Karlawish J. What features of stigma do the public most commonly attribute to Alzheimer´s disease dementia? Results of a survey of the U.S. general public. Alzheimer´s &Dementia. 2018-1-8 https://doi.org/10.1016/jalz.2018.01.006
21. Agar M. Philips J. l. Palliative Medicine and care of the elderly. Palliative Medicine and care of the elderly. In: Oxford Textbook of Palliative Medicine. Edited by N.I. Cherny, M.T. Fallon. St. Kaasa. R.K. Portenoy y D. Currow, Oxford University Press, 2015,1042-1055
22. Abordaje de la demencia. Guia de actuación en la coordinación Atención Primaria- Neurología.Servicio Navarro de Salud, Departamento de Salud. 2008
23. Mitchell S.L. Clinical Practice. Advanced Dementia. N. Engl J Med 2015; 372:2533
24. Mitchell, S., Care of patients with advanced dementia. UpToDate, Last updated Apr.05,2023
25. Hines S., McCrow J, Abbey J. et al. The effectiveness and appropriateness of a palliative approach to care for people with advanced dementia: a systematic review. JBI Libr Syst Rev. 2011:9(26):960-1131, doi10.11124/02938924-201109260-00001
26. Volicer L, McKee A., Hewitt, Demencia. Cllínicas neurológicas de Norteamérica, Cuidados Paliativos. Vol.4 , 2001, 863-881.

27. Watson M. Campbell R., Vallath N., Ward S, Wells J. Dementia and Frailty, Oxford Handbook of Palliative Alzheimer´s Disease International Third Edition 2019, 579-611, Oxford University Press.
28. Caprio T.V. Kosier B.Z., Dementia en Neuropalliative care. Edited by C. Creutzfeld, Kruger B.Z., Holloway R. Springer 2019,73-87
29. Astudillo W., Zabalza R. Cuidados de los pacientes con demencia. En: Los valores del cuidado, editado por W. Astudillo, A. Salinas, C. Mendinueta. Paliativos sin Fronteras, 2021, 265-281
30. Press D., Management of neuropsychiatric symptoms of dementia. UpToDate, this topic last updated Apr. 07-22
31. Petersen R., Envejecimiento, deterioro cognitivo leve y Enfermedad de Alzheimer. Clínicas Neurológicas de Norte América. Vol 4/2000,845-863
32. Steinberg Martin, Lyketsos C., Trastornos psiquiátricos en personas con demencia. En: Manual de Enfermedad de Alheimer y otras demencias, editado por Myron F. Weiner, A. Lipton. Editorial Médica Panamericana, 2010, 263-281,
33. MacRae R., Brown M. Tolson D. Dementia.In: Hospice Palliative Home Care and Bereavement, Edited by L. Holtslander, Peacok S. J. Bally. Springer Nature. AG 2019
34. Post SG., The Moral Challenge of Alzheimer Disease: Ethical Issues from Diagnosis to Dying. Baltimore, MD Jhon Hopkins University Press, 2000, 2n Ed.
35. Van der Steen, J., Lemos N., Gijsberts M.J., et al. Palliative care for people with dementia in the terminal Phase: a mixed-methods qualitative study to inform service development. BMC palliative care (2017) 16:28
36. Cohen-Mansfield., J. Nonpharmacologic interventions for inappropriate behaviors in Dementia; a A review. Summary and Critique. American Journal of Geriatric Psychiatry 9:361-381-.
37. Nonpharmacological therapies for the treatment of behavioural symptoms in people with dementia. https://www.alzheimers.org.uk/
38. Martin G, Sabbagh M. Preface. Palliative care for advanced Alzheimer´s and dementia. Springer Publishing Co. Alzheimer association. Desert Southwest chapter,2011
39. Lindstrom K.B, Bosh R. Cohen R, et al. Caregiving en; Palliative care for advanced Alzheimer´s and dementia. Springer Publishing co. Alzheimer asocciation. Desert Southwest chapter,25-40,2011
40. Martin G., Sgrillo J., Horton A. Creating the optimal milieu for care. In: Palliative care for advanced Alzheimer´s and dementia. Springer Publishing Co. Alzheimer Association. Desert Southwest Chapter,55-64,2011

41. Martin G, A, McCarthy M. Managing behavior problems associated with advanced dementia. In: Palliative care for advanced Alzheimer´s and dementia. Springer Publishing co. Alzheimer asocciation. Desert Southwest chapter, 65-80,2011
42. Simard J. The End Of life Namaste care Program for people with dementia. Baltimore M. B. Health Profession Press, 2007
43. Stacpoole, M., Hockley J. Thompsell A., Simard J, Volicer, L. The Namaste Care programme can reduce behavioural symptoms in care home residents with advanced dementia. International Journal of Geriatric Psychiatry, 2015, 30 (7),702-9
44. Santos R.L., B de Sousa M.F., Ganem A.C., Silva T, Douradod M. Cultural aspects in dementia: differences in the awareness of a Brazilian caregivers. Trends, Psychiatry Pssychother. 2013:35(3).191-197
45. Martorell M.A. Paz R., L., Montes, M.J., Jiménez H. M. F., Burjalés. M.D. Index Enferm Vol.19. nº2-3- Granada Abr/sept. 2010.
46. Lecanemab for Alzheimer´s disease: tempering hype and hope. www.the lancet.com, vol 40 ,Dec., 3,2022

23

Palliative Care, Supportive Care, Dignity, and Spirituality in People Suffering from Dementia and their Families

Loredana Buonaccorso, Ph.D.[1], Carla Ida Ripamonti, M.D.[2] and Monica Gandelli, M.D.[3]

Abstract

Supportive therapies and palliative care for people suffering from dementia were adopted in the last decades, in a cultural change that occurred over time. In every stage of all types of dementia, both care teams and society must pay attention to the dignity of the patient and the caregivers' resources, from diagnosis onward.

The chapter is organized as follows: the first section aims to focus on the main supportive care and palliative care interventions for people suffering from dementia and their family members. The treatment of all forms of dementia requires a multidisciplinary and multidimensional approach, including pharmacological and non-pharmacological interventions, and involves the caregiver, from the diagnosis onward. Scientific research continues to be mainly focused on pharmacological therapy, while randomized control trial

---

[1] Psycho-Oncology Unit, Azienda USL-IRCSS di Reggio Emilia, Reggio Emilia, Italy

[2] Palliative Medicine Chair, Department of Medical and Surgical Specialties, Radiological Sciences and Public Health, University of Brescia, Brescia, Italy

[3] Internistic and Geriatric Supportive Care Unit, Department Onco-Heamatology, Fondazione IRCCS Istituto Nazionale dei Tumori Milano, Milan, Italy

studies relating to non-pharmacological strategies, supportive care, and palliative care in patients with dementia are far fewer, with small sample sizes.

The last segment is dedicated to the discussion of dignity and spiritual dimensions related to dementia from the perspective of patients, family members, and healthcare professionals. Taking care of a patient with advanced dementia is highly complex and is accompanied by the risk of depersonalizing patients by making them morally equivalent to a "list" of signs and symptoms. Acknowledgment of the individual's life projects and life history is a crucial, dignifying component of care. Personal dignity can be reinforced by allowing individuals with dementia to talk about past achievements and significant events in their lives, allowing them to confirm their identity to themselves and others. Moreover, spiritual care offers several quality-of-life benefits for persons with dementia and their family members, including enhancing meaning and purpose in life, maintaining relationships, providing comfort and hope, and coping strategies.

Keywords: dementia, palliative care, supportive care, dignity, spirituality, care relationship

Abbreviations

Palliative care: PC
Randomized control trial (RCT)
Supportive care: SC
Healthcare professionals: HPs
World Health Organization: WHO
Global Dementia Observatory: GDO
Alzheimer's disease: AD
Clinical dementia rating: CDR
Health and care excellence: NICE
Non-pharmacological treatments: NPTs
Functional Assessment Staging Scale: FAST

Introduction

> "In fragility are hidden values of sensitivity and delicacy, of exhausted kindness and dignity, of intuition of the unspeakable and the invisible that are in life, and that allows us to identify more easily and with more passion in the moods and emotions, in the ways of existential being, of others from us"
>
> Eugenio Borgna

Supportive therapies and palliative care (PC) for people suffering from dementia were adopted in the last decades, in a cultural change that took place over time. In every stage of all types of dementia, both care teams and society must pay attention to the dignity of the patient and the caregiver's resources from diagnosis onward. The therapeutic alliance with the multidisciplinary care staff requires careful attention to the psycho-social aspects of the patients and their family members, as well as to the spiritual/existential dimension as a resource for coping with the disease. Each intervention must be well-balanced to evaluate the risks and benefits for the patient and the caregiver in the treatment setting.

Scientific research continues to be mainly focused on pharmacological therapy, while randomized control trial (RCT) studies relating to non-pharmacological strategies, supportive care (SC), and PC in patients with dementia are far fewer, with small sample sizes. The future challenge is to evaluate the effectiveness of non-pharmacological interventions and support strategies in each stage of the disease, with particular attention to accompaniment in the advanced stage of the disease.

The "Rights of People with Dementia" (Alzheimer Europe, 2014), details the human rights of dementia patients. The declaration affirms the following six rights: the right to a timely diagnosis; the right to access quality post-diagnosis support; the right to quality, person-centered, coordinated assistance throughout the illness; the right to equal access to treatment and therapeutic interventions; and the right to be respected as an individual in one's community.

1. Dementia: classification and epidemiology

The Diagnostic and Statistical Manual of Mental Disorders (DSM-V) defines dementia as "a disorder characterized by memory impairment and at least one more symptom such as aphasia, apraxia, agnosia, or executive functioning disorders combined with difficulties in social and occupational functioning" (Reisberg B, 2006). Dementia is, therefore, a chronic, progressive, cognitive deterioration of acquired origin that is manifested in the loss of cognitive functions, with a significant impact on autonomy in the patient's daily life (World Health Organization,1992). In Table 1, we present the classifications for dementia (World Alzheimer Report, 2020).

Table 1. Etiological Classification of Dementias (adapted from Columbus 2001)

Primary dementias	**Secondary dementias**
• Cortical dementias (without predominant motor signs) • Alzheimer's disease (AD) • Frontotemporal dementia (FT) • Subcortical dementias (with predominant motor signs) • Dementia with Lewy bodies (DLB) • Parkinson dementia • Huntington's chorea • Progressive supranuclear palsy • Cortico-basal degeneration	• Vascular dementia • Tumors and expansive processes of the central nervous system (CNS) • Normotensive hydrocephalus • Infectious and inflammatory diseases of the CNS (multiple sclerosis, encephalitis, neurosyphilis, HIV) • Head trauma • Endocrine disorders (e.g., hypothyroidism) • Metabolic diseases • Deficiency states (e.g., vitamin B_{12}, folate) • Toxic and drug encephalopathies • Miscellaneous

Neurodegenerative diseases represent a phenomenon on a large scale, especially in the most developed countries: there is an estimated 24.3 million cases of dementia in the world, with an estimated 4.6 million new cases annually. In other words, a patient is diagnosed with dementia every seven seconds (World Alzheimer Report, 2020).

The World Health Organization (WHO) began organizing its activities on this matter at the world conference in Geneva, held in March 2015, with the report "Dementia: A Public Health Priority." The WHO undertook to set up a "global dementia observatory" (GDO) to monitor the prevalence of dementia and support member countries in their strategic choices. Consequently, the GDO identified five areas in which to collect data—policy, resources, research and innovation, burden, and impact—which formed the basis for the construction of a set of indicators. Data from the WHO Global Action Plan 2017–2025 indicate that dementia affects 47 million people worldwide, a figure that is projected to rise to 75 million by 2030 and 132 million by 2050, with around ten million new cases per year. According to data from the WHO, Alzheimer's disease (AD) and other dementias are the seventh-leading cause of death in the world. Costs are estimated to be over $1 trillion per year, increasing progressively and continuing to challenge healthcare services (World Alzheimer Report, 2020).

Scientific research over the past thirty years has focused on therapies that can slow down but also change the course of the disease. In addition, the effectiveness of care models and case management still require years of study, and further research is needed to determine whether the proposed systems are effective for people with dementia and caregivers, in terms of clinical outcomes (World Alzheimer Report, 2020).

Finally, after the health emergency due to the SARS-CoV-2 pandemic, the hypothesis of permanent cognitive deficits post-infection has been proposed, which according to some authors could increase dementia diagnoses in the coming decades (Carlos AF, 2022).

The current diagnostic criteria for AD, known as the NIA-AA criteria, was published in 2011 by Guy McKhann (Jack CR, 2018). The strength of this criteria lies in having integrated the basic clinical diagnosis with the anamnestic interview, the evaluation of the typical signs of the disease, and the search for biomarkers. The average duration of AD is now estimated to be between 8 and 20 years; the division into stages is intended to guide the patient and caregivers as to the evolution of the pathology to adequately plan the care and life of the patient and his loved ones.

Among the tools adopted to define the severity of the disease is the Clinical Dementia Rating instrument (CDR) (Chaves F, 2007). The CDR scale evaluates the cognitive and functional performance of the patient in six areas: (1) memory, (2) orientation, (3) judgment and solution of problems, (4) social activities, (5) home and leisure, and (6) personal care. The scores of each area are summed to obtain a composite score ranging from 0 to 3 (7). With the CDR scale, dementia patients are classified into five progressive severity levels: CDR 1 (mild dementia), CDR 2 (moderate dementia), CDR 3 (severe dementia), CDR 4 (very severe dementia), and CDR 5 (terminal dementia). CDR 4 indicates very serious dementia: the patient has a severe speech or understanding deficit, difficulties in recognizing family members, inability to walk alone, and serious problems in eating independently and in controlling intestinal or bladder function. At this stage, SC is crucial. CDR 5 defines terminal dementia: the patient is completely unable to express himself and communicate, bedridden, totally incontinent, a vegetative state; PC is adopted at this stage.

2. The treatments

The treatment of all forms of dementia requires a multidisciplinary and multidimensional approach, including pharmacological and non-pharmacological interventions, and involves the caregiver, from the diagnosis onwards (Mitchell SL, 2004; European Foundations' Initiative on Dementia, 2016; Pink J, 2018). Also, society must integrate and facilitate the patient and the caregiver in daily life, as indicated in the international, dementia-friendly communities project (European Foundations' Initiative on Dementia, 2016).

The most used and recent recommendations for the diagnosis and treatment of dementia are from the National Institute for Health and Care Excellence (NICE) (Pink J, 2018). The NICE recommendations are based on systematic reviews of the best available evidence and explicit consideration of cost-effectiveness. When available evidence is limited, recommendations are based on the experience of the guideline development group, and the standards of good clinical practice. The strength of the NICE guidelines lies in the consideration of the fundamental aspects of the disease, from diagnosis to the terminal phase, and in the emphasis placed on the caregiver, as confirmed also by the studies of the Italian network of dementia (Cartabellotta, 2018).

2.1. Pharmacological therapies in the advanced stages of dementia

AD is a progressive neurodegenerative disorder that represents the most common form of dementia worldwide. AD is characterized by two major pathological lesions in the brain, amyloid plaques and neurofibrillary tangles (NFTs), composed mainly of amyloid-β (Aβ) peptides and hyperphosphorylated tau. The physiopathology of AD remains unknown. However, new imaging techniques such as positron emission tomography (PET) and single-photon emission tomography (SPECT) can provide valuable, new, in vivo data from the early course of the disease.

Currently, there are no disease-modifying drugs available, and AD treatment is based on three acetylcholine esterase inhibitors, namely donepezil, rivastigmine, and galantamine. Memantine is an N-methyl D-aspartate (NMDA) receptor antagonist that is also used for AD. PDE inhibitors are considered useful drugs in the treatment of memory deficits (Yu TW, 2021; Alzforum Networking for a cure, 2023). Side effects include nausea, diarrhea, increased salivation, abdominal cramps, hypotension, bradycardia, anxiety, tremors, lacrimation, rhinorrhea, and bronchial hypersecretion. It is important to monitor the parameters and the electrocardiogram. Anticholinesterase therapy is stopped when dementia becomes severe, whereas memantine can be continued in the severe phase of the disease.

The American Food and Drug Administration approved a specific anti-beta monoclonal antibody called aducanumab in 2021. It is a human IgG1 monoclonal antibody that acts by reducing deposits of amyloid beta protein, the accumulation of which in the brain is believed to be the cause of the neurodegeneration process (Alzforum Networking for a cure, 2023). The European Medicines Agency has chosen not to approve the use of aducanumab, considering the need for further studies on its risks, benefits, and sustainability (European Medicines Agency, 2022).

The target of therapy in the advanced stages of dementia is represented by non-cognitive, and above all, behavioral manifestations, which represent the greatest source of stress for the family and caregivers, including HPs (Abraha I, 2017).

Antipsychotic drugs, antidepressants, mood stabilizers, and memantine are the most widely used therapies in the moderate and advanced stages of dementia for the control of psychotic disorders, anxiety, depression, insomnia, and physical and/or verbal aggression. Side effects must be monitored constantly, and the minimum effective dose must be used for short periods to monitor the target symptom (Nawzad S, 2022).

2.2. Non-pharmacological treatments in the advanced stages of dementia

SC in dementia also includes interventions implemented to improve the quality of life of the patient as well as of the informal and formal caregivers. In dementia care, SC takes a holistic approach, oriented toward the protection of the human and social values of the person, based on their clinical, cultural, social, and spiritual condition. Support interventions, which are also rehabilitative in the broad sense, and psychosocial interventions are generally defined as non-pharmacological treatments (NPTs). NPTs can be adopted in different care settings and all stages of the disease. NPTs require the active involvement of formal and informal caregivers; therefore, the training of the caregiver is a fundamental aspect of care. The objectives of NPTs are aimed at the different needs of the patient (e.g., psychological, cognitive, behavioral, functional, social, and spiritual) (Duncan E, 2020; Guazzarini AG, 2022; Livingston G, 2014). Among the supportive NPTs adopted in the advanced stage of dementia (CDR 4), the following are emphasized:

1. Motor and/or cognitive support rehabilitation interventions
2. Global interventions (Gentlecare, validation therapy, person-centered care, and the enabling approach).
3. Specific interventions (music therapy, doll therapy, pet therapy).
4. Support interventions for HPs and informal and formal caregivers (information, psychoeducational interventions, psychological support, and psychotherapy).

2.2.1. Rehabilitative interventions and occupational therapies

In the advanced stages of the disease, the care team evaluates and adopts interventions aimed at fall risks, postural comfort, prevention of tendon muscle retraction, reduction of the risk of pressure sores, and control of pain from muscle stiffness (secondary parkinsonism) (Woodbridge R, 2018). In addition, interventions include custom activities of active and passive mobilization, massages, and global relaxation techniques (Lorusso LN, 2018).

For the cognitive rehabilitation aspects, occupational therapists play an essential role (Guazzarini AG, 2022). They work to reduce behavioral disorders and improve the patient's quality of life, enhancing the possibility of global expression compatible with the disease, while acting on the environment and the training and behavior of caregivers (Woodbridge R, 2018; Miller PA, 2000,22). Moreover, they involve caregivers in the management of the patient's behavioral manifestations, propose meaningful activities for the patient, and evaluate solutions to create a protective physical and relational environment at home and in different care settings (Woodbridge R, 2018; Miller PA, 2000).

In general, occupational therapists evaluate the following:

- accessories adapted to the patient's deficits (cutlery, plates, glasses, etc.)
- specific clothing for the patient with dementia (e.g., pajamas and overalls to avoid fecal handling)

- means of protection to reduce the risk of falling (e.g., sheets for Alzheimer's, non-slip mats)
- safe furnishings designed for cognitive deficits
- areas to simulate virtual realities in residential settings (areas resembling a station, a shop, or a workplace)
- garden areas and areas outside of the care setting for meaningful activities (vegetable garden and Alzheimer's garden)
- choice of technologies and home automation to facilitate patient monitoring and allow the patients to express themselves in safety

2.2.2. Global interventions

Gentlecare

Gentlecare, proposed by the Canadian occupational therapist Moyra Jones, focuses on the well-being of the patient and the caregiver by adopting the method of a "prosthetic" care environment, characterized by physical space, people, and activities suitable for the patient (Jones M, 1999). The physical space must be simple, safe, familiar, and comfortable and must facilitate the activities of people with dementia. Caregivers must be trained and motivated in behavior, language, and communication appropriate and adapted to the behavior of the patient.

The activities to ensure the well-being of the patient are the following:

- “primary” (eating, washing, dressing)
- “necessary” (rest, sleep, moments of privacy)
- “essential” (move, communicate)
- “significant” for the patient (activities reminiscent of work, home life, hobbies)

Gentlecare within Alzheimer's care units has been shown to reduce behavioral disturbances and stress for formal and informal caregivers (Jones M, 1999).

Validation therapy

Validation therapy, formulated by Naomi Feil, began as a communication technique with dementia patients (Neal M, 2000). The validation method uses empathy and trust to connect with the inner reality of disoriented patients. The hypothesis underlying validation is that dementia brings patients back to episodes of their past and relational conflicts with relatives or other significant figures. The caregiver must, therefore, follow the patients into their world to try to understand the subjective feelings, emotions, and behaviors that derive from reliving their past conflicts and engage with them empathetically (Neal M, 2000).

The Person-Centered Care Model

Tom Kitwood, an English social psychologist and gerontologist, proposed the person-centered care model, arguing that in the treatment of dementia, it is essential to maintain personhood, which means being a person in its most complete sense of feelings, emotions, culture, and habits, despite the decay of cognitive functions (Bissolo G, 2009). The purpose of this model is to satisfy the five basic psychological needs of every human being: comfort, identity, attachment, occupation, and inclusion. To achieve this goal, appropriate reports and personalized activities are needed. The caregiver must avoid engaging in devaluing behavior toward the fragile, sick person (malignant psychology) and adopt behaviors to enhance the person (benign psychology) (Bissolo G, 2009, vans-Roberts CEY, 2011).

The Enabling Approach

"Enabling" is a technique for creating conditions whereby the person with cognitive deficits can carry out the activities of which one is capable without feeling wrong. The objective of enabling is for the sick person to be happy doing what one does, as one does it, in the context in which one finds oneself. The enabling approach leads professionals to listen to the patients' words, even if seemingly meaningless, and to apply specific conversation techniques by entering the world of the forgetful patient to seek a relationship without prejudice (Vigorelli P, 2011).

The conversational techniques are also extended to the formal caregiver, through specific courses. The patients are recognized as people able to express themselves even in the advanced stages of the disease, where the para-verbal and non-verbal actors have a possible relationship with the person with dementia, recognizing the healthy ego and not only the sick ego. The dialogs conducted during the conversations with the patient are recorded, transcribed, and reflected upon and form the basis of training in the enabling approach (Table 2) (Vigorelli P, 2011).

Table 2. The Enabling Approach and the Twelve Steps for the Caregiver

1. Don't ask questions
2. Don't correct or complete sentences
3. Don't interrupt
4. Listen and concentrate on the words spoken. Respect silence and slowness
5. Accompany the relative with Alzheimer's with words in the "possible world"
6. Answer the questions
7. Communicate also with gestures and tone of voice
8. Recognize emotions: spot them, name them, legitimize them, reflect them with your words
9. Respond to requests: accept the negotiation and take into consideration the choices, even when we know that we will not be able to satisfy them
10. Accept that the subject does what one does, as one does it, and says what one says, as one says it
11. Accept the disease and the patient, including their quirks
12. Recognize that you need help and let yourself be helped

2.2.3. Specific interventions

Music therapy

Music therapy is used to promote the sleep-wake rhythm to reduce anxiety and apathy. Environmental, group, and individual interventions are distinguished. The music therapist can use the reproduction of sounds of nature, instruments including Orff instruments, and environmental music while monitoring the patient's response. In various care settings, the response of the patient and the caregiver is positive. Studies of the use of music therapy for patients with dementia are the most numerous and promising (Svansdottir HB, 2006).

Doll therapy

Doll therapy has its roots in the attachment theory of John Bowlby, a child psychologist who considered the search for contact between parent and child a primordial instinct (Cai X, 2021). The therapeutic doll represents a transitional object that recalls the dynamics of primordial care. Therapeutic dolls are used with somatic, weight, and material characteristics, specifically designed to facilitate the patient's embrace, touch, and sensory stimulation. The doll is given to the patient for short periods to reduce anxiety, aimless motor activity, and apathy. The effects must be monitored by the caregiver. The data relating to the testing of this therapy are still not validated, although the experiences in nursing homes are positive (Cai X, 2021).

Pet Therapy

Many international researchers have verified the possibility of using animal-assisted interventions as supportive therapy in subjects suffering from AD (Kanamori M, 2001). The data collected, although heterogeneous and still in need of further confirmation, indicates that individuals with dementia respond positively to animal-assisted therapy, with a general improvement in their psychophysical state. In addition, caregivers also derive indirect benefits from the interactions between patients and animals (Cepero JL, 2020). Several RCT studies have evaluated the effects of this intervention on people with dementia, but none of them assessed the harm of these interventions; these are studies with small sample sizes and a critical risk of bias (Cepero JL, 2020).

2.2.4. Support interventions for the caregiver

The impact of dementia on the caregiver is termed “caregiver burden,” which refers to the overall pressure on the caregiver’s physical, psychological, and social needs as a result of providing care (Zafra-Tanaka JH, 2019, Young Tu JY, 2022). It is essential to determine the level, type, and cause of the burden to propose and optimize correct interventions to prevent and reduce it (Zafra-Tanaka JH, 2019). Studies show that the consequences for the physical and mental health of the caregiver, particularly the formal caregiver, can be dire: in addition to a decreased quality of life, the caregiver may suffer from sleep disturbances, anxiety disorders, and depression (Zafra-Tanaka JH, 2019, Young Tu JY, 2022).

Caregivers face “separation” when they discover that their loved one’s mental functions are gradually diminishing. Some authors have defined this experience as “ambiguous mourning”: the person is perceived by the caregiver as physically present but psychologically absent, no longer emotionally and cognitively available due to the pathology (Young Tu JY, 2022). The Caregiver Burden Inventory quantifies the loads in the various aspects of a caregiver's life, and the influence of the characteristics of patients and caregivers (Van den Kieboom R, 2020). The scale has proven to be an effective multidimensional tool for evaluating the impact of burden on many aspects of the lives of caregivers (Marvardi M, 2005). For informal caregivers, studies on the effects and dangers of stress related to dementia care are on the rise. The risk of burnout is high and can lead to aggressive behavior (verbal or physical) toward the patient or abandonment.

Interventions to promote the knowledge of dementia

The WHO invited to inform and train the entire population about dementia to avoid the isolation of patients and family members (World Health Organization, 2021). Printed material, videos, tutorials, and dedicated social networks have become information channels in the world. The global action plan for the public health response to dementia 2017-2025, adopted by WHO member states during the 70th World Health Assembly in May 2017, has the primary objective of improving the quality of life of people with dementia and their family members and caretakers. The plan proposed the following actions:

- raise awareness and prioritize the issue of dementia
- reduce the risk of dementia
- ensure diagnosis, treatment, and assistance
- support family members
- strengthen information systems for dementia
- promote research and innovation.

Psychoeducational interventions

Psychoeducational interventions can be conducted both individually and in groups, using structured meetings. The goals are to know the pathology, to understand what happens to the patient, to accept the patient's behavior, to learn to manage behavioral disorders, to improve communication with the patient, and to provide activities that the patient can perform. Caregivers are advised not to neglect themselves either and to allow moments of pleasure outside their role while delegating to others the care of their loved one.

Over the years, places for meetings, information, training, and psychoeducational interventions have arisen around the world, including Alzheimer cafés (Miesen B, 1997) and meeting centers (Dröes RM, 2006). Alzheimer cafés and meeting centers are models of a global approach for the initial and moderate stages of the disease; they also help to start a pathway for support even in the advanced stages of dementia and assist in raising awareness of the disease among the population.

Psychological support and psychotherapy

In some cases, individual psychotherapy is required for the caregiver. The first step is to encourage the caregiver to start therapy to overcome the difficulty of accepting the disease and to contain emotional suffering, anxiety, depression, and other symptoms of mental distress. The following paragraphs describe other interventions for caregivers that are dedicated to dignity and spirituality.

3. Palliative care in the terminal phase of dementia

In the course of treatment of dementia, it is difficult to define the terminal phase temporally (van der Steen JT, 2017). The patient may remain for years in an advanced stage of the disease, characterized by severe hypokinetic-rigid syndrome (secondary parkinsonism), progressive impoverishment of speech, increasing difficulty in swallowing, calorie-malnutrition protein, and loss of urinary and fecal continence, until reaching the terminal stage, which resembles a vegetative state (Browne B, 2021). Therefore, in terminal dementia, the patient may suffer from cachexia; total dependency with fetal posture and limbs in quadruple flexion mutism; severe dysphagia, leading to high risk of choking; fecal and urine incontinence; decubitus injuries; severe infections; thromboembolic events; and fragility fractures (van der Steen JT, 2017; Browne B, 2021).

The difficulty of defining life expectancy in people with advanced dementia poses a problem with the criteria for access to PC. Over the years, different scales have been proposed to guide the prognosis of these patients. Among the assessment scales adopted in PC for dementia, there is the Functional Assessment Staging Scale (FAST), which is part of the National Hospice Organization medical guidelines for determining prognosis in dementia (Sclan SG, 1992).

According to the literature, treatment settings in the different stages of dementia are heterogeneous, and consequently, clinicians who deal with severe dementia in hospices require significant educational intervention (Table 3) (van der Steen JT, 2017; Giulio P, 2008; Walsh SC, 2021). Knowing the symptoms and characteristics of patients during the terminal stage of the disease can help improve the process of decision-making and avoid improper access to the emergency room (Table 4) (Erel M, 2022; Toscani F, 2015; Van der Steen JT, 2017). Both the Holmes and the Beers criteria, for example, can guide physicians in choosing appropriate therapies at an advanced stage (American Geriatrics Society, 2019).

Table 3. Appropriate procedures for terminal patients with dementia

1. Identify symptoms and target signs 2. Target evaluation of pain with specific scales 3. Implement drug deprescription 4. Choose routes of administration of less invasive drugs (e.g., subcutaneous as well as continuous, for analgesics and symptomatic management?) 5. Adopt homogenous and small boluses for comfort feeding and do not implement artificial nutrition or gradually reduce it 6. Reduce or adjust oral hydration with thickeners and/or for hypodermoclysis (comfort hydration) 7. Reduce the suspension of diagnostic and routine investigations and examinations 8. Plan procedures of dressing, overall hygiene, and comfortable oral cavity toilet 9. Assess postural comfort with suitable aids 10. Improve ambient comfort (brightness, temperature, noise, odors) by adopting specific strategies (ambient music, aromatherapy, appropriate lights) 11. Facilitate the presence of family members and affective figures and give them support 12. Involve and support the professional team in choices 13. Decide and make explicit to NOT hospitalize the patient in acute settings and not to undergo resuscitation maneuvers and implement terminal sedation 14. Ensure respect for religious rituals and spirituality 15. Plan post-mortem choices 16. In community care settings, consider roommates to evaluate travel or privacy assurance

Table 4. The main signs and symptoms in the terminal stage of dementia

1. Delirium—apathetic, agitated, or mixed (treated, if necessary, with allopurinol, trazodone, benzodiazepines, orally in droplet formulations or via IV or subcutaneous, also continuous) 2. Discomfort and dyspnea (treated with oxygen if necessary, carefully avoiding pressure relief lesions related to goggles and masks, evaluate therapy for bronchial secretions with scopolamine butylbromide below) 3. Hyperpyrexia (check with paracetamol and steroids and do not implement antibiotic therapy) 4. Alterations of the intestine (modulate the use of microclisms) 5. Decubitus lesions of stages III and IV (medicate carefully, taking into account the patient's comfort and provide for antalgic therapy before dressing with correct timing) 6. Severe muscle hypertonia (fetal-like posture) requiring adequate posture and aids to prevent pressure injury

3.1. Pain and dementia

In people with dementia, pain is underdiagnosed and undertreated. In people no longer able to communicate verbally, the pain from symptoms becomes a sign that must be carefully sought out, with the observation shared with all professional figures and family members. Pharmacological strategies must be integrated while taking into consideration that pain has a physical component as well as psychological and social ones. We propose a summary table with the most important signs for identifying pain in people suffering from dementia (Table 5) (Bullock L, 2020).

Table 5. How to identify pain in people suffering from dementia

Observe facial expression	Sad and frightened face, grimace, wrinkled forehead, closed or narrow eyes, any new distorted expression
Listen to vocalizations	Sighs, groans, grunts, shouts, noisy breaths

Monitor postures	Stiffness, tense body posture, rocking, continuous postural changes, new abrupt motor activities
Assess behavioral changes	Aggression, resistance to treatment, decreased social interactions, socially inappropriate acts, fatigue
Observe changes in habitual activities	Refusal of food, changes in appetite, increased rest or sleep periods, changes in the pattern of rest, sudden cessation of common habits
Acknowledge changes in mental state	Crying, increased confusion, irritability, anxiety, apathy

3.2. Assessment scales and therapy for pain in severe dementia

The most widely used observational scale, involving different members of the treatment team, is the Non-communicative Patients Pain Assessment Instrument (Snow AL, 2004). This scale was structured to highlight the presence of pain in patients unable to verbally communicate their suffering to the nursing staff. It is administered in patients with Mini-Mental State Examination Test scores below 15 and is limited by its numerous items (Folstein MF, 1975). Contrary to this, the Pain Assessment in Advanced Dementia Scale is a simple and short measure (Costardi D, 2007). The scale analyzes five patient aspects, with scores ranging from 0 to 2 as follows: (1) The patient's breathing (0 if it is normal, 1 if slightly altered, 2 if presents with continuous hyperventilation or periodic central breath); (2) Vocalization (0 if no complaining, 1 if occasionally complaining, 2 if continuously weeping or complaining); (3) Facial expression (0 if serene or smiling, 1 if sad or contracted, 2 if grimaces are present); (4) Body language (0 if relaxed, 1 if restless, 2 if rigid/particularly agitated); (5) Patient consolation (0 if does not need to be consoled, 1 if consoles through voice or touch, 2 if inconsolable). The scores on each item are summed to obtain an overall score between 0 and 10, in which 0 represents the complete absence of pain, and 10 a severe pain. A score of 5 indicates a need for monitoring (Costardi D, 2007).

Pain therapy in the sick with dementia is often ex juvantibus. It is important to understand if the patient consoles himself with relationships and/or with non-pharmacological strategies. If such strategies are ineffective, then the next step might be to adopt drug therapy for pain, which encourages the use of appropriate formulations of analgesic (drops, formulas hormonal, subcutaneous, transdermal, rectal), while considering the weight of the patient. Examples include paracetamol (rectally or in hormonal formulations), morphine (orally and subcutaneously), and the use of transdermal opioid patches (dose-based) (Albert L, 2017).

If surgery seems to provide relief, the pain can be considered the most likely cause of the abnormal behavior and signs/symptoms observed, but only after serious observations, recorded by the staff at an appropriate time. In patients with severe dementia, malnutrition with reduced fat mass and lean mass with hypoalbuminemia, hepatorenal framework, dehydration state, and comorbidity are to be considered in order to avoid adverse events from overtreatment. Therefore, the minimum effective dose should be used, slowly increasing doses and closely monitoring side effects. In particular, constipation, nausea, and behavior may worsen (Williams ML, 2022; Wei YJJ, 2022). Due to the difficulty of recognizing nausea, the use of ex-adjuvan drugs may be appropriate. For each drug used, the team must evaluate the chosen route of administration, the risks and benefits, and the objective, while paying careful attention to the ethics of personal care in compliance with the anticipated wishes of the patient, whether known directly or learned and shared by reference caregivers (Wei YJJ, 2022).

4. Dignity and spirituality in the care relationship

Humans have an intrinsic need for dignity as a basic element of well-being, especially in assistance care (Chochinov HM, 2007). Dignity is defined as a "moral nobility that belongs to the nature of man, his skills, and the respect he has of himself and arouses in others because of his condition" (Chochinov HM, 2007; Johnston B, 2017). Dignity is personal, subject to changes depending on one's experience and path in life, and linked to a person's individual goals and social context. In healthcare, some patients feel that their dignity is directly related to the disease, such as the management of symptoms (pain, physical and mental), and dependent on the highest level of autonomy that they can maintain in physical, cognitive, and social terms. Others believe that it is linked to the continuity of the self, the perception of being oneself in confronting the disease, or the possibility that after death there is another life (Buonaccorso L, 2022).

Dignity in care is linked to spirituality, if we consider it a human need for "attraction to beauty, to the knowledge of reality and the good life" (Buonaccorso L, 2022; Agora Spiritual Care Guideline Working Group: Spiritual care, 2013; Firshein J, 1997). Attention to the spiritual dimension is recognized as an integral part of high-quality care, so it has been proposed to consider spirituality as one of the "vital signs" of the patient, to be constantly evaluated and cared for (Agora Spiritual Care Guideline Working Group: Spiritual care, 2013). Moreover, in medicine, it is described as "the forgotten factor" (Firshein J, 1997). We hope to emphasize patient dignity by integrating spirituality into students' curricula.

HPs should promote patient dignity and spirituality in each phase of the treatment, even when the patient is no longer in a position to recognize the care relationship, or when they have lost hope for a meaningful end-of-life experience. In every moment of care assistance, it is possible to support an image of the patient among HPs that restores dignity and gives meaning to the care relationship, even when this image is not consciously recognized by the patient (Buonaccorso L, 2023).

Dementia represents a challenge from the ethical point of view of respect for the person and the recognition of their value (The Lancet Commission, 2017; van der Steen JT, 2014). The progressive deterioration of the brain and the consequent functional impairment cause substantial changes to the patient's personality, leading to the consideration of the person with dementia—especially in advanced stages of the illness—as a "non-person", an "empty shell", due to the perception that there is no longer any possibility of interaction (The Lancet Commission, 2017; van der Steen JT, 2014). Consequently, family members often struggle to maintain the emotional bond, resulting in a real sense of loss. Taking care of a patient with advanced dementia is highly complex and is accompanied by the risk of depersonalizing patients by making them morally equivalent to a "list" of signs and symptoms. This depersonalization does not take into account that the essential core of personhood remains and ignores the ability of the patient with dementia to feel emotions, feelings, and desires.

A qualitative, cross-sectional study on the perspective of personal dignity, conducted among fourteen individuals with mild to moderate dementia who lived at home, reported three major categories of potential dignity-related distress: (1) the individual self, (2) the relational self, and (3) the societal self (van Gennip IE, 2016). While changes in identity and the loss of autonomy diminished patients' dignity, participants generally described their dignity as still reasonably intact and reported that they generally still found meaning in their lives. In particular, a key factor in the preservation of their dignity was their engagement in meaningful activities within the safety and security of their homes. "Living in the moment" was an effective method of coping with the consequences of the disease and maintaining their dignity, as described in other studies (Chochinov HM, 2002; Donmez ÇF, 2020). Discussing with the patients the most important things in their lives helps them to find meaning in life and live in the moment. This can be supplemented by talking with them about issues that are non-illness related, encouraging them to partake in various activities, supporting them with carrying out their daily routines, and helping them set realistic goals (The Lancet Commission, 2017; van der Steen JT, 2014).

The opportunity for reciprocation is also considered a key element in maintaining personal dignity, as a perceived inequality in the relationship between the caregiver and the patient was experienced by the patients as emotionally painful. In particular, patients said their dignity was not diminished by having to call on the help of others, if they felt like they could offer something in return, resulting in a reciprocally beneficial relationship (van Gennip IE, 2016). Many studies on dignity-in-care have shown that when facing the loss of autonomy, through cognitive or functional decline, supporting the patients' sense of being a person with values, emotions, desires, and lessons to be transmitted can improve their sense of dignity (Chochinov HM, 2002; Östlund U, 2019; Chochinov HM, 2004).

Finally, participants also reported the fear of losing one's dignity in front of strangers (van Gennip IE, 2016). While most of them felt dignified when among family and close friends because they felt understood and accepted, many participants felt ashamed of their behavior around strangers. It appears that individuals with dementia feel highly self-conscious, helpless, and ashamed of their perceived deviations from social norms, especially during the earlier stages. The way others view and treat individuals with dementia has a significant impact on their sense of personal dignity. As such, the magnitude of the decline in personal dignity depended largely on the individual's social context. The data highlight the difference between the impact of the inner circle (partner, relatives, close friends) compared to that of the outer, external world in terms of shaping the experiences and perceptions of individuals with mild to moderate dementia (Chochinov HM, 2002; Donmez ÇF, 2020; Östlund U, 2019).

Personal dignity is first and foremost a relational concept that is highly dependent on interpersonal interactions. Thus, the way that patients are reflected in the eyes of the care provider must ultimately affirm their sense of dignity. At least in part, dignity appears to be a subjective understanding of the self, based on the perception of interpersonal interactions (Chochinov HM, 2004). Many studies conducted in different care settings, from palliative to emergency and intensive care, have shown that personal dignity is innate in personhood and is an inalienable right that ought to be prioritized in the healthcare setting (Chochinov HM, 2004; Su A, 2018; Díaz-Cortés MDM, 2018; Tanzi S, 2020).

An empirically based model of dignity in the terminally ill has been developed from several quantitative and qualitative studies conducted with patients (Chochinov HM, 2002). This model identifies three main dimensions around which patients construct a perception of their dignity and which can be observed, assessed, and appreciated by HPs: (1) illness-related concerns, (2) dignity-conserving repertoire, and (3) social dignity inventory. Within each dimension, subthemes are identified that can support HPs' efforts to assist patients in enhancing their dignity, provide caregivers with a therapeutic map, and incorporate a broad range of physical, psychological, social, and existential considerations that may affect individual perceptions of dignity. In recent years, other studies have expanded on this model and integrated some new themes, based on specific cultural contexts (Donmez ÇF, 2020; Östlund U, 2019; Chochinov HM, 2004; Su A, 2018; Díaz-Cortés MDM, 2018; Tanzi S, 2020).

4.1. Dignity therapy for people with dementia: a promising intervention

Acknowledgment of the individual's life projects and life history is a crucial, dignifying component of care. Personal dignity can be reinforced, for example, by allowing individuals with dementia to talk about past achievements and significant events in their lives, allowing them to confirm their identity to themselves and others (van Gennip IE, 2016; Chochinov HM, 2002). This awareness can be of particular importance to HPs, who may not have prior knowledge of the individual.

A broad review examining the intersection of dementia, spirituality, and PC demonstrated that all the studies assessing spiritually oriented PC interventions were designed for persons with dementia, such as dignity therapy (Palmer J, 2020). Dignity therapy is a brief psychotherapy developed in response to evidence regarding the prevalence of psychological and existential factors such as hopelessness, the burden on others, and dignity among PC patients (Chochinov HM, 2012). This therapy has an intensive format, where HPs interact with the patients to collect a direct narration of their lives and the most significant moments or important thoughts they wish to preserve. These therapy sessions are transcribed and edited, and the resulting "generativity document" is returned to patients, who can share it with their families, friends, and HPs. This intervention protocol features nine standard questions as prompts for the patients to begin their recollections about what they want to say. The questions help guide a conversation with HPs trained in dignity therapy (Table 6) (Chochinov HM, 2012).

Table 6. Dignity therapy questions

1	Tell me a little about your life history, particularly the parts that you either remember most or think are the most important. When did you feel most alive?
2	Are there specific things that you would want your family to know about you, and are there particular things you would want them to remember?
3	What are the most important roles you have played in life (family roles, vocational roles, community service roles, etc.)? Why were they so important to you, and what do you think you accomplished in those roles?
4	What are your most important accomplishments, and what do you feel most proud of?
5	Are there particular things that you feel still need to be said to your loved ones, or things that you would want to take the time to say once again?
6	What are your hopes and dreams for your loved ones?
7	What have you learned about life that you would want to pass along to others? What advice or words of guidance would you wish to pass along to your (son, daughter, husband, wife, parents, others)?
8	Are there words or perhaps even instructions you would like to offer your family to help prepare them for the future?

9	In creating this permanent record, are there other things that you would like included?

Generativity is a process where patients nearing the end of life invest in the loved ones that they will soon leave behind. HPs can promote generativity by encouraging patients to reflect on the essential things in their lives, shaping how they will be remembered. Sharing these reflections may benefit those who will grieve their loss (Chochinov HM, 2012; Buonaccorso, L, 2021). Dignity therapy has been extended to those with cognitive impairment. One study provided dignity therapy to twelve nursing home residents with none to mild cognitive impairment and eleven family members of those residents, using a mixed-methods approach (Chochinov HM, 2012). Residents characterized the intervention as helpful to themselves, whereas family members characterized it as helpful to both themselves and the resident. Providers reported that the intervention informed their perceptions of the resident and increased their knowledge of the resident. From the qualitative analysis of completed dignity therapy documents, common themes pertained to life lessons, the importance of relationships, sources of pride or accomplishment, and delights or joys (Chochinov HM, 2012).

Two other studies were conducted among community-dwelling persons diagnosed with early-stage dementia (n=7), using a mixed-methods approach (Johnston B, 2017; 2016). The findings showed that the intervention was feasible, acceptable, and potentially effective (Johnston B, 2017). The associated sub-study analyzed the dignity therapy documents qualitatively and found three themes: (1) the origin of values, (2) the essence and affirmation of self, and (3) forgiveness and resolution (Johnston B, 2016).

The application of dignity therapy in people with dementia showed that the intervention process offered an opportunity for patients to feel honored and worthy, despite their deteriorating physical condition. For the caregivers, this was an opportunity to shift from "this is not who my loved one is" and become more comfortable with the patient in their current condition. For the HPs, this was an opportunity to better understand their role, honoring and bearing witness to what was happening to both caregiver and patient (Aspiras D, 2019). Recognition of patients' personhood can move clinicians toward deeper inquiry, awareness, and connectedness in the clinical encounter. Although it is rare for clinicians to ask for details about patients' core values, these are the very values that sustained them throughout their disease. Unfortunately, it is also equally rare that patients are encouraged to discover new meanings in their life and disease (Buonaccorso L, 2021). Dignity therapy questions can address these issues to elicit responses that embrace the meaning of life, regardless of health condition, and therefore support both patients and professionals in opening a dialog that is not solely centered on suffering (Buonaccorso L, 2021). Dignity therapy can be an intervention that supports patients' sense of being a person who can transmit their values to those around them (Chochinov HM, 2012; Johnston B, 2017; 2016; Aspiras D, 2019). In this journey, patients, family members, and HPs can construct together a caring relationship centered on values and important choices for the future.

4.2. Spiritual support in dementia disease: a vital sign

"Spirituality" is a dynamic and intrinsic aspect of humanity through which persons seek ultimate meaning, purpose, and transcendence, and through which they experience relationships with the self, family, others, community, society, nature, and the significant or sacred. Spirituality is expressed through beliefs, values, traditions, and practices (Puchalski CM, 2014).

Research increasingly demonstrates how vital spiritual care (i.e., professional efforts to promote improved spiritual outcomes) is to PC among patients with serious illnesses, yet prior work has focused primarily on the spiritual component of PC among patients with cancer (Daly L, 2019). Spiritual care offers several quality-of-life benefits for persons with dementia and their family members, including enhancing meaning and purpose in life, maintaining relationships, providing comfort and hope, and coping strategies (Daly L, 2019). Notably, the data demonstrate that cognitive decline is slower for those with expressed spirituality and private religious practices, that personal spirituality correlates with the quality of life in AD, and that levels of spirituality do not decrease in the early stages of dementia (Daly L, 2019; Howorth P, 2003).

A meta-synthesis of how persons with dementia and caregivers view spiritual care in persons with dementia found three principal forms of spiritual care: (1) performing religious rituals that provide a sense of comfort; (2) getting to know the person, which provides opportunities to understand a person's meaning and purpose; and (3) attending to basic needs, which provides an opportunity to appreciate others' vulnerability and humanness (Ødbehr LS, 2017). Religious and spiritual frameworks provide benefits in the forms of resilience, peace, and serenity for the residents. The residents said that trust in God helped them cope with the vulnerability of not being able to remember. In general, participating in religious rites can represent a form of reminiscence therapy, as the words, the sacred hymns, and the reading of the sacred scriptures refer to situations learned in youth (Candlelight Group, 2014). Additionally, the multi-sensory experience in these situations evokes different types of memory: the colors of sacred vestments, the light of candles, and the smell of wax and incense, along with the music and hymns that are associated with experiences of the past (Candlelight Group, 2014). This is particularly important in the advanced stages of dementia when abstract thinking is disrupted and sensory modalities (hearing, sight, smell, etc.) become fundamental for the evaluation of the surrounding world.

These data suggest that with the decline of cognitive faculties, the spiritual aspects of the person can represent an important dimension of experiencing religiosity that brings hope and purpose amid the illness. These aspects help to reinforce feelings that generate a sense of belonging and, therefore, social identity. In particular, religious symbols can elicit thoughts, memories, and experiences that give coherence and unity to the life of persons with dementia by corroborating their identity (De Vanna M, 2005; Kim SK, 2015; Mitchell G, 2015). Recent research has focused on the relationship between dementia, identity, and spirituality, under the assumption that spiritual identity can be threatened by the dementing process (De Vanna M, 2005; Kim SK, 2015). However, it must be stated that in persons with dementia, social identity is primarily lost due to the lack of interaction with others, while personal identity can remain until more advanced stages of the disease. It has also been stated that when persons with dementia feel like part of a community of the faithful, this strengthens their sense of belonging and helps promote social interaction.

A recent study investigated the prevalence and predictive power of specific types of religious/spiritual struggles for mental health outcomes among 156 informal dementia caregivers, through the stress process framework model (MacDougall EE, 2022). Religious/spiritual struggles were defined as "implying that something in a person's current belief, practice, or experience is causing or perpetuating distress" (Exline, JJ, 2014). The study used the Religious and Spiritual Struggles Scale to measure six dimensions of religious/spiritual struggle: (1) divine struggle, which addresses problems in one's relationship with God; (2) demonic struggle, which addresses problems with a supernatural evil being; (3) interpersonal struggle, which addresses problems with religious people or groups; (4) moral struggle, which addresses problems with or perceptions of not living up to personal ethical standards; (5) ultimate meaning struggle, which addresses problems with one's sense of personal significance/meaning in life; (6) doubt struggle, which addresses confusion and uncertainty about one's religious/spiritual beliefs. The religious/spiritual struggles appeared to operate as a secondary stressor for informal dementia caregivers, adding predictive power to background/contextual factors and to primary stressors concerning the measured outcome of self-reported depression.

Recent qualitative research has aimed to assess the potential "what" of spiritual needs and the "who" and "when" of implementing spiritual care for people with dementia and their caregivers (Palmer JA, 2022). Data from twenty-four interviews with HPs revealed two themes: (1) spiritual experience in dementia differs from that of other medical conditions (subthemes: fear, profound loss of self, progressive and incurable nature, and impacting the ability to access faith), and (2) the need for spiritual intervention in the mild stage of dementia (subthemes: awareness in mild dementia and its influence on spiritual distress, and a window of opportunity). The implications of this research include the need for dementia-specific spiritual assessment tools, interventions targeting fear and loss of self early in symptom progression, and stakeholder training.

4.3. Compassionate community approach

Not all individuals suffering from dementia have a partner or other family members who are willing and able to care for them. Moreover, based on personal history and the burden of assistance, not all partners or other caregivers can provide sensitive and supportive care. Consequently, home care is not always the best solution for individuals with dementia (Gómez-Batiste G, 2018; Librada-Flores S, 2020). Furthermore, for many of those suffering from dementia, institutionalization is ultimately inevitable, as the disease progresses. Therefore, it is particularly relevant to determine how dignity can be maintained within the institutional social context (Öhlander M, 2009). Special dementia care units using a "homelike" framework that is highly individualized and relationship-oriented care seem promising in sustaining the dignity of patients with dementia. In particular, the most important dignity-sustaining factors include demonstrating an attitude of acceptance, always being available for support to prevent feelings of inferiority, and protecting the residents from disrespectful treatment by others (Öhlander M, 2009).

Recent studies proposed considering a *compassionate community approach* to improve psycho-social and spiritual support for patients and families with chronic and terminal diseases (Mallon A, 2021; Kellehear A, 2013; Kellehear A, 2016). The compassionate community movement is a population-based theory of practice that calls on society to intentionally contribute to caring for its citizens, especially those experiencing indicators of vulnerability. In this model, citizens are purposefully mobilized as volunteers in health and social care institutions to help people in need, while identifying their own person-centered goals for living well (Kellehear A, 2016). People are then connected with community resources and empowered to act on their goals and needs. With collective engagement, a compassionate community can become an interplay of caring actions with and among a community, its citizens, and health/social care organizations.

Compassionate communities can address the holistic, personalized, and client-centered needs of people who are homeless, living in low-income households, and those in social isolation. Citizen volunteers are often untapped health and social care capital that can be mobilized to promote the health of vulnerable persons within a community. Student volunteers in particular may benefit from experiencing and responding to the needs of a community's most vulnerable members. The compassionate community approach can be helpful for persons with dementia and their caregivers, especially for those who do not have an extended family and social network, or lack the potential for long-term assistance.

We conclude our contribution by reporting the Advanced Directive Treatments for people suffering from dementia and their caregivers (Walsh E, 2020; Gaster B, 2017).

Dementia and Advanced Directive Treatments

At the time of diagnosis, information related to the disease should be presented comprehensively and gradually, but at the same time without waiting for a cognitive deterioration that will make it difficult to express one's will
Identify early on a reference caregiver for the patient

Identify religious and cultural orientations and share with the caregiver
Address fears and desires pertaining to end of life
Conduct targeted interviews with the patient and the caregiver about supportive and palliative care and the care setting
Share the step-by-step decision journey for supportive and end-of-life care with the interdisciplinary care team
The physician has an obligation at an early stage to clarify for the patient and family members the nature of the disease, define the patient's goals, and translate these goals into specific interventions in order to provide adequate care for individuals with advanced dementia
A balanced perspective, in which the doctor takes into account both previously expressed wishes (respecting autonomy) and current reality (respecting charity)

References

1. Glasgow Declaration 2014 | Alzheimer Europe, https://www.alzheimer-europe.org
2. Reisberg B. Diagnostic Criteria in Dementia: A Comparison of Current Criteria, Research Challenges, and Implications for DSM-V. Geriatr Psychiatry Neurol. 2006 September. doi:10.1177/0891988706291083
3. World Health Organization (1992). The ICD-10 classification of mental and behavioural disorders: clinical descriptions and diagnostic guidelines. World Health Organization. https://apps.who.int/iris/handle/10665/37958
4. World Alzheimer Report, Alzheimer's Disease International 2020. https://www.alzint.org/resource/world-alzheimer-report-2020
5. Carlos AF, Poloni TE, Caridi M, et al. Life during COVID-19 lockdown in Italy: the influence of cognitive state on psychosocial, behavioral and lifestyle profiles of older adults. Aging Ment Health. 2022 Mar; 26(3):534-543. doi: 10.1080/13607863.2020.1870210.
6. Jack CR, Bennet DA, Blennow K, et al. NIA-AA Research Framework: Toward a biological definition of Alzheimer's disease. Alzheimer's Dement. 2018 Apr; 14(4): 535–562. doi: 10.1016/j.jalz.2018.02.018
7. Chaves F, Camozzato ML, Luiza A, et al. Validity of the Clinical Dementia Rating Scale for the Detection and Staging of Dementia in

Brazilian Patients. Alzheimer Dis Assoc Disord. 2007 Jul-Sep;21(3):210-7. doi: 10.1097/WAD.0b013e31811ff2b4

8. Mitchell SL, Morris JN, Park PS, et al. Terminal Care for Persons with Advanced Dementia in the Nursing Home and Home Care Settings. J Palliat Med. 2004 Dec;7(6):808-16. doi: 10.1089/jpm.2004.7.808
9. European Foundations' Initiative on Dementia. Mapping dementia-friendly communities across Europe: A study commissioned by European Foundations' Initiative on Dementia (EFID) 2016. http://www.efid.info/wp-ontent/uploads/2016/05/Mapping_DFCS_across_Europe_final_v2.pdf
10. Pink J, John O'Brien J, Robinson L, et al. Dementia: assessment, management and support: summary of updated NICE guidance. BMJ. 2018 Jun 20;*361*:k2438. *doi*:10.1136/bmj. k2438
11. Cartabellotta A, Eleopra R, Simone Quintana S, et al. Guidelines for the diagnosis, treatment and support of patients with dementia. Evidence 2018;10(10). e1000190 doi:10.4470/E1000190
12. Yu TW, Lane HY, Lin CH, et al. Novel Therapeutic Approaches for Alzheimer's Disease: An Updated Review Department of Psychiatry. Int J Mol Sci.2021Jul 30;22(15):8208.doi: 10.3390/ijms22158208
13. https://www.alzforum.org/news/research-news/us-fda-gives-green-light-leqembi-aka-lecanemab
14. https://www.ema.europa.eu/en/medicines/human/summaries-opinion/aduhelm
15. Abraha I, Rimland JM, Trotta FM, et al. Systematic review of non-pharmacological interventions to treat behavioural disturbances in older patients with dementia. The Senator-On Top series. BMJ open. 2017 Mar 16;7(3): e012759. doi: 10.1136/bmjopen-2016-012759
16. Nawzad S, Cahn W, Abdullah-Koolmee H, et al. The efficacy of antipsychotics in the treatment of physical aggressive behavior in patients with dementia in nursing homes. Ther Adv Psychopharmacol. 2022 May 16;12:20451253221097452. doi: 10.1177/20451253221097452. eCollection 2022.
17. Duncan E. Foundations for practice in occupational therapy. 6th Edition - May 22, 2020. Elsevier
18. Guazzarini AG, Casanova G, Buchholz F, et al. The Special Care Unit for People with Behavioral and Psychological Symptoms of Dementia (SCU- B) in the Context of the Project "RECage-Respectful Caring for Agitated Elderly": A Qualitative Study. Int J Environ Res Public Health. 2022 Dec 16;19(24):16913. doi: 10.3390/ijerph192416913
19. Livingston G, Kelly L, Lewis-Holmes, et al. A systematic review of the clinical effectiveness and cost-effectiveness of sensory, psychological

and behavioral interventions for managing agitation in older adults with dementia. Health Technol Assess. 2014 Jun;18(39):1-226, v-vi. doi: 10.3310/hta18390

20. Woodbridge R, Sullivan M, Harding EM, et al. Use of the physical environment to support everyday activities for people with dementia: A systematic review. Dementia (London). 2018 Jul;17(5):533-572. doi: 10.1177/1471301216648670. Epub 2016 Aug 4
21. Lorusso LN, Bosch SJ. Impact of multisensory environments on behavior for people with dementia: A systematic literature review. Gerontologist. 2018 May 8;58(3):e168-e179. doi: 10.1093/geront/gnw168
22. Miller PA, Butin D. The role of occupational therapy in dementia-C.O.P.E. (Caregiver options for practical experiences). Case Reports Int J Geriatr Psychiatry. 2000 Jan;15(1):86-9. doi: 10.1002/(sici)1099-1166(200001)15:1<86::aid-gps124>3.0.co;2-8
23. Jones M. GentleCare. Charging the Experience of Alzheimer's Disease in a Positive. 1999 Editor Hartley and Marks
24. Neal M, Briggs M. Validation therapy for dementia. Review Cochrane Database Syst Rev. 2000;(2):CD001394. doi: 10.1002/14651858.CD001394.
25. Bissolo G, Fazzi L, Gianelli M. Caring relationships. Introduction to Malignant Social Psychology. 2009 Carocci Faber Editor, Rome
26. vans-Roberts CEY, Turnbull OH. Remembering Relationships, Preserved Emotion-based Learning in Alzheimer's Disease. Case Reports Exp Aging Res. 2011 Jan;37(1):1-16. doi: 10.1080/0361073X.2011.536750
27. Vigorelli P., Bonalume M., Cocco A., Lacchini C., Maramonti A., Negri Chinaglia C., Peduzzi A., Pezzano D., Riedo E., Sertorio S., (2011), L'Approccio Capacitante nella cura degli anziani fragili e delle persone con deficit cognitivi. 10 anni di esperienza, Psicogeriatria, 2: 58-70
28. Svansdottir HB, Snaedal J. Music therapy in moderate and severe dementia of Alzheimer's disease: a case-control study. Int Psychogeriatr. 2006 Dec;18(4): 613-21. doi: 10.1017/S1041610206003206.Epub 2006 Apr 18
29. Cai X, Zhou L, Han P, et al. Narrative review: recent advances in doll therapy for Alzheimer's disease. Ann Palliat Med. 2021 Apr;10(4):4878-4881. doi: 10.21037/apm-21-853
30. Kanamori M, Suzuki M, Yamamoto K, et al. A day care program and evaluation of animal-assisted therapy (AAT) for the elderly with senile dementia. Am J Alzheimers Dis Other Demen. 2001 Jul-Aug;16(4):234-9. doi: 10.1177/153331750101600409

31. Cepero JL. Current Status of Animal-Assisted Interventions in Scientific Literature: A Critical Comment on Their Internal Validity. Animals (Basel). 2020 Jun 5;10(6):985. doi: 10.3390/ani10060985
32. Zafra-Tanaka JH, Barrios KP, Tellez WA, et al. Effects of dog-assisted therapy in adults with dementia: a systematic review and meta-analysis. BMC Psychiatry 2019 Jan 24;19(1):41. doi: 10.1186/s12888-018-2009-z
33. Young Tu JY, Jin G, Chen JH, et al. Caregiver Burden and Dementia: A Systematic Review of Self-Report Instruments. J Alzheimer's Dis. 2022;86(4):1527-1543.doi:10.3233/JAD-215082
34. Van den Kieboom R, Snaphaan L, Ruth M, et al. The Trajectory of Caregiver Burden and Risk Factors in Dementia Progression: A Systematic Review. J Alzheimer's Dis. 2020;77(3):1107-1115. doi: 10.3233/JAD-200647
35. Marvardi M, Mattioli P, Spazzafumo L, et al. The Caregiver Burden Inventory in evaluating the burden of caregivers of elderly demented patients: results from a multicenter study. Aging Clin Exp Res. 2005 Feb;17(1):46-53. doi: 10.1007/BF03337720
36. Global status report on the public health response to dementia World Health Organization 2021. ISBN 978-92-4-003324-5 (electronic version) ISBN 978-92-4-003325-2 (print version)
37. Miesen B, Blom M. Alzheimer Café Guide. https://www.alzint.org/what-we-do/policy/dementia-friendly-communities/alzheimer-cafes/
38. Dröes RM, Meiland FJM, Schmitz M, et al. Effect of the Meeting Centers Support Program on informal carers of people with dementia: Results from a multi-center study. Aging Ment Health. 2006 Mar;10(2):112-24. doi: 10.1080/13607860500310682
39. van der Steen JT, Dekker NL, Gijsberts MJHE et al. Palliative care for people with dementia in the terminal phase: a mixed-methods qualitative study to inform service development. BMC Palliat Care. 2017 Apr 28;16(1):28. doi: 10.1186/s12904-017-0201-4
40. Browne B, Kupel N, Moore KJ, et al. Defining end of life in dementia: A systematic review. Palliat Med. 2021 Dec; 35(10):1733-1746. doi: 10.1177/02692163211025457. Epub 2021 Jun 17
41. Sclan SG, Reisberg B. Functional assessment staging (FAST) in Alzheimer's disease: reliability, validity, and ordinality. Int Psychogeriatr. 1992;4 Suppl 1:55-69. doi: 10.1017/s1041610292001157

42. Giulio P, Toscani F, Villani D, et al. Dying with advanced dementia in long-term care geriatric institutions: a retrospective study. J Palliat Med. 2008 Sep;11(7):1023-8. doi: 10.1089/jpm.2008.0020
43. Walsh SC, Murphy E, Devane D, et al. Palliative care interventions in advanced dementia. Cochrane Database Syst Rev. 2021 Sep 28;9(9):CD011513. Doi: 10.1002/14651858.CD011513.pub3
44. Erel M, Marcus EL, Heyman SN, et al. Do Perceptions about Palliative Care Affect Emergency Decisions of Health Personnel for Patients with Advanced Dementia? Res Public Health. 2022 Aug 17;19(16):10236. doi: 10.3390/ijerph191610236
45. Toscani F, Van der Steen JT, Finetti S, et al. Critical decisions for older people with advanced dementia: a prospective study in long-term institutions and district home care. J Am Med Dir Assoc. 2015 Jun 1;16(6): 535.e13-20. doi: 10.1016/j.jamda.2015.02.012. Epub 2015 Apr 2
46. Van der Steen JT, Lemos Dekker N, Gijsberts MJHE, et al. Palliative care for people with dementia in the terminal phase: a mixed-methods qualitative study to inform service development. BMC Palliat Care. 2017 Apr 28;16(1):28. doi: 10.1186/s12904-017-0201-4
47. American Geriatrics Society 2019 Updated AGS Beers Criteria for Potentially Inappropriate Medication Use in Older Adults. By the 2019 American Geriatrics Society Beers Criteria® Update Expert Panel. J Am Geriatr Soc. 2019 Apr;67(4):674-694. doi: 10.1111/jgs.15767. Epub 2019 Jan 29
48. Bullock L, Chew-Graham CA, Bedson J, et al. The challenge of pain identification, assessment, and management in people with dementia: a qualitative study. BJGP Open. 2020 Jun 23;4(2): bjgpopen20X101040. doi: 10.3399/bjgpopen20X101040. Print 2020
49. Snow AL, Weber JB, O'Malley KJ, et al. NOPPAIN: A Nursing Assistant-Administered Pain Assessment Instrument for Use in Dementia. Dement Geriatr Cogn Disord. 2004;17(3):240-6. doi: 10.1159/000076446. Epub 2004 Jan 27
50. Folstein MF, Folstein SE, McHugh PR. Mini-mental state. A practical method for grading the cognitive state of patients for the clinician. J Psychiatr Res. 1975 Nov;12(3):189-98. doi: 10.1016/0022-3956(75)90026-6.
51. Costardi D, Rozzini L, Costanzi C, et al. The Italian version of the pain assessment in advanced dementia (PAINAD) scale. Arch Gerontol Geriatr. 2007 Mar-Apr;44(2):175-80. doi: 10.1016/j.archger.2006.04.008. Epub 2006 May 30

52. Albert L, Ulrich HG, Benjamin M, et al. Pain assessment in advanced dementia. Validity of the German PAINAD—a prospective double-blind randomised placebo-controlled trial. Pain. 2019 Mar;160(3):742-753. doi: 10.1097/j.pain.0000000000001430
53. Williams ML, Payne S. Can multidisciplinary guidelines improve the palliation of symptoms in the terminal phase of dementia? Int J Palliat Nurs. 2002 Aug;8(8):370-5. doi: 10.12968/ijpn.2002.8.8.10680
54. Wei YJJ, Chen C, Wintersteinet AG. Discontinuation of Long-Term Opioid Therapy in Patients with Versus Without Dementia. Am J Prev Med. 2022 Feb;62(2):270-274. doi: 10.1016/j.amepre.2021.07.020. Epub 2021 Oct 24
55. Chochinov HM. Dignity and the essence of medicine: the A, B, C, and D of dignity conserving care. BMJ. 2007 Jul 28;335(7612):184-7. doi: 10.1136/bmj.39244.650926.47
56. Johnston B, Papadopoulou C, Östlund U, et al. What's dignity got to do with it? Patients experience of the dignity care intervention: A qualitative evaluation study. SAGE Open Nurs. 2017;3:1– 12. community nurse
57. Buonaccorso L, Miccinesi G, Ripamonti CI. Enhancing Dignity and Hope in Caring for Cancer Patients through Palliative Care, Italy. In: SILBERMAN M, BERGER A: Global Perspectives in Cancer Care: Religion, Spirituality, and Cultural Diversity in Health and Healing. Oxford University Press, 133-148, Oxford 2022
58. Agora Spiritual Care Guideline Working Group: Spiritual care. Nation-wide guideline, Version: 1.0, 2013. https://cupdf.com/document/spiritual-care-nation-wide-guideline-version-10.html?page=1
59. Firshein J. Spirituality in medicine gains support in the USA. Lancet, 1997;349:1300
60. Buonaccorso L. La dignità in medicina, in "Assistenza alla persona malata: aspetti spirituali". Poletto Editore, febbraio 2023. A cura di Guido Miccinesi
61. The Lancet Commission. Dementia prevention, intervention, and care. www.thelancet.com Published online July 20, 2017 http://dx.doi.org/10.1016/S0140-6736(17)31363-6
62. van der Steen JT, Radbruch L, Hertogh CM, et al. White paper defining optimal palliative care in older people with dementia: a Delphi study and recommendations from the European Association for Palliative Care. Palliat Med 2014; 28:197e209
63. van Gennip IE, Pasman HRW, Oosterveld-Vlug MG, et al. How Dementia Affects Personal Dignity: A Qualitative Study on the

Perspective of Individuals With Mild to Moderate Dementia. Gerontol B Psychol Sci Soc Sci, 2016, Vol. 71, No. 3, 491–501 doi:10.1093/geronb/gbu137

64. Chochinov HM, Hack T, McClement S, et al. Dignity in the terminally ill: A developing empirical model. Soc Sci Med. 2002;54:433–443
65. Donmez ÇF, Johnston B. Living in the moment for people approaching the end of life: A concept analysis. *Int J Nurs Stud Adv.* 2020;108:103584.
doi: 10.1016/ j.ijnurstu.2020.103584 (PMID:32450405)
66. Östlund U, Blomberg K, Annika Söderman A, et al. How to conserve dignity in palliative care: Suggestions from older patients, significant others, and healthcare professionals in Swedish municipal care. BMC Palliat Care. 2019;18:10. https:// doi.org/ 10.1186/ s12904- 019- 0393-x
67. Chochinov HM. Dignity and the eye of the beholder. J Clin Oncol. 2004 Apr 1;22(7):1336-40. doi: 10.1200/JCO.2004.12.095
68. Su A, Lief L, Berlin D, et al. Beyond Pain: Nurses' Assessment of Patient Suffering, Dignity, and Dying in the Intensive Care Unit. J *Pain Symptom Manage*. 2018 Jun;55(6):1591-1598.e1.
doi: 10.1016/j.jpainsymman.2018.02.005. Epub 2018 Feb 17
69. Díaz-Cortés MDM, Granero-Molina J, Hernández-Padilla JM, et al. Promoting dignified end-of-life care in the emergency department: A qualitative study. *Int Emerg Nurs* 2018;37:23-28
70. Tanzi S, Buonaccorso L. Enhancing patient dignity: Opportunities addressed by a specialized palliative care unit during the coronavirus pandemic. *J Palliat Med.* 2020; doi: 10.1089/ jpm.2020.0661
71. Palmer JA, Smith AM, Paasche-Orlow RS, et al. Research Literature on the Intersection of Dementia, Spirituality, and Palliative Care: A Scoping Review. Pain Symptom Manage. 2020 Jul;60(1):116-134. doi: 10.1016/j.jpainsymman.2019.12.369. Epub 2020 Jan 7
72. Chochinov HM. Dignity Therapy: final words for final days. Oxford text, 2012
73. Buonaccorso L, Tanzi S, De Panfilis L, et al. Meaning Emergin From Dignity Therapy Among Cancer Patients. *J Pain Symptom Manage.* 2021 Oct;62(4):730-737.
doi: 10.1016/j.jpainsymman.2021.02.028. Epub 2021 Feb 20
74. Chochinov HM, Cann B, Cullihall K, et al. Dignity therapy: a feasibility study of elders in long-term care. Palliat Support Care 2012;10:3e15
75. Johnston B, Lawton S, Pringle J. "This is my story, how I remember it': in-depth analysis of Dignity Therapy documents from a study of Dignity

Therapy for people with early stage dementia. Dementia (London) 2017;16:543e555

76. Johnston B, Lawton S, Mccaw C, et al. Living well with dementia: enhancing dignity and quality of life using a novel intervention, Dignity Therapy. Int J Older People Nurs 2016; 11:107e120
77. Aspiras D, Empeno J, Lori, P. Et al. To honor and bear witness: a clinician's reflection on dignity therapy for people living with dementia. Case Rep. J. Palliat. 2019 Med. 22, 1007–1008. doi: 10.1089/jpm.2019.0018
78. Puchalski CM, Vitillo R, Hull SK, et al. Improving the spiritual dimension of whole person care: reaching national and international consensus. J Palliat Med. 2014 Jun;17(6):642-56. doi: 10.1089/jpm.2014.9427
79. Daly L, Fahey-McCarthy E, Timmins F. The experience of spirituality from the perspective of people living with dementia: a systematic review and meta-synthesis. Dementia (London) 2019;18:448e470
80. Howorth P, Saper J. The dimensions of insight in people with dementia. Aging Ment Health 2003;7(2):113-22
81. Ødbehr LS, Hauge S, J Danbolt LJ, et al. Residents' and caregivers' views on spiritual care and their understanding of spiritual needs in persons with dementia: A meta-synthesis. Review Dementia (London). 2017 Oct;16(7):911-929. doi: 10.1177/1471301215625013. Epub 2015 Dec 30
82. Candlelight Group: a pilot project for people with dementia 2004. Royal College of Psychiatrist (Spirituality and Psychiatry Special Interest Group). www.rcpsych.ac.uk/PDF/higgins
83. De Vanna M, Carlino D, Aguglia E. Conceptual and Interpretative Aspects of Insight in Alzheimer's Disease. Journal Psychopathology 2005;11(1)
84. Kim SK, Park M, Effectiveness of person-centered care on people with dementia: a systematic review and meta-analysis. Clinical Interventions in Aging 2017:12 381–397
85. Mitchell G and Agnelli J. Person-centred care for people with dementia: Kitwood reconsidered. Nurs stand. 2015 Oct 14;30(7):46-50. doi: 10.7748/ns.30.7.46.s47
86. MacDougall EE. Predicting depression in dementia caregivers: do religious/spiritual struggles play a role? Aging & Mental Health, 2022, 26:11, 2270-2276, DOI: 10.1080/13607863.2021.1961124
87. Exline, JJ, Pargament, K. I., Grubbs, J. B., & Yali, A. M. (2014). The Religious and Spiritual Struggles Scale: Development and initial

validation. Psychology of Religion and Spirituality, 6(3), 208–222. https://doi.org/10.1037/a0036465

88. Palmer JA, Hilgeman M, Balboni T, et al. The Spiritual Experience of Dementia From the Health Care Provider Perspective: Implications for Intervention. Gerontologist. 2022 Apr 20;62(4):556-567. doi: 10.1093/geront/gnab134
89. Gómez-Batiste G, Mateu S, Serra-Jofre S, et al. Compassionate communities: design and preliminary results of the experience of Vic (Barcelona, Spain) caring city. Ann Palliat Med 2018;7(Suppl 2):S32-S41
90. Librada-Flores S, Nabal-Vicuña M, Forero-Vega D, et al. Implementation Models of Compassionate Communities and Compassionate Cities at the End of Life: A Systematic Review. Int. J. Environ. Res. Public Health 2020, 17, 6271; doi:10.3390/ijerph17176271
91. Öhlander, M. Dignity and dementia: An analysis of dignity of identity and dignity work in a group dwelling. In L. Nordenfelt (Ed.) Dignity in care for older people. Hoboren, NJ: Wiley-Blackwell, 2009.
92. Mallon A. Compassionate community structure and function: a standardised micro-model for end-of-life doulas and community members supporting those who wish to die at home. Palliative Care & Social Practice 2021, Vol. 15: 1–14. DOI: 10.1177/ 26323524211052569
93. Kellehear A. Compassionate communities: end-of-life care as everyone's responsibility. QJM 2013;106:1071-5
94. Kellehear A. The compassionate city charter: inviting the cultural and social sectors into end of life care. In: Wegleitner K, Heimerl K, Kellehear A. editors. Compassionate Communities: case studies from Britain and Europe. Abingdon, UK: Routledge, 2016;76-87
95. Walsh E. Cognitive Transformation, Dementia, and the Moral Weight of Advance Directives. Am J Bioeth. 2020. PMID: 32757910
96. Gaster B, Larson EB. Advance directives for dementia: meeting a unique challenge. JAMA. 2017;318:2175-2176

24

THE IMPACT OF CULTURE AND SPIRITUAL PERSPECTIVES ON DEMENTIA CARE IN TURKEY

TESLIME ATLI, MD[1]

Abstract

The impact of cultural and spiritual perspectives on dementia care in Turkey is significant, as these factors shape the way that individuals with dementia and their families understand and manage the condition. The traditional family structure plays a large role in the care of individuals with dementia. Long-term care is generally understood to be the responsibility of the family in Turkey. Women are the primary providers of family-based care services in Turkey. Therefore, the great majority of the long-term care burden in families is shouldered by women to a large extent. The limits of providing care in the family are becoming apparent as the prevalence of dementia increases. The number of long-term care services are increasing but they are still very limited in capacity and concentrated only in large cities. Religion plays a significant role in shaping the culture and attitudes toward elderly care in Turkey, with family and religious institutions being central to the care of older adults.

Keywords: Dementia, spiritual care, culture, family-based care, Turkey

Turkey's population is still relatively young compared to many countries; however, rapid population aging is anticipated along with a rising life expectancy and low fertility rates during the upcoming decades. Turkey's total population was 84.6 million in 2021. The proportion of people 65 years and older was 9.8% and is expected to increase to 12% by 2030 and to 21%

[1] Ankara University Department of Geriatric Medicine, Ankara TURKEY

by 2050 (1). Life expectancy at birth was 81.3 years for women and 75.9 years for men, with an average of 78.6 years for both genders for the years 2017-2019. Furthermore, according to population projections, the share of very old individuals in the older population will increase within the next two decades. For example, 62.8% of the older population in 2019 was 65–74 years old, 28.2% was 75–84 years old, and 9.1% was aged 85 years and over. However, it is estimated that 55.3% of the older population will be in the age range of 65–74 years in 2040, 34.1% will be in the age range of 75–84 years, and 10.6% will be 85 years old and over. Among people 70 years of age or older, the leading causes of mortality are cardiovascular conditions, Alzheimer's disease, and chronic obstructive pulmonary disease. Among people 60 years and older, the prevalence of dementia was about 4% in 2018 (2,3).

Long-Term Care in Turkey

Turkey is going through a very serious restructuring of the health system. Besides the sustained health system reforms, there have been significant steps in establishing a long-term care system. The Directorate-General for Disabled and Elderly Care Services, with responsibilities for organizing and implementing long-term care services, was created in 2011 as part of the establishment of the Ministry of Family, Labor, and Social Services. The new structure integrates formerly independent units in order to organize and provide care services for older people and people with disabilities, pursuing the mission of "coordinating national policies and strategies for the social participation of disabled and older people" (4). Shortly after the creation of the ministry, a National Plan for Action was adopted, highlighting the importance of improving the social integration of older people, developing long-term services (LTC), and improving access to health care (5).

Long-term care in Turkey includes residential care, home care, palliative care, and community services. Community-based care for older people who need social support and social inclusion is very limited in capacity (6). Private providers, notably the Alzheimer Association, operate a few centers in large urban areas (Istanbul, Eskisehir, Mersin, and the Konya province). Nongovernmental organizations offer programs such as Neighbor from the Heart and My Patient is Safe, which are devoted to providing unpaid caregiver services. However, such private initiatives are isolated and small in scale (7). Mental health services are provided in psychiatric hospitals and the mental health wards of public and research-and-training hospitals. Such services are covered under the public system, but capacity is insufficient to meet the needs of the population (8). Outpatient mental health care services are subject to co-payments. Palliative care is traditionally provided within hospitals, while private care services have only recently emerged in the long-term care system (9).

Strong family ethics and related values can lead to family-provided care, with the attendant benefits. However, the limits of providing care in the family are becoming apparent as the prevalence of dementia increases and a growing number of older people live with functional impairments and multimorbid conditions, requiring specialized and formalized care provision. Informal care is essential for the sustainability and future development of a long-term care system, but it cannot substitute for the development of accessible and high-quality formal long-term care.

The most important factor to grasp regarding the future of family caregiving is family size. As family size decreases, the incidence of solitary living is anticipated to rise for the older population. In 2019, fertility in Turkey finally remained below population replacement level (2.1 children per woman), indicating an irreversible declining trend for the next several decades. Delayed age of marriage is another trend, which results in a decreasing number of children in families and an expanded age disparity between parents and children. Such strong trends toward "childlessness" are among the main constraints on the supply side of family care. Another trend is the decreasing number of marriages and the increasing number of divorces, signaling changes in traditional household formations, family structures, and family ties. This slow but substantial loosening of family structures and household patterns is leading to a decline in the proportion of older people living with their adult children.

Immigrant care workers are becoming increasingly relevant in providing long-term care services. Although no official data exist on their numbers or profile, their importance is generally believed to be increasing. Immigrant caregivers are mostly women from Azerbaijan, Georgia, the Republic of Moldova, Turkmenistan, and Uzbekistan (10). The lack of statistical information and a legislative framework in the field render this workforce invisible and impossible to monitor in terms of quantity, quality, and the type of care provided.

Family-Based Long-Term Care in Turkey

Because of the existing legislation, the dominant patriarchal culture, and the religious values embedded in extended kinship relations and inter-generational and intra-generational family ties, the concept of older parents receiving care in an institutional care facility is usually stigmatized as shameful. Moreover, older people mostly prefer to stay and age in their own homes or co-reside with their adult children (11). Consequently, many older people receive care from their family (often from a spouse or child) in the home. However, recent demographic and economic trends are generating fewer family care providers than before. Since it is primarily women who shoulder the care burden of older family members, the size of the female population in caregiving ages relative to the older population is one of the crucial indicators to understand the future supply of family caregiving.

Long-term care is generally understood to be the responsibility of the family in Turkey (12). A 2011 survey of people 40 years of age and older found that 83% of individuals consider caring for older relatives a responsibility of the family, and 11% place that responsibility on the government. When asked about their projections for old age, 62% of adults anticipate living with their spouse, 21% expect to co-reside with adult children, and 5% to live in a nursing home (13). Another factor leading to the increased demand for family-based long-term care is the strong desire and preference of older persons to remain with the family and be cared for at home by adult children. The unwritten, intergenerational contract for reciprocal help, deeply embedded in cultural and religious values, leads older people in Turkey to see their children as "inseparable" family members and obligates such adult children to fulfill the traditional filial duties.

Both the penal and the civil codes in Turkey specify the obligation of relatives to care for dependent individuals within the family (13). Overall, women overwhelmingly bear the responsibility for caring for older people (12). The 2011 Turkish Family Structure Survey found that 32% of older people received care from a daughter-in-law, 27% from a spouse, 22% from a son, and 20% from a daughter. Other studies have found similar findings and reported that taking care of older people is a significant barrier to full-time employment (14).

While families are legally and traditionally expected to care for older relatives, there is no structured strategy to understand the needs of unpaid caregivers. Cash benefits for low-income households (Cash-for-Care service), provided by the Ministry of Family, Labor and Social Services, are currently the only form of support for unpaid caregivers (4).

Cash-for-Care service

The Cash-for-Care service enacted in Turkey targets people who live under an income level predetermined by law and provide care services for older and disabled members within their own families. To be eligible for this scheme, the per capita income in the household where the disabled person is living must be less than two-thirds of the monthly minimum wage, and the person being cared for must have at least 50% severe disability, confirmed by a medical board report (14; 15). Accordingly, the monthly regular cash payments are publicly known as “wage for home-based care” and the recipients of these payments are formally represented as “employed” but “uninsured” care workers. As of October 2020, more than half a million family caregivers (primarily women) were active beneficiaries of this scheme. Around 30% of them provide long-term care for older people (16,17). The scheme’s design leads to the continuity of the conservative familistic welfare regime, which ultimately aims to keep the long-term care provision of older people within the family sphere.

Women are the primary providers of family-based care services in Turkey. Therefore, the great majority of the long-term care burden in families is shouldered by women to a large extent. However, the shift of women from unpaid care work to paid market work is expected to accelerate, resulting in a reduced availability of women to provide care for family members in need of assistance (18).

Although the state’s role in sharing care responsibilities has expanded in the recent decade compared to the past, the capacity of institutional long-term care services appears to remain limited to covering only the care needs of low-income older people who have no family ties. Similarly, the number of private, long-term care facilities has increased simultaneously, but they are too expensive to afford and concentrated only in Turkey’s large cities (14).

Given all these trends, it is highly likely that family-based caregiving will remain the mainstay of the long-term care regime in Turkey. However, there are rising concerns about the supply of family caregivers. Again, the interplay of changing economic and demographic trends is expected to have a potentially decisive effect on the supply side of family care.

Spirituality and Spiritual Care in Turkey

An increasing body of work has focused attention on the religious and spiritual aspects of dementia care. A belief in God or some other form of "Supreme Being" provides a sense that all is not lost, a sense that someone else "out there" is in control and that everything will work out in the end. Religion and spirituality remain crucial coping strategies for living with Alzheimer's for both the diagnosed individual and family caregivers. Consequently, everyone involved in dementia care, including the diagnosed individual, the family, the clinician, and the social service worker, should consider the role of religion and spirituality in a comprehensive and holistic dementia care plan.

In 2017, Turkey developed a 'National Plan for Aged Care' and a 'National Dementia Care Plan' (NDCP) (19,20). Both of these plans endorse a 'system of care' approach that is person-centered and aims to enable independent living in the community for as long as possible. The plans, especially the NDCP, recognized the need to develop well-organized and culturally sensitive residential care services with nursing for older people with severe conditions and at advanced stages of dementia. The primary mode of support is to provide means-tested cash benefits to older people, pensioners, and people with disabilities. Another type of support includes in-kind benefits such as the provision of care-at-home, retirement homes, and assistance for admission to care homes. In particular, home care has been viewed as a culturally appropriate option when the immediate family cannot provide such care (21). In addition, palliative care services in Turkey have undergone considerable development since 2010 through the implementation of the "Pallia-Turk Project," which is a new, national, community-based palliative care program initiated by the Turkish Ministry of Health.

In Turkey, as in many other countries, the cultural and spiritual beliefs of the individual and their family can greatly influence the way that dementia is understood and managed (22,23). Thus, in Turkish culture, older individuals are often viewed as wise and worthy of respect, shaping the treatment received by individuals with dementia. Also, formal titles are commonly used when referring to individuals with dementia, and efforts are spent asking about their opinions and wishes, even when they are not fully able to communicate or make decisions for themselves.

Spirituality can play a vital role in dementia care in Turkey, providing a sense of meaning, connection, and support for not only individuals with dementia but their caregivers as well. By incorporating spiritual practices and traditions into care routines, families and caregivers can help create a sense of peace and purpose for those affected by dementia. For example, singing spiritual songs or hymns may help trigger memories and emotions, provide a sense of connection to a person's faith tradition, stimulate the brain, and bring joy and engagement to those with dementia. It is important for care providers to be aware of these cultural and spiritual influences and to work with caregivers to provide care in a way sensitive to beliefs and values. This may include incorporating spiritual practices, such as prayers and Qur'an recitation, into care plans or respecting the wishes of caregivers about certain types of care.

In terms of spiritual perspectives, Islam is the dominant religion in Turkey, and this can influence the way in which a diagnosis of dementia is approached (24). For example, some individuals may believe that dementia is a punishment from God or that it is caused by spiritual or supernatural forces (25). These beliefs may affect how individuals with dementia are treated, as well as affecting the types of treatment and support that are sought (26). Many old individuals in Turkey turn to religious institutions, such as mosques, for support and assistance. Mosques often provide social and religious activities for older adults, as well as assistance with practical needs such as transportation and healthcare. Additionally, many old Turkish individuals rely on religious leaders, such as imams, for guidance and support in their daily lives. Imams may offer spiritual counseling, guidance on religious practices, and assistance with accessing healthcare and other services (27).

Religion plays a significant role in shaping the culture and attitudes toward elderly care in Turkey, with family and religious institutions being central to the care of older adults. Some studies have revealed that old individuals believe more firmly in Allah, the Hereafter, Paradise, and Hell. According to Research on Religious Life in Turkey by the Turkish Presidency of Religious Affairs (Diyanet), old individuals have a great interest in religious issues. Compared to the younger population, more individuals over 65 years of age shape their lives according to religion and perceive themselves as religious. Religious belief is an important mechanism that fulfills the desire for forgiveness. Religious integration, surrendering to God, and feelings of peace, trust, and well-being may come to the fore in old age. Religious beliefs become the most important element that will keep old individuals lively and give them a life force, helping them to discover new meanings in life and improve their quality of life. Moreover, religious belief provides people with explanations about their creation, death, and the afterlife (27).

Spiritual counseling and care is relatively new in Turkey, though in essence it is not a novel concept. Today's changing social conditions and societal needs do necessitate the institutionalization of services in the field of spiritual counseling and care both theoretically and practically. Therefore, the Center for Values Education, a division of the Turkish Presidency of Religious Affairs (Diyanet), aims to establish a theoretical basis for the field of spiritual counseling and care by developing a body of literature around it. The Center has organized research projects, workshops, seminars, and two international conferences in this field. Indeed, during this period, the interest in the subject in Turkish academic circles has increased. However, spiritual counseling and care services are still not prevalent in Turkey.

Summary

In Turkey, the traditional family structure plays a large role in the care of individuals with dementia. Additionally, the concept of filial piety, or respect for one's elders, is deeply ingrained in Turkish culture. This can cause caregivers to feel a strong sense of responsibility for caring for their elderly relatives with dementia and may lead them to prioritize the needs of their relatives over their own. The impact of cultural and spiritual perspectives on dementia care in Turkey is significant, as these factors shape the way that individuals with dementia and their families understand and manage the condition. Caregivers and healthcare professionals need to be aware of these cultural and spiritual influences in order to provide culturally sensitive and appropriate care to individuals with dementia in Turkey.

References

1. Turkish Statistical Institute; 2019 http://www.turkstat.gov.tr (accessed 7 February 2023)
2. Elderly statistics, 2016. Ankara: Turkish Statistical Institute; 2017 https://data.tuik.gov.tr/Bulten/Index?p=Istatistiklerle-Yaslilar-2016-24644 (accessed 9 February 2023)
3. Health at a glance: Europe 2020. Paris: OECD Publishing; 2020
4. Özmete E, Hussein S. Best practice examples from Europe and designing a model for Turkey. Report on services for older people in Turkey; Ankara: Ministry of Family and Social Policies; 2017

https://www.ailevecalisma.gov.tr/media/9334/tuerkiye-de-yaşlı-bakım-hizmetleri-avrupa-dan-en-iyi-uygulama-oernekleri-ve-tuerkiye-için-bir-model-tasarımı-proje-kitabı.pdf (accessed 11 February 2023).

5. Okem ZG, Cakar M. What have health care reforms achieved in Turkey? An appraisal of the "Health Transformation Programme". Health Policy. 2015;119:1153–63.
6. Karadeniz O. Pensions, health care and long-term care, Turkey; 2014. Annual national report 2014 http://ec.europa.eu/social/BlobServlet?docId=12985&langId=en (accessed 10 February 2023).
7. Tufan I. Pflegebedürftigkeit und pflegerische Versorgung in der Türkei – dargestellt am Beispiel des Alzheimer-Zentrums in Nazilli [Care in Turkey – illustrated using the example of the Alzheimer Centre in Nazilli]. Migration Soziale Arbeit. 2016;38:331–6.
8. Tatar M, Mollahaliloğlu, S, Şahin B, Aydin S, Manresso A, Hernández-Quevedo C. Turkey: a health system review. Health Syst Transition. 2011;13:1–186.
9. Adaman F, Aslan D, Erus B, Sayan S. ESPN thematic report on challenges in long-term care: Turkey. Brussels: European Commission; 2018 https://ec.europa.eu/social/main.jsp?pager.offset=30&catId=792&langId=en&moreD ocuments=yes, (accessed 3 February 2023).
10. Oglak S. Long-term care in Turkey: challenges and opportunities. In: Christiansen K, Pilling D, The Routledge handbook of social care work around the world. London: Routledge; 2017
11. Kagitcibasi C, and Ataca B. Value of children and family change: A three-decade portrait from Turkey. Applied Psychology, 54(3), 317–337. https://doi.org/10.1111/j.1464-0597.2005.00213.x
12. Aran M A, and Aktakke N. Women's invisible contribution: Quantifying the economic value of women's unpaid care activities in Turkey and policy options to reduce women's care burden. Research Paper Series No. 1601. Development Analytics.
13. Eryurt MA. The elderly population in Türkiye and preferences for elderliness. Research on family structure in Türkiye: findings and recommendations. Istanbul: Çizge Tanıtım Publishing; 2014 https://ailevecalisma.gov.tr/uploads/athgm/uploads/pages/indirilebilir-yayinlar/research-on-family-structure-in-turkiye-2013-findings-and-recommendations.pdf (accessed 8 February 2023).
14. Adaman F, Aslan D, Erus B, and Sayan S. ESPN thematic report on challenges in long-term care: Turkey. European Social Policy Network,

Directorate-General for Employment, Social Affairs, and Inclusion. 2018

15. Atasü-Topcuoğlu R. Gender inequality, the welfare state, disability, and distorted commodification of care in Turkey. New Perspectives on Turkey, 1–31. https://doi.org/10.1017/npt.2020.35
16. Akkan B. The politics of care in Turkey: Sacred familialism in a changing political context. Social Politics: International Studies in Gender, State & Society, 25(1), 72–91. https://doi.org/10.1093/sp/jxx011
17. Ministry of Family and Social Services (MFSS). Disability and ageing statistical bulletin. General Directorate of Services for Persons with Disabilities and the Elderly. 2020 https://www.aile.gov.tr/media/46090/bulten_en_200508.pdf
18. Buğra A, and Yakut-Çakar B. Structural change, the social policy environment and female employment in Turkey. Development and Change, 41(3), 517–538. https://doi.org/10.1111/j.1467-7660.2010.01643.x
19. Healthy Aging Action Plan and Implementation Program 2015–2020. Ankara: Ministry of Health; 2015 https://extranet.who.int/countryplanningcycles/sites/default/files/planning_cycle_repository/turkey/turkey_health_aging_action_plan_and_implementation_program_2015-2020.pdf (accessed 9 February 2023)
20. Sumer S, Shear J, Levent Yener A. Building an improved primary health care system in Turkey through care integration. Washington (DC): World Bank; 2019 http://documents.worldbank.org/curated/en/895321576170471609/Building-an-Improved-Primary-Health-Care-System-in-Turkey-through-Care-Integration (accessed 11 February 2023) https://ec.europa.eu/social/BlobServlet?docId=19872&langId=en
21. Aybars A İ, Beşpınar F U, and Kalaycıoğlu H S. Familialization of care arrangements in Turkey: Questioning the social inclusion of 'the invisible.' Research and Policy on Turkey, 3(2), 115–137. https://doi.org/10.1080/23760818.2018.1517447
22. Yazıcı B. The return to the family: Welfare, state, and politics of the family in Turkey. Anthropological Quarterly,2012. 85(1), 103–140. http://www.jstor.org/stable/41427090
23. Yılmaz Z. "Strengthening the family" policies in Turkey: Managing the social question and armoring conservative–neoliberal populism. Turkish Studies, 16(3), 371-390. 2015 https://doi.org/10.1080/14683849.2015.1067863

24. Kaya A. Islamization of Turkey under the AKP rule: Empowering family, faith and charity. South European Society and Politics, 20(1), 47–69.
https://doi.org/10.1080/13608746.2014.979031
25. Agli O, Bailly N, Ferrand C. Spirituality and religion in older adults with dementia: a systematic review. Int Psycho- geriatr 2015;27:715e725.
26. Daly L, Fahey-McCarthy E, Timmins F. The experience of spirituality from the perspective of people living with de- mentia: a systematic review and meta-synthesis. Dementia (London) 2019;18:448e470.
27. Huzurevi, yaşlı bakım ve rehabilitasyon merkezlerinde manevi danışmanlık ve rehberlik hizmetleri. Sevde Düzgüner, Serap Telek.Diyanet İşleri Başkanlığı Yayınları, 2020.

25

DEMENTIA CARE AND RELIGION, SPIRITUALITY, CULTURE-BASED NURSING IN JAPAN

SAYURI SUWA[1] AND TOMOKO MAJIMA[2]

Abstract

Given the expected increase in the number of older people with dementia in the future, it is important to build a stronger comprehensive community care system to support the lives of older people with dementia living in the community. The basic idea of the "Principles for Promoting Dementia Policies" is that "Dementia can happen to anybody and is becoming a familiar illness to many people. Japan has provided the following support: early diagnosis and consultation of dementia, and support by citizens. Also, It will become increasingly important to provide emotional and cultural support the person with dementia themselves and families regarding bereavement and living alone in Japan. Not many people in Japan formally belong to traditional religious institutions or regularly participate in required activities of religion. However, spirituality is interpreted as "exploring the meaning of one's own existence, and cognitive changes associated with aging are regarded as natural. Further, to provide care in the family and community that uses the individual strengths of aging people, it is important to provide nursing that considers

[1] Ph.D., R.N., P.H.N., Dean and a Professor at Chiba University Graduate School of Nursing, Community Health Nursing in Japan. Her research interests include dementia care, gerontological care and care robots.

[2] Ph.D., R.N., P.H.N., Professor at Chiba University Graduate School of Nursing, Advance Practice Nursing in Japan. Her research interests include palliative care and cardiovascular nursing.

the individual's background and culture, as well as spiritual care, such as looking back on daily enjoyment and memories.

Keywords: Dementia care, Culture-based nursing, Japan, spirituality

1. Prevalence of Dementia in Japan and the Daily Life of Older Adults with Dementia

The Japanese population is ageing at a considerably higher rate than in other countries. According to a Japanese epidemiological study in 2012, the prevalence of dementia in older adults aged 65 years and older is estimated to be about 15% (Ikejima 2012,120-123). (Ministry of Heath, Labour and Welfare 2013). With these projections, the number of older adults with dementia is expected to increase to about 1 in 5 by 2025 (Cabinet Office, Japan 2016). Older adults with dementia use medical and long-term care insurance within their community-based comprehensive care systems as they live their daily lives.

The community-based comprehensive care system is a system that provides integrated housing, medical care, long-term care, prevention, and lifestyle support so that older adults can live to the end of life in their own homes in the neighborhood they are accustomed to living in, even with severe disabilities (Ministry of Health, Labour and Welfare 2012).

Given the expected increase in the number of older people with dementia in the future, it is important to build a stronger comprehensive community care system to support the lives of older people with dementia living in the community. Local comprehensive care systems are created by municipalities and prefectures, which act as the insurers, according to the community characteristics, depending on the autonomy and independence of the local community.

2. Basic Approaches to Dementia Care in Japan

In Japan, various dementia measures have been implemented. In particular, in January 2015, the "Comprehensive Strategy for the Promotion of Dementia Measures (New Orange Plan) - Toward the Establishment of Communities Friendly to Older Adults with Dementia" was announced (Ministry of Health, Labour and Welfare (2015). The basic idea of the "Principles for Promoting Dementia Policies" (Ministry of

Health, Labour and Welfare 2019) is that "Dementia can happen to anybody and is becoming a familiar illness to many people, including those who have patients in the family or among their acquaintances". With the aim delaying the onset of dementia and of creating a society where people can live with hope even if they develop dementia, we will promote measures on the two axes of "coexistence" and "prevention" while emphasizing the perspective of people and families with dementia. Based on this concept, we will implement the following measures by 2025: (1)disseminate information and support individuals to increase awareness on dementia, (2)prevent (i.e., delay the onset of dementia, and slow the progression of dementia), (3)provide support for medical care, long-term care services, and caregivers, (4)promote a barrier-free society for people with dementia, support for young people with dementia, and services to increase social participation, and (5)research and development, industry promotion, and their international promotion. The importance of planning and promoting the measures so that they truly respond to the needs of people with dementia and their families is emphasized.

The concept of "co-existing" with people with dementia is of particular importance in this guideline promoting dementia measures. The aim is to realize a barrier-free society for people with dementia by eliminating the impediments in their living environment such that they can continue to live in the community they are accustomed to. For example, people with dementia are more likely to experience difficulty of accomplishing tasks such as making payment at ATMs and supermarkets and using public transportation such as trains and buses. Breaking the systematic barriers to these services which collectively translate to difficulty of living should improve the lives of people with dementia. It should be noted, however, that people with dementia may also feel concerned that such attempts would only highlight their disabilities as well as wonder who should make the judgement as to exactly what constitutes barriers to people with dementia.

3. Support for People with Dementia and Family Caregivers in Japan

In light of these developments, Japan has provided the following support (Ministry of Health, Labour and Welfare 2005).

3.1 Early Diagnosis of Dementia

Early consultation and diagnosis of dementia and the differentiation of the causative disease are important for anybody with suspected dementia. In doing so, visiting medical institutions with specialists in geriatric psychiatry in the community, a Dementia Medical Center, or dementia support physicians who play a central role in the establishment of a community health care system for dementia is recommended. In addition to serving as a consultant and advisor to family physicians regarding dementia diagnosis, etc., dementia support physicians also play a role in establishing a collaborative system with other dementia support physicians. However, as these medical institutions are still limited, medical associations and dementia support physicians of various prefectures should cooperate to provide training to family physicians in the local communities on knowledge and skills related to dementia, and how to cooperate with local resources.

3.2 Early Consultation

Family members continue to provide care for a long period of time while worrying about various issues such as the differential diagnosis of dementia, which medical institution to visit when suffering from physical illness, how to treat older adults with dementia, and how to use the long-term care insurance system. Therefore, it is important for families to obtain information on where to consult about long-term care.

The main organizations that families can consult about long-term care for dementia include the local comprehensive community support center, dementia medical center, call centers established by prefectures and major designated cities, and the Association of Persons with Dementia and their Families.

3.3 Support by Citizens

Families that attempt to care for a dementia patient alone results in excessive stress and fatigue, which makes it difficult for them to handle the speech and behavior of older adults with dementia. For this reason, knowing that there are people in the community who can help older adults with dementia can ease the burden of the caregiving families and give them a sense of comfort. We train dementia supporters in cities designated by prefectural ordinances as people who can support older adults with dementia and their families in their communities and workplaces. Dementia supporters have knowledge of dementia, and "caravan mates" who have received training hold dementia supporter training courses in their communities and workplaces to train them (National Caravan Mate Liaison Council 2005). There were 14.05 million dementia supporters as of 2022. In the future, it is important to increase the number of dementia supporters in the community and to create a community that supports each other as a care system for older adults with dementia and their families.

In addition, support is provided by Dementia Cafes and the SOS network System for Wandering Elderly, which cooperates with local residents to find older adults with dementia who have left home and are no longer aware of their whereabouts. Staff from these services also pay visits to the homes of older adults with dementia to ensure their safety and spend time with them (but not providing home-visit care services), and watch them while their families are away from home or when they need a break. It is desirable to obtain such information so that it can be utilized at any time depending on the care conditions of the person with dementia.

4. Passage of the Basic Law for Dementia

Furthermore, the Japanese government has been aiming to pass the Basic Law for Dementia by 2023 on the assumption that a society that is friendly for people with dementia is friendly for people of all other demographics. And in June 2023 the Basic Low Dementia was passed ahead of the rest of the world. The purpose of this Act is to establish the basic principles of dementia measures, identify the responsibilities of the national and local governments, and promote dementia measures comprehensively and systematically.

5. Understanding and Care for Symptoms of Dementia

5.1 Daily Life Difficulties and Care

Our daily life consists of activities such as eating, excretion, bathing, sleeping (going to bed), awakening (waking up), shopping, and cleaning. And these lifestyle behaviors are repeated constantly over the 24-hour days, creating a so-called daily routine. When dementia is present, it increases the difficulty in carrying out these daily living activities independently due to cognitive dysfunctions such as memory and attention deficit, disorientation, aphasia, agnosia, apraxia, and executive dysfunction. Examples of such disorders include the inability to recognize a pair of chopsticks, spoon, or fork (agnosia) and the failure to hold them in hand, mistaking the patterns on a plate for food and attempting to pick it up with chopsticks repeatedly, which makes the person unable finish their meal, forgetting how to strain during a bowel movement, and inability to wash their face thoroughly because they wash only the right side, and neglect the other side. These disorders are collectively referred to as daily life difficulties. However, daily life difficulties are often observed when the person with dementia is placed in new, unfamiliar environments. This is because procedural memory (movements and skills that the body remembers) is more likely to be activated in familiar environments, thereby preventing from escalating to a full daily life difficulty.

These daily life difficulties can therefore be eased by communicating in ways that are easy to be understood by people with cognitive dysfunction and adjusting the physical environment to support the autonomy and independence of older adults with dementia as much as possible. The ingenuity and implementation of care for those with daily life difficulties will lead to a well-managed daily routine and reassurance for older adults with dementia (Suwa S, 2019, 2021).

5.2 Guidelines for Respecting the Decisions of Older Adults with Dementia who Require Medical and Long-Term Care

It is desirable for older people with dementia to be able to live at the homes they are accustomed to within a comprehensive community care system until the end of their lives. However, in Japan, a super-aging society, older people with dementia often suffer from diseases such as hypertension, diabetes, cancer, fractures, and infectious diseases, or see these complications worsen. In that case, they are admitted to a general hospital (acute care hospital) that provides acute care, receive treatment, and aim for recovery and discharge back to their homes. However, if their ADL does not recover to conditions pre-admission and caring for them by family members alone is deemed difficult, usually the older adult with dementia have no choice but to be discharged to a nursing home, despite their wish to be discharged home. Three guidelines for decision-making support have been developed in Japan to respect the autonomy and independence of older people with dementia in such conditions.

The first of these is the Ministry of Health, Labour and Welfare (MHLW) "Guidelines on the process of decision-making on end-of-life healthcare and care." (The Ministry of Health, Labour and Welfare 2018).

This revised "Guideline of the decision-making process for terminal care," compiled in 2007, takes into account the need to respond to build community-based comprehensive care to meet the needs of a progressively aging death-ridden society and the widespread adoption of research and initiatives based on the concept of Advance Care Planning (ACP), mainly in the United Kingdom and the United States.

In Japan, artificial hydration and nutrition has been implemented as a standard medical treatment when eating and swallowing disorders appear in older adults with dementia at the end-of-life. However, there was no evidence that older adults who receive artificial hydration and nutrition live longer; instead, it seemed to prove that it may cause, worsen, or prolong physical and mental pain and harm. Medical and long-term care costs for older adults also continued to increase, leading to greater social problems.

To address this issue, the Japan Geriatrics Society formulated the Guidelines for Decision-making Processes for Elderly Care on the Introduction of artificial hydration and nutrition in 2012 (Ouchi Y. 2012, Ouchi Y, 2018). This guideline refers to the assumption that people should live for as long as possible regardless of their condition at the end of life. It raises the importance of medical, nursing, and welfare workers to determine whether not medical and care interventions should be provided to maintain and improve their quality of life through communication with the patient himself or their family and proxy decision-makers.

In 2018, the Ministry of Health, Labour and Welfare (MHLW) issued the "Guidelines to Support Decision-making in the Daily and Social Lives of Persons with Dementia." (The Ministry of Health, Labour and Welfare, 2018). This guideline summarizes the basic concepts, attitudes, methods, and matters that should be considered for decision support provided by people around the supporters of people with dementia and aims to allow people with dementia to live their daily and social lives in a way that respects their own will.

5.3 New Problem of Dementia Care in the Super-Aging and Death-Ridden Society

The super-aging society is simultaneously a death-ridden one. Although older people with dementia were conventionally assumed to die before their caregiving families, we are finding an increasing number of older people with dementia who outlive their similarly-aged spouses and aging children. The number of older people with dementia living alone will also increase in Japan. Many family members of older adults with dementia worry whether the person with dementia will understand when they learn of the loss of a loved one, how the bad news should be conveyed to them, and how to interact with them after sharing such information. This concern may also trouble professionals in medical and long-term care.

Therefore, it will become increasingly important to support family caregivers of older people with dementia who are bereaving the loss of a spouse, as an example.

Based on the model of Worden's mourning process (Worden J.W. (2010), the mourning process of older adults with Alzheimer's dementia who have been separated from their spouses, which corresponds to FAST 4-6 as shown in Fig. 1, goes back and forth through four stages: "Inability to remember the spouse's death and repeatedly re-experiencing loss," "Living in confusion and anxiety in a world without the spouse," "Finally recognizing the spouse's death after about a year," and "Finding an eternal connection with the deceased on the process of starting a new life" (Watanabe A., 2017). For older adults with dementia to follow through these four stages, it is essential to support them by decorating objects and other memorabilia that remind the death of their spouse in visible places, attending memorial services, and repeatedly conveying their grief in an easy-to-understand manner.

In addition, an analysis of the diaries of an older Japanese woman living alone during four years after she was diagnosed with Alzheimer's disease revealed that although she faced many challenges due to cognitive dysfunction, she encouraged herself and gradually accepted the support of her caregivers (Table 1). (Suwa S, 2018).

It will become increasingly important to provide emotional and cultural support the person with dementia themselves and families regarding bereavement and living alone in Japan.

Table 1 Linguistic analysis: Expressions repeated ≥3 times, 2010 to 2013

		2010	2011	2012	2013	Total
Emotions about daily life	I'm lonely by myself	23	10	49	16	98
	I'm miserable	10	7	14	15	45
	I'm sad	1	0	8	4	13
Memory loss experience	I don't know	28	56	89	65	228
	Miserable	11	66	34	50	161
	Foolish	10	14	35	32	91
	Shameful	16	20	21	22	79
	I've become stupid (I understand my stupidity. Silly)	7	16	22	26	71
	Embarrassing	3	17	22	7	49
	My mind is foggy	9	6	8	9	32
	Senile	8	13	3	8	32
	Sad	5	11	12	3	31
	Vexed	1	3	13	6	23
	I'm distressed	5	5	4	3	17
	I no longer understand myself	0	2	8	4	14
	Lonely	4	6	0	1	11
	It can't be helped.	2	2	0	1	5
Self-evaluation	Silly human	16	8	12	19	55
	I'm appalled	1	4	10	3	18
	Useless human	2	2	5	0	9
	I've become unsteady, sloppy	4	1	1	0	6
	I'm upset	1	2	0	0	3
Resignation	It can't be helped, it's because I'm old.	4	14	4	1	23
Positive coping	Take care of myself	19	2	28	31	80

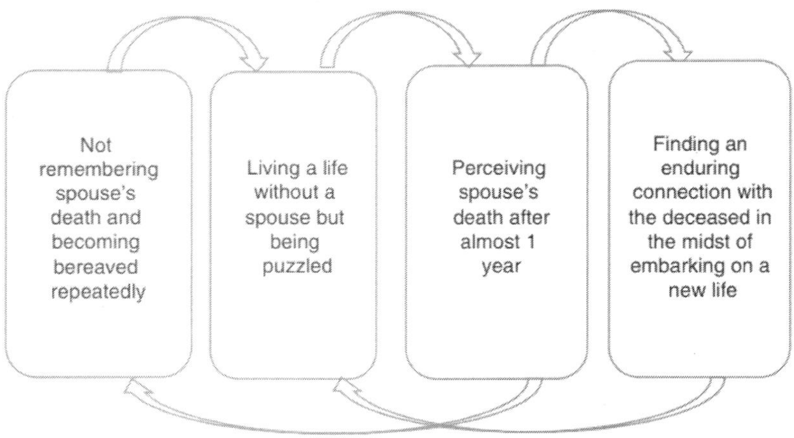

Figure 1 The mourning process of people with dementia in FAST4–6.

5.4 Religion and Spirituality in Japan

The 2022 Religious Almanac of Japan reveals a diverse mix of religious cultures: 49% Shinto, 46% Buddhism(Religious Almanac 2022), 1%

Christianity, and 4% other religions (Religious Almanac 2022). The NHK survey in October 2018 revealed that: ① Although the traditional values of Japanese are, "the SUN is watching," "the existence of power beyond human understanding," and "God living in nature," the number of people having these beliefs is decreasing. ② The number of people who expect religion to play a role such as "healing" is decreasing、③It indicates that more people perceive religion as dangerous than those who do not(NHK, 2019).

Spirituality is a concept that is difficult to understand for the Japanese people who do not have religious backgrounds. However, in recent years, spirituality has been explored as an aspect of spiritual needs that all humans have and the meaning of searching for the ``meaning of self-existence." Moreover, providers of spiritual care are not only religious experts but also people who surround the person. Caring for the spiritual aspects of individuals (groups) in a crisis, such as illness or difficult experiences, is an important purpose and function of nursing. In Japan, many studies have been conducted on how to provide spiritual care to terminally ill cancer patients.

Takeda (Takeda.S, 2006) explored the conceptual structure of spirituality in the Japanese elderly. The reason is that the elderly are in a crisis situation, facing the loss of physical function, bereavement of family and friends, and retirement from social roles. According to this research review of spiritual care for the Japanese elderly, the spirituality of the Japanese elderly comprises the following six concepts: [meaning and purpose of life], [attitude toward death and dying], [self-transcendence], [harmony with others], [reliance], [harmony with nature]. In particular, "attitudes toward death and dying" and "harmony with others" are important concepts for the elderly.

As spiritual needs include the search for the meaning of self-existence, attitudes toward death and dying, and harmony with others, it has become possible to verbalize the necessity and importance of spirituality and spiritual care.

5.5 Culture-Based Nursing in Japan

Ishigaki explained that although the Japanese nursing education system strongly reflects Western-style thinking in education, many nurses adopt nursing methods based on Japanese culture. She and her research team of the Chiba University Graduate School of Nursing have identified the following four key concepts that represent culture-based nursing: "relationship," "embodiment," "society/organization" culture and “values”. Thereafter, the Society of Cultural Nursing Studies was established in 2007 to explore nursing science based on the Japanese culture (Chiba University 21st Century COE Program,2008).Based on the key concepts of culture-based nursing, it is possible to understand the following backgrounds of the elderly: an unstable mind, old friends and people around them, shame about physical problems such as assistance with excretion and comfort care, lifestyle habits, regional climate, pleasant memories of the past recalled by eating events of the past, and social resources that can be selected.

Moreover, in the case of the elderly with dementia, it is possible to determine the power that the person has and a method of support that uses the person's strengths.

When we consider the key concepts of culture-based nursing, we find the perspective of nursing necessary for individualized care because there are problems that cannot be solved by medical thinking centered on natural science alone. Therefore, thinking in terms of key concepts of culture-based nursing, will enable us to understand how to support the elderly with dementia.

Hirakawa interviewed care workers and nurses who care for the elderly with dementia, and indicated the necessary concepts for them. The results suggest that, even if cognitive impairment is more severe, it is important to find joy in independent activities of daily living, remembering the past, and finding simple pleasures daily. It has been indicated that support for elderly people's independence and daily enjoyment is implemented in rehabilitation and activities in the Japanese day service system (Hirakawa, Y.2020). Masaki et al. developed dementia prevention classroom programs in the target regions of China and Japan and examined the development process between the two countries. Consequently, in China, “the need for care owing to the deterioration of the autonomic capacity of dementia patients is the premise," and “the need for concern from the entire society is coordinated." In Japan, dementia is common owing to aging and “Nursing care is considered to be in natural circulation in the community." In addition, it was revealed that people around them did not understand the closeness of the parent-child relationship and the burden of care when considering dementia care. (Masaki,H.2009)

Thus, not many people in Japan formally belong to traditional religious institutions or regularly participate in required activities. However, spirituality is interpreted as "exploring the meaning of one's own existence, and cognitive changes associated with aging are regarded as natural. Further, to provide care in the family and community that uses the individual strengths of aging people, it is important to provide nursing that considers the individual's background and culture, as well as spiritual care, such as looking back on daily enjoyment and past memories.

Bibliography

Ikejima, C., A. Hisanaga, K. Meguro, T. Yamada, S. Ouma, Y. Kawamuro, K. Hyouki, K. Nakashima, K. Wada, S. Yamada, I. Watanabe, T. Kakuma, Y. Aoyama, K. Mizukami and T. Asada: Multicentre population-based dementia prevalence survey in Japan: a preliminary report, Psychogeriatrics 12(2): 120-123,2012.

Cabinet Office, Japan: Annual report on the aging society, 2016. Retrieved from https://www8.cao.go.jp/kourei/english/annualreport/2016/2016pdf_e.html

Chiba University 21st Century COE Program Kazuko Ishigaki: Preface to Japanese Cultural Nursing -Establishment and Development of Nursing Based on Practical Wisdom—Establishment and Development of Nursing Science Based on Practical Wisdom 2008. (in Japanese)

Hirakawa, Y.,Chiang, C.,Yasuda, K.,Iwaki, Y.,Andoh, H.,Aoyama, A.: Spirituality in older men living alone near the end-of-life, Nagoya J Med Sci,81, 2019,557-570. DOI :10.18999/nagjms.81.4.557

Ministry of Health, Labour and Welfare (2013). "Grant-in-Aid for Scientific Research: Comprehensive research project on dementia prevention. Dementia prevalence in urban areas and response to functional disorders in activities of daily living associated with dementia. FY2011 to FY2012 Summary Research Report. Retrieved from http://www.tsukuba-psychiatry.com/wp-content/uploads/2013/06/H24Report_Part1.pdf

Ministry of Health, Labour and Welfare: Comprehensive strategy for promoting dementia measures. New Orange Plan,2015. Retrieved from

https://www.mhlw.go.jp/stf/seisakunitsuite/bunya/0000064084.html
Ministry of Health, Labour and Welfare:Community-based integrated care system. 2012 Retrieved from https://www.mhlw.go.jp/stf/seisakunitsuite/bunya/hukushi_kaigo/kaigo_koureisha/chiiki-houkatsu/

Ministry of Health, Labour and Welfare (2015). Comprehensive strategy for promoting dementia measures. New Orange Plan,2015. Available from https://www.mhlw.go.jp/file/06-Seisakujouhou-12300000-Roukenkyoku/nop1-2_3.pdf

Ministry of Health, Labour and Welfare : Outline for the Promotion of Dementia Measures, 2019. https://www.mhlw.go.jp/content/000522832.pdf

Ministry of Health, Labour and Welfare: Main Dementia Policies, 2005, (https://www.mhlw.go.jp/stf/seisakunitsuite/bunya/0000076236_00006.html).

National Caravan Mate Liaison Council, 2005. (https://www.caravanmate.com/).

Kobayashi T. (NHK survey): How has Japanese religious awareness changed?, 2019, https://www.nhk.or.jp/bunken/research/yoron/pdf/20190401_7.pdf. (2019) (in Japanese)

Ouchi Y.:The Japan Geriatrics Society:Guidelines for the decision-making processes in medical and long-term care for the elderly: focusingon the use of artificial hydration and nutrition." Nihon Ronen Igakkai Zasshi 49: 632–645、2012 (in Japanese).

Ouchi, Y., K. Toba, K. Ohta, I. Kai, T. Shimizu, N. Higuchi, S. Shimazono, S. Iijima, S. Suwa, M. Nishimura, H. Ninomiya and K. Aita,Guidelines from the Japan Geriatrics Society for the decision-making processes in medical and long-term care for the elderly: Focusing on the use of artificial hydration and nutrition." Geriatr Gerontol Int 18(6): 823-827,2018.

Suwa, S., S. Otani, M. Tsujimura, K. Nogawa and Y. Shiya : The diary of a nonagenarian-centenarian woman with dementia: Memory loss, life changes, and community care in Japan, Int J Nurs Pract 24 Suppl 1: e12655,2018 https://doi.org/10.1111/ijn.12655.

Suwa, S., A. Yumoto, M. Ueno, T. Yamabe, Y. Hoshishiba and M. Sato Characteristics of care methods for daily life disabilities in Alzheimer's

type dementia that respect autonomy and independence. Nurs Open 6(3): 930-941,2019.
https://doi.org/10.1002/nop2.283.

Suwa, S., A. Yumoto, M. Ueno, T. Yamabe, Y. Hoshishiba and M. Sato: Practitioners' identification of informal caregivers' difficulties with activities of daily living interventions for older people with dementia in Japan, Psychogeriatrics 21(4): 466-477,2021.
https://doi.org/10.1111/psyg.12689).

Takeda K., Futoyu Y.:Conceptual framework of spilituality in Elderly Japanese, Kawasaki Medical Welfare Journal,161),2006,53-66. (in Japanese)

The Ministry of Health, Labour and Welfare,2018.
https://www.mhlw.go.jp/file/04-Houdouhappyou-10802000-Iseikyoku-Shidouka/0000197701.pdf). (in Japanese)

The Ministry of Health, Labour and Welfare,2018.
https://www.mhlw.go.jp/file/06-Seisakujouhou-12300000-Roukenkyoku/0000212396.pdf

Watanabe, A. and S. Suwa:The mourning process of older people with dementia who lost their spouse, J Adv Nurs 73(9),2017: 2143-2155,2017. DOI: 10. 1111/jan. 13286

Worden J.W.: Grief Counselling and Grief Therapy: A Handbook for the Mental Health Practitioner. Routledge, London,2010.

Masaki H., Zhang P., Zhou Y., Torita M., Takahashi Y., Tanimoto, M., Xiao H.: Comparison Between Japan and China Trough the Process of Developing Culturally Congruent Dementia Prevention Class" Journal of Cultural Nursing Studies, 1(1)22-30,2009.
https://www.jstage.jst.go.jp/article/bunkakango/1/1/1_1_22/_pdf/-char/ja (in Japanese)

26

THE JEWISH APPROACH FOR GRANTING MEANING, BELONGING, AND SELF-WORTH TO PEOPLE WITH DEMENTIA AND THEIR FAMILIES IN THE COMMUNITY- THE MELABEV EXPERIENCE IN ISRAEL

DR. ZEEV FRIEDMAN,PH.D[1]
AND DR. LIORA COHEN, PH.D[2]

> "Do not cast me away from your presence, and do not take your holy spirit from me"" (Psalms 51:13)

Melabev: Providing meaning, belonging, and a sense of value to people with dementia and their families in the community

According to data from the Israeli Central Bureau of Statistics, persons 65-years old and above will constitute 15% of the population in Israel in 2025. Furthermore, in less than two decades, the average life expectancy in Israel will be 84.8 for men and 89.5 for women (ICBS, 2016). If to this point we characterized the older population as representing "the third age", today older adults over the age of 80 are being characterized as belonging to "the fourth age"—as written in the Bible, "With the ancient is wisdom; and in length of days understanding" (Job 12:12).

The aging process is not homogeneous, and it is possible to refer to three types of aging: the first type, which comprises between 60% to 80% of the

[1] CEO of Melabev

[2] Director of Content and Training of Melabev

older adults is characterized by healthy, productive, active people, who volunteer, study, and are enriched by knowledge and hobbies; they are well aware of their rights and how to fully utilize them. As the Bible says, "They shall still bring forth fruit in old age; they shall be flourishing" (Psalms 92:14). And indeed, the artist Claude Monet painted the water lilies in his garden in his ninth decade; Giuseppe Verdi composed the Falstaff opera when he was 85 years old; Benjamin Franklin invented the bifocal lens at 78 years of age; the architect Frank Lloyd Wright designed the Guggenheim Museum of Art in New York when he was 92; Michelangelo, Matisse, and Picasso were all still creative in their ninth decade. In this spirit, there is a saying attributed to Henrietta Szold: "The young have better vision but the old see better."

Active aging has been defined by the World Health Organization (WHO, 2002) as based on three elements: participation, which refers to involvement in social, economic, cultural, and spiritual activities, as well as public affairs; maintaining health and reducing risk factors, engaging in physical activity and receiving proper nutrition; and security, which refers to rights and a secure living environment. Being active at an old age is critical for coping with the retirement crisis (in Israel, the retirement age for men is 67 and for women 62), as people who are active physically, mentally, and psychologically often abruptly find themselves in a reality of emptiness, passivity, low self-worth and self-image.

The second type of aging, which comprises between 15% to 30% of the older adults, is characterized by difficulties in functioning and dependency on institutions. Older adults in this group are exposed to dangers and risks, and they live in poverty and economic straits. Some suffer from food insecurity, loneliness, childlessness, and isolation. Some are victims of violence and exploitation, and some of them suffer from medical problems and are in psychological distress. In this regard, it is written in the Bible: "Cast me not off in the time of old age; forsake me not when my strength fails (Psalms 71:9).

The third type comprises between 10% to 15% of the older adults and is characterized by dementia and cognitive decline. In this regard, it is written in the Bible: "Do not cast me away from your presence, and do not take your holy spirit from me" (Psalms 51:13). This group will be the focus of this article and the study case of Melabev, a non profit association in Israel.[3]

[3] Melabev is a Hebrew acronym for "Community Clubs for Eldercare"

The association was founded in 1981 by Professor Arnold Rosin (1930-2018) and Leah Abramowitz, a social worker, in a reality that lacked dedicated frameworks for people with dementia who live in their homes, and out of a desire to provide a better quality of life to these people and their family caregivers. Melabev began as a unique day center in Jerusalem and in time expanded, operating additional day centers and developing services for family caregivers, professional bodies, and the general public throughout the country.

Melabev was founded out of a sense of social responsibility "Tikkun Olam" (a Hebrew term literally meaning "repairing the world"), a concept based on the Jewish bookshelf, while corresponding with contemporary conceptions. The phenomenon of dementia was discussed in the Jewish sources centuries ago. This is what the sage Maharal of Prague, a sixteenth-century Jewish theologian wrote about dementia: “The [spiritual] level acquired by a man by [studying] the Torah cannot be seen as eliminated … because he has forgotten what he had learned. It is not considered that the Torah leaves a person … because it is a matter of a person having a body and that body cannot have the Torah with it all the time … and also, even though the Torah has gone away because of the illness of the receiving body, it is not considered that the Torah has gone away from him” (Netivot Olam, Netiv Hatorah ch. 12). The words of the Maharal can be understood as meaning that the contents of memory still exist, it is just that our intellectual apparatus, our ability to retrieve “data”, has been damaged. In other words, it is possible to physically damage the body, but a person’s spiritual assets, gathered throughout an entire lifetime, remain preserved within them.

This conception, which emphasizes the parts that remain preserved in a person, accords with the question that engaged theoreticians in the 1990s: to what extent does a person’s identity persist alongside dementia? Until the 1990s, the dominant biomedical model defined dementia as a destructive neurological syndrome that causes a gradual deterioration of the individual to the point of becoming “a living dead” person. One of the pioneers of the change was Thomas Kitwood (1997), who advocated for “person-centered care,” according to which people with dementia must be viewed first and foremost as human beings, regardless of age and cognitive status. Indeed, it has been discovered that the emotional system remains intact even in the advanced stages of dementia, including the range of feelings that are at the foundation of human existence, such as the ability to experience happiness, enjoyment, pain, sadness, and a desire for intimacy and relationship (Magai et al. 2002). Therefore, we do not speak in terms of medical pathology: we

use the term "people with dementia" rather than "dementia patients", and we use the term "syndrome" rather than "disease". In practical terms, this means that we do not speak over the heads of thepersons with dementia; instead we provide empathy, attention, patience, and tolerance.
It is important to emphasize that viewing people with dementia as human beings does not mean denying the difficulties; rather, it means treatment from a point of view of including rather than excluding, as formulated in an ancient, sixth-century Jewish text, the Babylonian and Jerusalem Talmud: "And be careful to continue to respect an elder who has forgotten his Torah knowledge due to circumstances beyond his control (Sanhedrin Tractate 96)," as well as "Both the tablets of the Covenant and the broken tablets are placed in the Ark of the Covenant in the Temple" (Brakhot 8b). The message for a person with dementia is that your role in this world has not yet ended: you are not a lost case to be dismissed, since the broken tablets are placed next to the whole ones; they garner the same amount of respect, glory, and sanctity in the Ark of the Covenant in the Temple as do the whole tablets.

The sense of loss and absence experienced by people with dementia is not denied, and therefore the fundamental guiding principle of Melabev is to provide meaning in life alongside dementia. This is what we have learned from Rabbi Soloveitchik's book *Out of the Whirlwind* (2004) and from the science of logotherapy, developed by Viktor Frankl in his book *Man's Search for Meaning* (1946). They both address a reality of victimhood, where there is a loss caused by an external factor—as in dementia—and recommend that we do everything we can to channel ourselves into a path of meaning and fullness rather than to a path of victimhood or victimizing. They both argue that one must not search for reasons of victimhood; instead, one should direct and channel oneself toward meaning and destiny. This means not asking "Why" but asking "For what purpose?"

The goal of finding meaning in life alongside and despite dementia motivated the establishment of the day centers, which are at the heart of the caregiving activities offered by Melabev. Further, the heart at the root of the name itself—in Hebrew "melabev" means, literally, "heartwarming"—reflects the warm heart of the caregiving staff (Rosin and Abramowitz 1996).

We rely on the sustained personhood model for dementia care (Berenbaum et al. 2017a) in order to understand how to turn the act of finding meaning among people with dementia into a caregiving practice. According to this model, there are three levels of personhood that exist alongside dementia: (1) a *sociologic personhood*, which comprises one's reciprocal relations with the environment; (2) an *individual personhood*, which is manifested in one's uniqueness and personality, history, communication, spiritual dimension, and self-worth; (3) a *biologic personhood* that includes basic needs, pleasure, and management of pain. According to the model, these three levels of personhood exist throughout dementia with varying degrees of dominance, so that one's personhood appears as a "continuous I" as opposed to an increasingly vanishing one. Accordingly, caregiving has the power to awaken the vitality inherent in a person.

The preservation of the *sociologic personhood* takes place primarily through the group component, which enables alleviating the loneliness of people coping with dual social exclusion, both because of their age and the stigma of dementia. Furthermore, the day centers are meant to provide a framework of belonging and identity: Melabev's day centers are customized and adapted to varying levels of cognitive ability in order to allow group members to feel that they are among peers. In addition, there is a linguistic-cultural adaptation, reflecting the cultural layers of the State of Israel, with separate groups for Hebrew, English, French, Russian, and Arabic-speakers. Thus, for example, breakfast for the English-speaking groups includes toast with jam, apple juice, and oatmeal porridge, while the Hebrew-speaking group receives sandwiches with cheese and vegetables. The linguistic-cultural adaptation provides the participants with an anchor and strengthens their sense of belonging.

Additional components of the sociologic personhood in the day centers include sitting together in transportation, shared meals, and the activities, most of which are held in the group framework and which generate the group's unique power. One such activity, conducted by a group leader in a day center, included warming up the vocal cords, so that each participant was asked to produce any sound they wanted, and the others were asked to repeat it. The group leader related that the voices thus produced were free and contagious, such as laughter, and created an electrifying atmosphere in the group.

From another angle, a study conducted by Melabev's research team (e.g., Berenbaum et al. 2017b) established the importance of preserving the sociologic personhood through a discussion of the complex issue of giving participants the right to mourn the passing of another group member: do people with dementia have the ability to cope with death? And what is the best way to maintain their right to mourn? The study interviewed fifty-two staff members in Melabev's day centers, with the aim to understand their attitudes and beliefs regarding people with dementia's coping with the death of a group member. The study showed that most staff members believe that people with dementia have the emotional ability to mourn the death of another group member, as expressed in the following interview excerpts: "Even if the mind forgets, the heart doesn't", and "If you don't commemorate [the loss of a group member] and just ignore the death, participants see that someone's not there. They feel that when they pass away the same will happen to them—no one will care." The research findings show that preserving the sociologic personhood may be manifested in giving day center participants the right to mourn the end of a relationship due to someone's passing.

Preservation of the sociologic personhood is even more important for people with advanced dementia since their inner world is increasingly closed off to them; they find it difficult to access and even more so to mediate it to others. As Geiger wrote about his father's dementia in *The Old Man in His Exile*: "Since my father can no longer cross the bridge to my world, I must cross the bridge to his" (2013). Notably, preserving the sociologic personhood in advanced dementia is expressed in paying attention to minute signals. For example, any kind of response of a patients to something outside themselves (e.g., a staff member, another group member, the group activity itself) is considered a success (Abramowitz 2008).

The preservation of the *individual personhood* is manifested in many ways in the caregiving practices of Melabev's day centers. One such practice is maintaining the continuity of the participants' personal history between "who I used to be" and "what I am now." Examples include creating an "office" for a former psychologist, with books on the desk, stationary, and a pen—he observes from the desk, takes notes, and gives advice; a former meteorologist measures the amount of rain, notes the data in his diary, and reports his findings to the members of the group; a participant who was a legendary soccer player now assists the staff in conducting physical activities for the group. In one of the day centers, pictures of the participants' weddings displayed in a prominent location. These pictures encourage them to discuss and raise memories from the past. As dementia advances, it becomes more difficult to express and understand verbal messages, which challenges the use of verbal means to maintain continuity. In these cases, reciting prayers may be a ray of light that penetrates the fog, as they pass through the participants' lips effortlessly, even among those who have almost stopped talking (Abramowitz 2008).

Due to the prominent role of the emotional system in communicating with people with dementia, the preservation of the individual personhood is manifested in attention to the emotional truth that breaks through incoherent speech and challenging behaviors such as wandering, repetitiveness, and aggression. As a group leader in one of the day centers observed, a participant who repeats his home address most of the day is attempting to hold on to the sole piece of ground left to him; if he lets go of it, he will lose everything. This approach accords with the theory of need-driven behavior in dementia (Algase et al. 1991), which conceptualizes challenging behaviors as an expression of needs and distresses that, given the limited ability to articulate them verbally, erupt behaviorally. In addition, some of our staff have been trained in the validation method (Feil 1993), according to which challenging behaviors express the emergence of traumas that were repressed throughout the years, thereby creating an opportunity to initiate processes of resolution and healing. Also, we place a great emphasis on providing a pleasant experience during the participants' sojourn in the day centers, which according to the staff makes an impression that remains with the participants after they return home. Even if they do not recall the details of the experience, their hearts do not forget its imprint.

Other ways in which the Melabev day centers engage in the preservation of the individual personhood include boosting self-worth and a sense of control. One example is the smart games that are available for participants and that are intended to activate cognition. They are played with the guidance of a skilled therapist and include exercises in math, language, shapes, and memory that appear on a computer screen. Studies that examined the effectiveness of smart games found that people with dementia learn and improve their performance at a similar rate to those without dementia. Furthermore, working on cognitive functions helped increase participants' self-efficacy and self-confidence (Berenbaum et al. 2011; Tziraki et al. 2017).

The spiritual dimension is also manifested in the day centers, primarily through music, which has a primordial effect and is known to have therapeutic benefits for people with dementia. In fact, music dominates daily life in the day centers: pleasant, culturally-appropriate music is played in the room when participants are received in the morning, as well as at mealtime and before returning home. Beloved personal playlists, put together in consultation with family members, are played to the participants through earphones; these are intended mainly for participants who are withdrawn and rarely make contact with their environment, as well as for those who require calm and a significant reduction in stimulation. In addition, the day centers have sing-alongs facilitated by musicians and with live instruments; musical bingo with a board that features the names of the songs (sometimes accompanied by a drawing)—every participant marks a song and the entire group sings; and music therapy that includes working on rhythm and movement. Staff members have reported that people with advanced dementia who are withdrawn into themselves respond to the beat and sometimes make dance movements (Abramowitz 2008).

Finally, the preservation of the *biological personhood* takes place through attention to the physical space of the day centers. Activity rooms have natural sunlight, as well as plants and flowers in the room itself or in an adjacent garden. Multi-sensory stimulation is provided through individual work in Snoezelen rooms, access to furry pets, aromas from cakes being baked in the oven and from aromatherapy oils. Ice cream cones are held securely even by those who have lost the ability to eat independently, and great care is taken to serve food in an aesthetic and inviting way.

Despite its advantages and the effort to preserve people's personhood alongside dementia, the person-centered care approach may "lock" the person with dementia into passivity, as objects of care and support. Therefore, Melabev strives to create opportunities for participants to be *active partners and contributors*. This, based on the conception that the ability to give to others is an important component in the meaning that people see in life and in their sense of self-worth. Examples include participants preparing packages for Ukrainian war refugees and sandwiches for kindergartners; a participant who blesses the members of her group and the caregiving staff and recites stories from the Torah; a participant who serves as a cantor and leads prayers. In addition, multi-generational projects go beyond giving children a brief glimpse into the day center and involve creating something together. Thus, at the conclusion of a year-long multi-generational project, a twelve-year-old girl said: "The main thing is the privilege of learning from the older adults: stories, wisdom, Torah, and history."

In 2022, Melabev founded a new therapeutic initiative called "A Listening Heart", which enables day center participants to express empathy for others. In this initiative, people with dementia at relatively high cognitive levels volunteer at the call center to reduce loneliness among older adults. They call seniors living alone who need human conversation and warmth. Suitable candidates are asked directly, “Do you wish to call lonely people and converse with them? There are lonely seniors who do not have anyone who calls them; can you help us?” When people with dementia arrive at the call center, the project coordinator gives them a printed sheet with a list of phone numbers and the first sentence to start the conversation, written out clearly. The coordinator is in the same space as the person with dementia and enables a free conversation, while at the same time being prepared to intervene in case the participant gets stuck, confused or begins discussing issues that are not in the purview of the call center, such as giving medical advice. Assisting the participants with dementia requires maintaining a delicate balance between the autonomy of the volunteer and providing support when needed. Nonetheless, most of the time, unknowing observers would not notice that the volunteer is a person with dementia; they will just see one human being reaching out to another and offering a sympathetic ear.

The “Video-Feedback” workshop is another example that demonstrates the importance of allowing people with dementia to be worthy partners in communicating with their caregivers. This workshop was developed based on prior work that dealt with the promotion of emotional bonds in intimate caregiving relations (Cohen et al. 2022), and that was adapted to this population. In 2023, a pilot workshop was conducted with group leaders working at the Melabev day centers, focusing on promoting the emotional dyadic relationship between group leaders and participants, and emphasizing the reciprocal relations and effects within the dyad. Group leaders watched video segments of interactions with participants, meant to demonstrate moments of reciprocity in the interaction, moments of back-and-forth, of exchange and shared delight.

The three constructs of personhood also correspond with the **biopsychosocial model** formulated by the psychiatrist George Engel from Rochester University, which was introduced to the scientific community in an article published in *Science* in 1977. This model is manifested in three dimensions: **biophysical**, which includes maintaining the patients’ cleanliness, aesthetics, and security and serving two meals that emphasize both nutrition and a sensitive and dignified manner of serving them; **psychotherapeutic**, which refers to an array of treatments aimed at preserving the person's memory reserve, such as group discussions, memory and thinking activities, physical activities, art and music; **social**, which refers to the person's sense of belonging to the group and alleviating loneliness, to proactivity—from being to doing, from being supported to supporting—and to delaying dependence and preventing deterioration. The fact that the day centers areconnected to the environment and the community enables maintaining inter-generational relations with children and youths as well as the volunteer activities of the participants themselves.

Importantly, the establishment of Melabev's day centers was a result of the need to provide a framework and sense of belonging to people with dementia but also, and no less importantly, it was a result of the need *to support their family caregivers* (Rosin and Abramowitz 1996). Being in the day center for 6 hours allows caregivers respite, time to care for themselves, and somewhat alleviates the burden of care. As time passed, additional services were added such as individual therapy at people with dementia ' homes combined with counseling and support provided by social workers to family members. An evaluation study (Habib et al. 2021) examined the views of thirty-one primary family caregivers regarding the benefit of Melabev's home service to their dear ones who live with dementia and for themselves. The findings showed that most caregivers reported improved mood, alertness, and quality of life of their dear ones. They also reported that the service provided them with professional and emotional support when needed, and time free from the concerns of caregiving.

During the Coronavirus pandemic in 2020, a unique service was established that offeres Zoom meetings with family caregivers on topics relevant to the issues they are coping with. To date, forty five meetings have been held, reaching some 6,500 family caregivers. Thus, for example, the most recent meeting was on "who will caring for the caregivers?" Currently, the Zoom meetings have been expanded to emotional and professional support groups and individual counseling.

Dementia affects spouses, adult children, as well as the entire family. A unique pilot study conducted by Melabev's research unit (Berenbaum, in process) focused on the 8- to 18-year-old grandchildren of people with dementia, in an attempt to understand how they cope with their grandparents' dementia. The study found that the grandchildren wish to receive information about dementia, ways of coping, and behavior related to their grandparent's cognitive deterioration in order to maintain a warm and loving relationship despite the changes.

Melabev was founded as a response to the burning needs in the field, in a reality that had no dedicated frameworks for people with dementia who are living in their homes, and out of a desire to provide better quality of life for them and their family caregivers. The organization's services were developed based on the experience gained in the field over the years, while being accompanied by research (e.g., Berenbaum et al. 2017a,b). Therefore, at this stage, after the accumulation of clinical and research experience, we began a large-scale project in 2022 that focuses on mapping the day centers' activity units. The first layer includes a detailed syllabus of the activities, starting from the minibus ride to the day center, group activities (such as physical activity, art and music), meals, waiting for the minibus, and returning home. The description is detailed and refers to structural aspects (number of participants, manner of sitting, time of day, frequency of activity), as well as to the activity content, that will enable a description of the actual experience of staying at Melabev's day centers. A further layer we are aiming for is to find means to measurethe activities' effectiveness for the participants, based on observations, surveying and Interviewing group leaders, and the components of the sustained personhood model presented above.

The Melabev association is a unique organization ,it is a social factor and agent of change, with the social mission of "Tikkun Olam", to ***"repair the world"***Thus, one can say that the motivating force of Melabev are the social values embodied in the Jewish bookshelf. That is from where we draw our organizational and professional culture and also the conceptualization and proper language used to honor the dear people whom we serve.

The notion of Tikkun Olam shapes our mission. When we provide services to people with dementia and treat them with respect, we are actually repairing the world and turning it into a better, more enlightened place. Thus, we work to re-establish routine structured life with a clear daily routine for our participants and their family caregivers, inspired by the words of the renowned Israeli poetess, Leah Goldberg (1911–1970):

> And here you have aged, become old and white-haired,
> and your days are numbered, and ever more precious
> And you realize, each day may be the last under the sun
> And you realize, there *is* something new each day under the sun
> …
> Teach my lips to bless and sing a song of praise
> As your time begins anew, morn and night
> Lest today be as days gone by
> Lest my days settle into a rut

List of References

Israeli Central Bureau of Statistics. "Life Span in Israel 2016." December 11, 2017 (in Hebrew). https://www.cbs.gov.il/he/mediarelease/Pages/2017/%D7%AA%D7%95%D7%97%D7%9C%D7%AA-%D7%97%D7%99%D7%99%D7%9D-%D7%91%D7%99%D7%A9%D7%A8%D7%90%D7%9C-2016.aspx

Habib, J., Zikri-Segal, H., Friedman, Z., Berenbaum, R., Zemel, S., and Brent, Y. *Evaluation Study of the Effectiveness of Melabavev's Home Service* (in Hebrew). Jerusalem: Melabavev, 2021.

Abramowitz, L. (2008). Working with advanced dementia patients in a day care setting. *Journal of Gerontological Social Work, 50* (3-4), 25-35.

Algase, D. L., Beck, C., Kolanowski, A., Whall, A., Berent, S., Richards, K., & Beattie, E. (1996). Need-driven dementia-compromised behavior: An alternative view of disruptive behavior. *American Journal of Alzheimer's Disease, 11*(6), 10-19.

Berenbaum, R. *Grandchildren of people with Alzheimer's Disease and Dementia. How can we help them deal with the "ongoing funeral?* (In process).

Berenbaum, R., Lange, Y., & Abramowitz, L. (2011). Augmentative alternative communication for Alzheimer's patients and families' using SAVION. In *Proceedings of the 4th International Conference on PErvasive Technologies Related to Assistive Environments* (pp. 1-4)

Berenbaum, R., Tziraki, C., & Mazuz, K. (2017a). The enduring self: personhood, autonomy and compassion in the context of community-based dementia daycare centers. *Journal of Compassionate Health Care*, *4*(1), 1-10.

Berenbaum, R., Tziraki, C., & Cohen-Mansfield, J. (2017b). The right to mourn in dementia: to tell or not to tell when someone dies in dementia day care. *Death Studies*, *41*(6), 353-359.

Cohen, L., Sher-Censor, E., Dassa, A., Ayalon, L., Oppenheim, D., & Palgi, Y. Emotional availability in dyads of nursing aide-resident with dementia: Old tool, new perspective (2022). *Dementia,* 1-17.

Feil, N. (1993). *The Validation breakthrough: Simple techniques for communicating with people with" Alzheimer's-type dementia."*. Health Professions Press.

Kitwood, T. (1997). *Dementia reconsidered: The person comes first.* Buckingham, United Kingdom: Open University Press.

Magai, C., Cohen, C. I., & Gomberg, D. (2002). Impact of training dementia caregivers in sensitivity to nonverbal emotion signals. *International Psychogeriatrics, 14*(1), 25-38.

Rosin, A.J., & Abramowitz, L. (1996). Melabev - Transition from Concept to Reality: The History of the Development of the First Psychogeriatric Day Center in Jerusalem. *Gerontology: Special issue, Community Geriatrics and an outlook towards the 21st century.*

Tziraki, C., Berenbaum, R., Gross, D., Abikhzer, J., & Ben-David, B. M. (2017). Designing serious computer games for people with moderate and advanced dementia: Interdisciplinary theory-driven pilot study. *JMIR serious games*, *5*(3), 1-17.

World Health Organization. (2002). *Active ageing: A policy framework.* https://apps.who.int/iris/bitstream/handle/10665/67215/WHO_NMH_NPH_02.8.pdf?sequence=1&isAllowed=y

27

THE TREATMENT OF DEMENTIA IN THE GREEK CHRISTIAN ORTHODOX CONTEXT: A CULTURAL PERSPECTIVE

BEKIARIDIS-MOSCHOU DIMITRIOS PHD[1],
LAZAROU EFTYCHIA MSC MA[2],
OIKONOMOU VALENIA MA[3],
AND TSOLAKI MAGDALENE MD PHD[4]

1. Introduction

It is known that for many patients, suffering from chronic and life-threatening diseases, such as dementia, meeting their spiritual and religious needs is often as important as attending to their biological and physical needs. Spirituality is defined as the way in which man tries to give meaning and purpose to his life and to his experience of contact with himself, others, nature and supernatural forces[1]. Religiosity is defined as the acceptance of specific rituals and beliefs within a framework of organized and structured religion, either publicly or privately[2].

According to the World Health Organization, the extension of life expectancy of the population is one of the greatest advances of humanity,

---

[1] Psychologist, Alzheimer Hellas, "Agios Ioannis" Day Care Center, Thessaloniki, Greece.
[2] Philologist, Alzheimer Hellas, "Panagia Glykofilousa" Dementia Palliative Care Center, Thessaloniki, Greece.
[3] English Language and Literature, Greek Ministry of Education and Religious Affairs.
[4] Professor of Neurology, Alzheimer Hellas, "Panagia Glykofilousa" Dementia Palliative Care Center, Thessaloniki, Greece.

but at the same time one of the most important challenges, since aging places increased economic and social obligations on states. The development of science and medical technology has increased the number of people reaching old age and although old age does not cause disease, it is still associated with health problems, disabilities and dementia. Senile dementia with the main representative being Alzheimer's disease affects more than 10% of the world's elderly population, about 20,000,000 people in the world, with an increasing trend of this percentage, and is a serious public health issue with a huge economic burden on modern society[3]. Thus, it becomes apparent that supporting and helping these patients and their families in any possible way is of high importance for them and the community in general. In this respect a holistic approach has been proposed in approaching the treatment, prevention and alleviation of dementia patients their caregivers and the elderly population in general. In this holistic approach taking into account the spiritual needs and the effect of religiosity has been proven to be very useful, producing significant positive results[4,5,6,7,8].

2. Dementia and Mild Cognitive Impairment

2.1 Dementia and Mild Cognitive Impairment as a major problem of older adults in our days. Treatment and preventive measures

Dementia is a progressive neurodegenerative disease of the central nervous system. In its early stages, it is characterized by a gradual loss of memory and limitation of mental functions. As the disease progresses, daily functioning is gradually affected until the patient is completely dependent on others. The disease is often accompanied by behavioral disorders such as symptoms of depression, anxiety, aggression, etc. It mainly appears in the "elderly" and rarely at ages under 65 years old. Alzheimer's disease is one of the forms of dementia that have been identified. As long as the patient maintains daily functioning at a satisfying level despite the deterioration of mental functions, he is characterized as suffering from Mild Cognitive Impairment (MCI). Neurology has established specific international criteria for defining both dementia and MCI.

Although, in our days, there has not been found an effective treatment for this disease, early diagnosis as well as some preventive measures that limit possible risk factors in the development of the disease are important for its treatment. Prevention includes good cardiovascular performance, normal regulation of diabetes, regular physical exercise, socialization, healthy diet, keeping under control symptoms of anxiety and depression, limiting alcohol intake as well as exercising mental functions[9].

2.2 Cognitive training as a measure to prevent and treat MCI and dementia

It has been repeatedly found that the participation of elderly people in activities that stimulate brain functions helps them to strengthen and develop these functions, as well as to protect them from further worsening either due to age or neurodegenerative diseases[9,10,11,12].

There have been used memory, logic and speed processing training programs[13], psychomotor and cognitive function training programs[14] as well as techniques for developing cognitive skills through interactive computer programs[15]. All of these techniques have been successful in enhancing brain function and slowing down cognitive decline in MCI or normal ageing. As a matter of fact, the results of this cognitive training seem to apply to a wide range of brain functions and to be long-lasting[13]. Thus, these techniques are used in dementia prevention.

Smith et al.[16], studied elderly people over 65 during the implementation of an educational program (Brain Fitness Program; Posit Science, 2009) of strengthening cognitive functions using a computer program in which audio-visual material on history, art and literature were presented. Training would take place for 1 hour per day, five days per week for more than 8 weeks. The beneficiaries completed some cognitive tests on the educational material they were exposed to. Their neuropsychological assessment (Repeatable Battery for the Assessment of Neuropsychological Status) showed that the participants who attended the educational program had a greater improvement in the auditory subtests. Additionally, the improvement in performance was generalized to measurements of memory and attention which were not practiced in the program.

3. The contribution of Orthodox Christian counselling and church life to the prevention and treatment of dementia and MCI

In relation to dealing with problems, such as dementia, encountered in older adults, the contribution of religiosity, church attendance, devotional life and religious history, art and literature have all been studied. Although some decades ago scientific thinking tended to avoid the approach of religiosity for issues such as dementia, in the last decade or so, there is a shift and more and more scientific fields are investigating and promoting religiosity and issues related to it for the treatment of diseases and the enrichment of medicine and psychological practice. The emergence of specialties such as Biotheology, Neurotheology, Psychology of religion, etc are indicative of it. In addition, in 2009 almost 30 American medical schools include religiosity in their curricula[17]. Both Psychiatry and Gerontology recognize that the elderly are more inclined to receive psychological help from priests, and the church is asked to play a special supporting role for these age groups[17]. In palliative care centers where the aim is to improve the quality of life of patients with life-threatening illness as well as that of their families, the therapeutic team often includes a chaplain who provides care for the spiritual needs of the beneficiaries.

3.1 Mental health and religiosity

In recent years, there has been a lot of research in the field of religion - spirituality, mental health and psychotherapy. In most studies it is shown that there is a direct relationship between religion and mental health[18]. Those who believe appear to have better mental health indicators, because religiosity is associated with more hope, greater optimism and satisfaction with life, less depression and faster remission of it, lower suicide rates, reduced rates of delinquency, drug and alcohol use. In people suffering from schizophrenia, religiosity has been shown to influence patient adherence to treatment and the outcome of the disease [19]. According to the results of other research conducted between 2000 and 2012 in chronically ill patients, it has been shown that the religious activity of believers could be used as part of treatment to deal with or limit anxiety, substance abuse, suicidal ideation and depression. In particular, for depression, it has been shown in a recent study that religiosity has a protective effect mainly on the recurrence of the depressive episode and in fact where there was a genetic burden [19].

In Alzheimer's disease religiosity has been found to slow down the progress of the neurodegenerative symptoms more than quality of life[6]. Also, liturgical life has been found to have a protective effect in relation to cognitive decline due to age, especially for woman suffering from depression[7]. A systematic review of recent studies concludes that religiosity has a significant positive effect in cognitive function for the elderly[8]. A recent study investigated the relationship between religiosity and participation in religious practices with cognitive function, depression and anxiety for individuals with MCI in a Greek Christian Orthodox setting. Levels of depression and anxiety for individuals with MCI were found to be negatively related to religiosity, while preservation of measures of cognitive functioning such as selective attention was found to be positively related with participation to religious practices. Thus, better mental health and less cognitive decline were associated with increased levels of religiosity and participation in religious practices for a Greek Christian Orthodox sample of individuals with MCI[20].

Religiosity and religious practices in the Christian Orthodox Church have been found to support and help older adults by intervening on different and specific levels of their life.

3.2 Existential identity and meaning in church life as means of psychological support

Christian counseling can help people at the last stage of their life to rationalize the difficulties they face, to acquire an existential identity that gives them optimism and perspective, and to show patience and fortitude by eliminating anxiety and depression. A related study focused on the role of religiosity in offering meaning and an existential identity to patients with dementia as well as its contribution to better coping with this disease by enhancing hope and vigor while reducing fears and anxiety[21]. The findings confirm the results of other studies which conclude that the development of religiosity can delay the progress of the disease[4,6,7,8,17]. The International Alzheimer Society officially collaborates in many countries with local religious organizations to provide spiritual support to both patients and health care providers[17]. Research has shown that in most cases spiritual care was more effective than support provided by their family and social environment, including social services[17].

In the Orthodox Christian teaching of the Holy Bible and the Fathers of the Church there is another dimension that is given to mortality and fragility of man under the prism of repentance and the resurrection of Christ which entail hopeful messages and the encouragement to accept the trials of earthly life by remaining patient. In the paternal tradition, the spiritual benefit that a person can have from health and illness is emphasized[22,23]. According to Saint John Climacus, illness can take on an ascetic character and, by humiliating the body, it can help the patient to reach purification and completion[24]. Also, according to Gregory Palamas, illness can become an accomplice for the salvation of the patient, since it removes the passions of the soul. It is noteworthy that faith in God's providence calls the believer to deal positively not only with health but also with illness and pain. The Christian Orthodox Church sees man and life with an eternal perspective, which is not limited only to the maintenance of physical health and biological functions, but extends to the completion as a person[25].

3.3 Cognitive enhancement in the context of Christian Orthodox Church

Parish life which includes liturgical arts, liturgical life with a specific timeline, confession and asceticism provide what a very well organized and effective day center for the elderly would offer. Additional studies on dementia emphasize on the fact that it is essential to take into account all the patient's needs including his religiosity[26]. It is becoming apparent that an emphasis on faith and religious worship related issues can help patients at many different stages of coping with this disease. It has been shown that despite memory problems, patients respond to religious hymns, vocal prayer and recitations of the Holy Bible as well as images of saints[27]. Also, religious narrative and literature, liturgical life and church arts can be an excellent exercise of brain functions which, besides the presentation and processing of many stimuli and the activation of verbal and visual memory, they also provide the possibility of practicing semantic memory and emotional processing[17].

3.4 Church life as a means of socialisation for the elderly

The social dimension of church life enables the integration of the elderly into society. Their participation in collective activities as well as the interaction and communication with others act protectively against loneliness, depression, dementia, mental disorder and other problems faced by the elderly. A study conducted in America confirms the above by resulting that participants who had an active religious life had a much slower rate of mental loss than those who did not[28].

3.5 The experience of church life promotes psychosomatic therapy

Within the Christian Orthodox tradition the experiential knowledge of church life through services, prayer and participation in the processes and life of church offers the elderly psychosomatic therapy. Joy, love and peace replace pessimism, anxiety and negative thoughts. The mysteries of the church stimulate people and help them face the difficulties they encounter in life more effectively. The spiritual life as it is promoted and developed through church life is the most effective antidote to mortality and corruption that man has inherited and is asked to overcome daily.

The Orthodox Church directs its interest towards people suffering from incurable diseases in three different and parallel directions: a. It is interested in providing psychological support and achieving a better emotional state for patients. Science often is not enough to alleviate human suffering and boost the patient's morale. The Church, with its simplicity and love for the suffering person and the sanctifying grace of the holy mysteries, can alleviate their loneliness and anxiety and make them feel safe. b. The Church is interested in ensuring the acceptance of the patient as a person with a personality by his/her intimate environment and by society. By every means, it tries to sensitize the faithful and convey the message that the patient is a holy and respected person, who needs prayer and support and is entitled at every stage of the illness to sympathy, care and love from everyone. c. The Church directs its interest and love to the relatives, who have assumed the responsibility of the care and custody of the sick. It supports them, comforts them, encourages them and helps them in various ways in the difficult task that they have undertaken.

3.6 Relationships within families are improved through the church teachings

Also, the Christian Orthodox church teaching contributes to the harmonious relationship between parents and children. This relationship is a factor that largely defines the progress of senility. Both the Old Testament and the New Testament are full of examples that incite children to take care of their elderly parents, tolerate and forgive them[29]. Christian faith and church life encourages understanding, acceptance and mutual help between parents and children, as well as every young person's towards their elders.

3.7 Death and loss in the church context of Christian Orthodox tradition

Death is a reality for all people. The mortality of human nature is an inevitable fact. Frailty as expressed through old age, sickness, pain is a part of earthly life. Both death and perishability are experienced by modern man as a loss and he seems to prefer avoiding their awareness[30]. The most certain fact, however, in our life is the mortality of human nature. One of the purposes of Christian ethics is for man to overcome the fear of death. In the teaching of the Holy Bible and the fathers of the church about death, illness, old age and pain we find an approach and understanding of these problems of human life that gives them meaning and utilizes them in a way that leads man to their acceptance, to hope and it transforms them into means to fight against sin and cultivate the virtues[31]. In the Christian Orthodox tradition divine providence utilizes these unpleasant situations for the benefit of human race, leading through them to repentance and the posthumous recompense of patience and faith during these trials. Death and corruption is a result but it also becomes a remedy for sin in many ways[32].

The memory of death as developed in the ecclesiastical context with the hope of resurrection helps man to recognize the real values of life, to avoid futility and to be prepared for the last stage of his life. The church takes care of people even during death with the funeral service and the prayers that are read, but also continues to help after death with memorial services, prayers for repose and almsgiving. In this way, the relationship among people still exists even after death and does not disappear. Often for older adults, the death of loved ones is a serious blow and often illnesses or even a new death occur as a consequence. The church contributes to giving meaning and coping more effectively with the loss that the elderly often experience after the death of a loved person.

4. Taking care of the elderly in ancient times, and in the history of the Greek Orthodox Church until today

In the context of church tradition and teaching, the value of respecting the elderly as people who contributed, offered and now need help and support is emphasized. We know that John the Evangelist was lovingly carried by his disciples to the church when he himself could no longer go alone due to his advanced age. Taking care of the elderly is considered to be a virtue and is realized through the operation of church institutions dedicated to it. Honoring and caring for older adults begins in Ancient Greece, continues in the times of the Macedonian Empire and has a special place in church tradition and teaching until today.

In the Iliad, Homer presents Nestor, the King of Pylos, as a model of wisdom and prudence, while in the Odyssey, the young Telemachus refuses to dispel his elderly governess despite the prompting of the suitors, showing his honor and respect to her[33]. It is characteristic that in the memoirs of Xenophon there is a reference to an Athenian law that if someone had not taken care of his elderly parents he had no right to hold public office: «Η πόλις, εάν τις γέροντας γονέας μη θεραπεύη, δίκην αυτώ επιτίθησι. και αποδοκιμάζουσα ουκ εά άρχειν»[33] Also, Plutarch mentions that among the cultural goods that Alexander the Great transported on his campaign, he carried the notion of respect and care for the elderly[33].

During the Byzantine period, the organized provision of social welfare in the form of institutions was established for the first time. Consequently, in addition to hospitals, orphanages and poorhouses, the institution of nursing homes was also developed. Following the example of Basil's the Great "Vasiliada", the church also developed social welfare[33]. In fact, for a period of time there were so many nursing homes in Byzantium that the Emperor Nikiforos Phokas in 964 AD was forced to prohibit the establishment of new ones[33]. This tradition continues until present time. The majority of the Metropolises in Greece have established and maintain nursing homes and care facilities for the elderly until today.

References

1. Koenig H.G. (2007). Religion and remission of depression in medical in patients with heart failure/pulmonary disease. *The Journal of nervous and mental diseases* 195(5): 389-95.
2. Koenig H.G (2012).Religion, Spirituality, and Health: The Research and Clinical Implications. *International Scholarly Research Network Psychiatry*.
3. Mok E., Wong F. & Wong D. (2010). The meaning of spirituality and spiritual care among the Hong Kong Chinese terminally ill. *Journal of Advanced Nursing* 66(2): 360–370.
4. Vaitsa Giannouli, Konstantinos Giannoulis, Gazing at Medusa: Alzheimer's dementia through the lenses of spirituality and religion, *Health Psychology Research* 2020; 8:8833
5. Bonelli MR., An Evidence-based Review on Religiosity in Psychiatry. *J Neurol Stroke,* 2017, 7(2): 00231.
6. Kaufman Y., Anaki D., Binns M., Freedman M., Cognitive decline in Alzheimer disease: Impact of spirituality. *Neurology* 68, May 1. 2007: 1509-1514.
7. Corsentino EA, Collins N, Sachs-Ericsson N., Blazer DG., Religious Attendance Reduces Cognitive Decline Among Older Women With High Levels of Depressive Symptoms. *J Gerontol A Biol Sci Med Sci,* 2009 Vol. 64, No. 12, 1283-1289.

8. Agli O., Bailly N., Ferrand C., Spirituality and religion in older adults with dementia: a systematic review. *International Psychogeriatrics,* August 2014.
9. Livingston G, Huntley J, Sommerlad A, Ames D, Ballard C, Banerjee S, Brayne C, Burns A, Cohen-Mansfield J, Cooper C, Costafreda SG, Dias A, Fox N, Gitlin LN, Howard R, Kales HC, Kivimäki M, Larson EB, Ogunniyi A, Orgeta V, Ritchie K, Rockwood K, Sampson EL, Samus Q, Schneider LS, Selbæk G, Teri L, Mukadam N, Dementia prevention, intervention, and care: 2020 report of the Lancet Commission, *The Lancet Commissions,* Volume 396, ISSUE 10248, P413-446, August 08, 2020.
10. Antoniou M. Gunasekera G. Wong P. Foreign language training as cognitive therapy for age related cognitive decline: A hypothesis for future research. *NeurosciBiobehav Rev.* 2013 Dec. 37 (10 0 2): 2689-2698.
11. Belleville S, Clément F, Mellah S, Gilbert B, Fontaine F, Gauthier S. Trainingrelated brain plasticity in subjects at risk of developing Alzheimer's disease. *Brain.* 2011;134:1623–1634.
12. Simon SS, Yokomizo JE, Bottino CMC. Cognitive intervention in amnestic Mild Cognitive Impairment: A systematic review. *NeurosciBiobehavRev*. 2012;36:1163–1178.
13. Willis SL, Tennstedt SL, Marsiske M, Ball K, Elias J, Koepke KM, Morris JN, Rebok GW, Unverzagt FW, Stoddard AM, Wright E. Long-term effects of cognitive training on everyday functional outcomes in older adults. *JAMA*. 2006; 296: 2805–2814.
14. Oswald WD, Rupprecht R, Gunzelmann T, Tritt K. The SIMA-project: effects of 1 year cognitive and psychomotor training on cognitive abilities of the elderly. *BehavBrainRes.*1996.
15. Barnes DE, Yaffe K, Belfor N, Jagust WJ, DeCarli C, Reed BR, Kramer JH. Computer-based cognitive training for mild cognitive impairment.Alzheimer *Dis AssocDisord.*2009;23:205–210.
16. Smith GE, Housen P, Yaffe K, Ruff R, Kennison RF, Mahncke HW, Zelinski EM. A cognitive training program based on principles of brain plasticity: Results from the improvement in memory with plasticity-based adaptive cognitive training (IMPACT) study. *J AmGeriatrSoc.* 2009; 57: 594–603.
17. *http://antifono.gr/portal/Πρόσωπα/Τσιτσίγκος/Αρθρογραφία/1354--alzheimer.html* Feb 2018.
18. Bonelli MR., An Evidence-based Review on Religiosity in Psychiatry. *J Neurol Stroke,* 2017, 7(2): 00231.

19. Ε. Τζούνης - Κ. Γουργουλιάνης, «Πνευματικότητα και πνευματική αξιολόγηση, ο ρόλος τους στην παροχή πνευματικής οροντίδας», Διεπιστημονική Φροντίδα Υγείας 5 (1) (2013), σ. 7-12.
20. Μπεκιαρίδης-Μόσχου Δ, *Ποιμαντικοψυχολογική προσέγγιση στην αντιμετώπιση της άνοιας και της Ήπιας Νοητικής Διαταραχής.* Τμήμα Κοινωνικής Θεολογίας και Χριστιανικού Πολιτισμού, ΑΠΘ, Διπλωματική Εργασία ΠΜΣ, 2023.
21. Snyder L, "Satisfactions and Challenges in Spiritual Faith and Practice for Persons with Dementia", *Dementia* 2/3 (2003) 299-313.
22. Rentsch T., 1997, «Aging as becoming oneself: A Philosophical Ethics of Late Life», Journal of aging studies, 1;4: 263-271.
23. Κουντουρά Ι., «*Ορθοδοξία και επιστήμη, Αναζητώντας νόημα στον πόνο*», Αθήνα 2001,σ.56-58.
24. Ορθοδοξία και Επιστήμη, Περιοδική Έκδοση Ενώσεως Ορθοδόξων Επιστημόνων Λεμεσού,Λευκωσία , 1995 / Γ. Μαντζαρίδης, «*Ο πόνος στην Ορθόδοξη παράδοση και θεολογία*», Σημειώσεις μαθήματος «Σύγχρονες Βιοηθικές αντιλήψεις και Χριστιανική Ανθρωπολογία», Θεσσαλονίκη, 2017.
25. Κ. Θ. Κιούλος - Ι. Δ. Μπεργιαννάκη, «Θρησκευτικότητα, πνευματικότητα και κατάθλιψη», Αρχεία Ελληνικής Ιατρικής 31(3) (2014), σ. 263-271. Κ. Κιούλος, «Θρησκευτικότητα, πνευματικότητα και ψυχοθεραπεία».
26. Lawrence R.M. "Dementia. A personal legacy beyond words", *Mental Health, Religion & Culture* 10/6 (2007) 553 – 562, St George's University of London, London 2007.
27. Ellor J.W. "Reaching Out to the Spiritual nature of Persons With Dementia", *Annual Meeting of NCOA.ASA* Washington D.C. 03/27/08, www.baylor.edu/gerontology
28. Fischer Th. *"Power of Prayer"*, December 2006/January 2007, www.aarp.org
29. Βάντσος Χ.Κ., *Θέματα Ποιμαντικής Ψυχολογίας,* Εκτύπωση: «Αϊβαζή», Θεσσαλονίκη, 1997.
30. Μαντζαρίδης Γ, «*Ο πόνος στην Ορθόδοξη παράδοση και θεολογία*», Σημειώσεις μαθήματος «Σύγχρονες Βιοηθικές αντιλήψεις και Χριστιανική Ανθρωπολογία», Θεσσαλονίκη 2017, σ. 107.
31. Χ. Ν. Τσιρώνης, Θρησκεία και κοινωνία στη δεύτερη νεωτερικότητα, Λόγοι, διάλογοι και αντί-λογοι στο έργο του UL. Beck,Μπαρμπουνάκης Χ., 2018.
32. Κατσιμίγκας Γ. Μαραγκούτη Αικ. Σπηλιοπούλου Χ. Γκίκα Μ. Νοσηλευτική και θεολογική Προσέγγιση του θανάτου, *ΝΟΣΗΛΕΥΤΙΚΗ* 2007, 46(4):441–452.

500 27

33. Π. Ζήσης Θ. *Ο θάνατος και τα μετά θάνατον.* (2015), Εκδ. Το Παλίμψηστον.

28

THE PHILOSOPHY OF DEMENTIA: A SPIRITUAL OPPORTUNITY?

LODOVICO BALDUCCI M.D.[1]

Abstract

Dementia is a syndrome characterized by cognitive impairment incompatible with independent living. In most case it is associated with progressive neurological degeneration and is irreversible from a medical standpoint. Dementia is universally considered an unconditional handicap. The author of this chapter has spent forty years managing demented patients with cancer and has developed an alternative vision of dementia. This chapter focus on two aspects of dementia: timelessness, and ability to experience simultaneously the most meaningful events of one's life. These aspects may make of dementia an anticipation of eternity and may indicate that the degeneration of some parts of the brain may allow previously neglected spiritual experiences to emerge. These assumptions may not be proven or disproven by experimental science and remain philosophical speculations that have nonetheless important management implications. They suggest that in lieu of benign neglect a direct interaction humoring the patient's narrative may foster the patient's trust and welfare, sooth the emotional loneliness, and at the same time my open the caregiver to the comprehension and acceptance of a spiritual reality. They indicate the necessity to create the most comfortable conditions for the development of the patient's new vision even at the price of physical safety. The iron-clad safety of assisted living may destroy the patient's creativity and anticipate his/her demise. They uphold the patient's right to be the owner of his/her medical decisions.

Keywords: Dementia; philosophy; spirituality; timelessness; eternity

---

[1] Senior Member Emeritus, Moffitt Cancer Center, Tampa, FL.

Introduction

Most readers may question what kind of business a medical oncologist has to explore the philosophy of dementia. Very reasonable question. My answer is contained in the following story.

A priest, a minister, and a rabbi decide to play a golf game, that in the USA is the most fashionable recreation for people of the cloth. Once on the course, they realize that they might not be able to conclude their game. The threesome in front of them seems unable to move. It takes 45 minutes for the clergies to reach the first hole. Disappointed and kind of miff they complain to the director of the course who is very understanding and apologetic "I am so sorry for you gentlemen, but you must understand that it is a miracle if the three people in front of you could play at all. They are blind!" Hearing this explanation, the priest exclaims: "blessed be God almighty for the gift of the will that allows these people to overcome their handicap with a strenuous training!" The minister exclaims "blessed be God almighty for the gift of intellect that allows these people to see the things their sight cannot reach." More practical, the rabbi asks: "why don't they play at night?"

The proposal of the rabbi enlightened my profession as geriatric oncologist. For forty years I have been dealing daily with deaths and disabilities, that are commonly considered unconditional existential losses. Since death is unavoidable, if it is a failure the whole humanity is doomed. To avoid this impending doom it behooves us to find an ultimate existential meaning of death and of functional decline. In this chapter I plan to share with the readers my vision of dementia that evolved over four decades of observation.

Of course, I am not a scholar of philosophy. My only acquaintance with this discipline was obtained from the curriculum of humanity in the Italian high school I attended more than sixty years ago. My knowledge is fragmentary and not updated. But I am a human being capable to frame emotions and thoughts with the knowledge and experience of a lifetime. For forty years I had the privilege to attend individuals made vulnerable and frail by diseases and disabilities. They have modulated my scientific knowledge, my humanistic culture and more in general my full experience of life.

Case Studies

Nona

"She is shepherding her flock on the hills of Scotland singing a Gaelic refrain" so Elizabeth described the last few hours of her 92-year-old grandmother. Nona, as her grandchildren called her, had left her native Scotland at age 13 and never went back. A fond and unselfish homemaker, she had raised five children in a working class neighbor of Brooklyn. When her husband's salary proved inadequate to support a growing family, she proudly accepted all types of menial engagements on top of her home-making tasks. After the death of her spouse of fifty years she had joined her older son in Florida and became the trusted confident of her two granddaughters during their embattled adolescence. "We loved her and trusted her as she has never been judgmental" Elizabeth remembered. Instead of making her fearful of a punishing God, her strict Presbyterian uprising had made her confident in a loving God who would have not allowed any of their children to get lost. "Nona was able to obtain a victory out of any defeat, Elizabeth remembered. "Think about this. Once I started sobbing and admitted to her an affair with a married man that I had revealed to no one. Instead of deprecating adultery, Nona hugged me and cried with me. "Your pain is the road through which a young person learns to love. Love has led Jesus to be crucified. As long as your love is blessed by pain you are assured that it is blessed by God, she told me" Few days later I found the strength to terminate my relation, armored with a new wisdom. Since my conversation with Nona I had grown to understand that the nature of love is the sacrifice of the self in a shared labor to give origin to new life."

The professor

Sitting on a Chippendale chair in the living room adorned with the trophies of a long and glorious career, the old professor of surgery in a three-piece suit and a newspaper in his hands still wore the imperious expression that subjugated with awe and fear hundred of coworkers. But when you talked to him his command would dissipate into the apologetic smile of a child who has failed to understand your words. No matter what the topic of the conversation was, his answer always would be: "O Jesus burning of love I wish I never offended you; my beloved and good Jesus I promise to offend you never more." This was probably the only Christian prayer he had learned as he was raised in an agnostic family and most of their acquaintances had no feelings for any deity, and loathed any form of religion. How many times we heard him bragging at a cocktail party, holding a tumble of expensive whisky, that "I have opened with my scalpels thousand of chests and of tummies and not once I had the opportunity to witness the release of the soul from the prison of the body." How many times had the walls of the operating room echoed his blasphemies! Indeed, he had claimed that his profanities were the keys of successful surgery. When a particularly challenging operation was scheduled, he tried to refine the curses of God's name. His ancestral family was from Tuscany, the Italian region that gave birth to Pietro Aretino,[1] a literate of the renaissance who made a poetic art out of blasphemy!

The literate and humanist

The people closed to him at the time of his death described the last few days of Alessandro Manzoni as an agony worth its name[2]. The world agony derives from the Greek *agòn,* fight, and is commonly intended as the ultimate fight with death of the dying person. In the case of Manzoni, it involved multiple lifelong fights. The fight between religious faith and rationalistic doubt, between Christian submission to God's will and human rebellion to suffering, between love-inspired peace and harmony, and hatred-inspired revenge and chaos. To the dismal of his children and his friends, the venerable old man uttered expressions of lasciviousness, cursed his closest friends, and even blasphemed the God he had worshipped for six decades.

Alessandro Manzoni[3] was and is still revered as the most consequential novelist of the Italian literature. His novel "I Promessi Sposi" ("The Betrothed") is considered a frame of reference of Italian style even by modern authors. Published in 1842, the novel incarnates the Catholic faith of the author, who confides in the intervention of a loving God in human events and mistrusts human justice enshrined by the American and French revolutions. In this respect "The Betrothed" challenged the culture of the times that suspected Christianity as a vehicle of ignorance and an instrument of popular oppression and hallowed reason as the only source of truth according to the enlightenment religion. Despite bucking the times "The Betrothed" gained universal consensus and admiration even among non-believers. The Jewish literary critic Attilio Momigliano[4] wrote one of the most compelling comments to the novel while concealed in a psychiatric hospital of Florence to escape the Nazis. "Though the writer of this comment may never profess any religious beliefs" he wrote" he cannot help being pervaded by the sense of peace emerging from Manzoni's faith." He wrote these words as his and his spouse's lives were under constant threat. But the peace emanating from his writing was founded on intimate struggles that at the end of life erupted, as dementia unleashed all intellectual and moral brakes.

A springboard to eternity

These cases were handpicked to highlight the communality of the human experience despite the unicity of each person. Let's examine the points of convergence in these three characters : a Scottish shepherdess turned American homemaker who ended ten decades of life at the beginning of the twenty-first century ; an agnostic and self-absorbed professor of surgery that modulated the medical culture with skepticism and blind worship of physical sciences in the middle of the past century; a revered ancient writer endowed with a unique humanistic education and a tormented soul, who has imprinted the culture of the Italian nation in the nineteenth century. Despite differences in sex, education, time, and space, at the end of their lives these three individuals experienced in common:

- Loss of the consciousness of time. They confirmed Simone Weil's remark that time is a delusion[5]. They lived an alternative reality, subtracted to the scanning of time, and inaccessible to even the closest people. The experience of most individuals allows an occasional taste of eternity. It includes dreams, contemplation of beauty and goodness, engagement in a wholesome activity. Perhaps the most significant of these experiences is the discovery of the world by an infant. A new life is greeted with a sip of eternity. But for our three characters timelessness represented a new and permanent condition. For this reason an Italian poet saw dementia and a springing board toward eternity[6].
- Loss of consciousness of physical dependence. The concern for survival did not seem to bother them. Absence of self-awareness may also be considered the effect-or the origin- of timelessness.
- Soaking the most meaningful moments they had distilled from their living experience in the form of an essence. For Nona the Scottish pasture conveyed the sense of freedom inspired by her simple faith. That sense of freedom allowed her to provide unconditional love to all members of her family and to her friends. It should not surprise anybody if she dwelt in the source of a lifelong fulfillment at the conclusion of her earthly life. It is more challenging to interpret the prayer the illustrious professor reiterated as a broken record, but it is

legitimate to make reasonable assumptions. As most successful people, he had experienced his liveliest emotions in the anticipation of incoming successes. Once the limelight had extinguished, the success had always proved less satisfactory than expected. This alternance of anticipation and delusion had fueled the hunger of more successes, the same way that the dissipation of the drug fuels the craving of more drugs. With age the professional skills wane and with them the arousal in anticipation of a reward. He had used his spouse as a platform for his promotion. He had incited his children to neglect family bonds in order of pursuing affirmation. Deserted by family and friends, deprived of the most powerful living stimulus, at a time of cognitive and physical decline he had gained a confused appreciation of a persistent reality underlying the swirling flow of his life. He perceived this reality as a safe harbor where he would have been enabled to love himself despite his decay, his shortcomings, and his rudimentary experience of love. The simple prayer he might have learned from a handmaid in his household or in the hospital or from a patient with whom he had shaken hands prior to surgery, stuck to his mind as a possible anchor to this mysterious reality promising to satisfy his hunger for love and to relieve his solitude. A world renown medical oncologist made paraplegic by a stroke recently described in a memoir a comparable recovery of faith[7].

Nona had experienced the Christian Faith as a light that had illuminated with transcendency all difficulties and joys of life. Manzoni had experienced the same faith as an ongoing agony, consistent with his rationalistic formation and his neurotic personality[2]: a battle between the worship of reason and the acceptance of mystery; between his addiction to vice and his aspiration to innocence; between the rebellion to sufferance and its acceptance as a redeeming currency, between his impetus and his inadequacy to love. In his writings Manzoni seems able to settle the contradictions of the living experience with the faith in a providential design. But the settlement required an ongoing struggle that was the very source of his faith. To fuel his faith up to the conclusion of his earthly life the struggle would not abandon him even throughout his death. More than for peace or joy he was looking for meaning.

- Most important of all, they claimed the dignity of the living even if they lived in a dimension inaccessible to their loved ones. They reminded the watchers that the worst experience of a desert entails a crowd that refuses to acknowledge your presence. Years ago an

> editorial of a major newspaper was entitled: "Tell the bitch I am still alive." A patient judged terminal had overheard a nurse telling a colleague during the report: "Ignore him; he is terminal and has a "do not resuscitate" order." Unexpectedly the patient survived his presumed terminality and was able to share his experience after leaving the hospital: he had felt carried to the morgue still sentient! It is very common to isolate dying patients and to treat them as if they were not with us anymore. For individuals considered demented this populated desert may last for years!

Unaware of time and of physical needs these individuals seemed able to visit many decades in a split instant and to bring to the forefront the events that had made their existence meaningful and unquenchable. They had distilled from their lives a precious essence of Bulgarian roses: each drop contains thousand of petals withered a long time ago. Was the alternative reality a result of organic brain changes or did it demonstrate the spiritual world taking over the material one, the Greek *pneuma* (spirit) substituting the *psuché* (that supports thoughts, mood, and feelings)? A definitive answer to this question cannot be provided by experimental science nor by philosophical investigations. It is legitimate to speculate about alternative answers, by reviewing what we do know about the clinical and neuropathological basis of dementia.

Dementia: clinical and pathological aspects.

Dementia is a clinical syndrome characterized by a degree of cognitive impairment incompatible with independent living[8]. Several degenerative diseases of the brain underlie dementia and explain the multifaceted manifestations of this syndrome[9]. Loss of inhibition, with lack of impulse control and episodic aggressiveness and loss of executive function are common to most forms of dementia and especially of fronto-temporal dementia[10-11]. Hallucinations are seen late in the course of Alzheimer dementia, but are common throughout the trajectory of Lewis Body and Parkinson's dementia [10-12]. And of course different manifestations may overlap because multiple simultaneous brain lesions may coexist[8]. A number of points need to develop this chapter.

First, the organic base of dementia should be acknowledged. Except in rare cases (such as normal pressure hydrocephalus[13] or hypovitaminosis[14-15]) the underlying pathology is a degenerative brain disorder unlikely to be reversed by medications, though medications may delay the progression of dementia and provide palliation. The only realistic hope to reverse neurodegeneration sits in regenerative medicine and may involve the use of stem cells[16]. This approach currently has no clinical applications. In most cases dementia should be considered an impairment leading to disability.

Second, environmental adaptations may improve the mood of individuals with dementia and facilitate their management. At a medical convention in Bogota (2010) the Colombian novelist Gustavo Alvarez Gardeazabal described how his demented mother who had grown in the open countryside became suddenly taciturn, surly, more confused, and agitated when she came to live in her son's apartment. When returned to the familiar environment of the open country she became joyful and gregarious again and regained the sweetness that had been the hallmark of her whole life. She had been transferred to town for safety, but it became clear that too much safety might have killed her sooner than the risks of living in a rural area with limited supervision and primitive medical resources. The environmental component should be emphasized when discussing the philosophy of dementia, as it may mandate a compromise of physical safety and even of ethical obligations in exchange for an enjoyable existential experience.

Third, this chapter took off with the description of conditions that are common to most individuals of dementia: timelessness and dwelling in the most meaningful experiences of one's life. These situations provide a cue to explore an alternative reality that might be constructed as anticipation or preview of eternity. The author is aware that they represent occasional and mostly unpredictable oasis in a very onerous, prolonged and unpredictable journey. In no way this chapter intends to minimize the physical, social, and economic burden dementia bestows on patients and their caregivers. The main goal of the chapter is to illustrate how occasional steps of this journey may enrich both patient and caregiver with a spiritual appreciation that may sooth fatigue and depression and may foster closeness, allegiance and affection among the individuals compelled to travel together. The additional goal includes the need to privilege the human aspect of the management even when it may contradict medical, legal, and even religious considerations. In Jewish Christian terms it is an invitation to privilege mercy over justice. Or even better to discover in mercy the supreme form of justice.

Philosophy of dementia

Almost every adult has met individuals who live in an alternative reality where time is irrelevant and physical needs are all but ignored. Three examples of this reality where provided in the initial case studies. From a medical standpoint these individuals are not just impaired but also disabled and handicapped[17]: in other words an impairment in activities of daily living or Instrumental activities of daily living does not allow them to survive without the assistance of caregivers. The hallucinations of Nona, the repetitive prayer of the old professor, and the ultimate struggles of Manzoni are expression of a brain dysfunction due to progressive and, as of now, irreversible degeneration. Yet these experiences are real for the individuals living them. And it is legitimate to ask how these experiences may influence human existence. Let us use this example: a paraplegic patient is certainly handicapped. And yet, the use of the wheel chair, the slowdown of his activities may provide to him a new appreciation of the world around him. As disabling as it is, the paraplegia may reveal to the patients for the first time the beauty of the flower beds around their house or simply give a new appreciation of independent life that previously was taken for granted, or allow the patients to visit dimensions of life that were foreign to them such as meditation. May one discover the same redeeming features in dementia? Is it a worthwhile task to escort Nona through the hills of Scotland, and to engage Manzoni in a religious argument?

Let's start saying that the Judeo-Christian history is filled with experiences that may be considered as hallucinations. We are told that the deity spoke repetitively to Abraham and Moses and in the case of Moses God's command prompted a well-documented historical event known as the Exodus. Are we to believe that these leaders did make up God's message in order of getting authority on gullible savages? It is certainly possible, but the account of the Exodus at least suggests otherwise. The leadership of the tribe proved burdensome to Moses, rather than rewarding. Were they hallucinations? If they were, they involved the activation of certain areas of the brain that allowed an anticipatory vision of reality. They revealed a reality more real than that most people were allowed to appreciate. It is legitimate to ask whether these ancient individuals possessed a way to talk directly with the deity that was lost by a brain whose circuits became overloaded with so called "scientific information."

Closer to our days, Paul of Tarsus experienced a temporary blindness as he was riding a horse toward Damascus and heard the voice of Christ asking why he was persecuting him[18]. A modern interpretation considers this event a temporal lobe seizure. But does it mean that the voice was unreal? Is it not possible that a temporary dysfunction of the temporal lobe allowed Paul to hear the real voice of the resurrected Christ? Eventually a reliable historical account tells us that Paul followed the recommendations of the voice and regained his sight.

The Roman Catholic tradition entails many examples of individuals who felt privileged to communicate with Christ and with the Virgin Mary. In the middle of the nineteenth century, in the Pyrenean town of Lourdes, in South West France a peasant girl, Bernadette Soubirous, had a number of visions of a Lady considered the Blessed Mother. Following the indication of the vision Bernadette dug a fount of water that since that time up to our days proved capable to heal incurable diseases including metastatic cancers and neurodegenerative disorders[19]. Even somebody who does not partake of the Judeo Christian faith or of any faith cannot help acknowledging that Bernadette was privileged with some type of communication denied to her neighbors[20].

The discussion of religious faith is beyond the scope of this chapter. These examples are intended to acknowledge that the extratemporal or supernatural experiences reported by demented individuals are also apanage of individuals considered normal. Even if they are ascribed to the abnormal function of some portion of the brain, these experiences may convey a message more insightful than that transmitted by a brain functioning normally. This constatation begs the question to which realm these unexplainable experiences belong. It is certainly legitimate to consider them the result of a chain of not yet identified natural causes. Certainly, some specific components of the Lourdes water (that has been tested repeatedly for almost two centuries), might have caused the brain of an uneducated young woman to generate a vision that revealed the therapeutic power of the water. It is likewise legitimate to speculate that these experiences, largely disregarded throughout a person's life time, become predominant at the life end thanks to progressive neuro-degeneration.

Two constructs are germane with transcendence: spirituality and eternity. These constructs are intertwined like the two helices of the DNA, because a spiritual substance is subtracted to the control of time. As these constructs escape the sensorial experience they are described with metaphors.

To distinguish the *pneuma* from the *psuche* it may be helpful to try to imagine music without instruments. Is it possible that human consciousness be able to contain at the same time all possible musical expressions? This capability is beyond the limited power of the brain connections. Human consciousness may be endowed with this capability. In this case the audition of music will only activate through the brain the musical consciousness. This possibility was conceived by Marcel Proust in "Le Temps Retrouvè" where he claims that the artist is a translator rather than a creator[21]. According to Proust the task of the artist is to translate in temporal terms the content of the timeless spirit. Alternatively human consciousness may develop as a timeless secretion of time-rooted experiences. In this case the audition of different pieces of music enables human consciousness to distillate and store the essence of music. Whether a spirit is a full coffer that needs to be opened by the brain or an open and empty coffer that needs to be filled by the brain, the coffer may subsist independently from the nervous system, that exercise an irreplaceable function in the management of the coffer during a person lifetime. In other words the spirit may be constructed as the capability to live simultaneously all the meaningful experiences of one's life, the way Nona went back to her native Scotland or Manzoni struggled with his faith. In the Judeo-Christian view the vision of God after death will enlighten with joy these meaningful experiences.

After talking about timelessness if may be time (no pun meant) to spend a few words about eternity. From the concepts we have exposed one is entitled to exclude eternity as a persistent present. Present is a virtual reality. As soon as it exits the future it becomes a component of the past. At most, Faust's ambition to nail the instant[22] would lead to a recurrent torment similar to that of Prometheus[23]. In the Greek mythology Prometheus was punished by the gods for having comparted with humankind the fire that was considered a divine prerogative. He was enchained to a rock and every day a crow would chomp his liver, that regenerated during the night to allow the crow to devour it again day after day. Likewise, the scholastic philosophy holds the eternity as an undisturbed contemplation of the truth (that for both Christian and Islamic scholars coincide with the almighty eternal God)[24]. This vision may imply the dissolution of the individual spirit, a "nirvana" that ends all suffering rather than an inexhaustible source of individual joy. It also assumes that the contradictions of human nature will be smoothed out. This assumption begs the questions: "is it possible to remain human and enjoy the good without a conscience of the evil? Perhaps the best way of affording this problem was offered by the German philosopher Georg Wilhelm Friedrich Hegel[25], who proposed the triad of thesis, antithesis, and synthesis as the structure of human thought, that reflects the universal reality. The ongoing execution of this process may represent the source of eternal joy.

On a practical standpoint eternity may comprehend the simultaneous enjoyment of the riches of every individual spirit. Kind of a cyclorama or a virtual exposition that brings to life without interruption the meaningful experiences occurred in each personal life.

Management Implications of the spiritual hypothesis

The spiritual hypothesis entails important management implications. It suggests a fruitful interaction between the demented person and the caregiver. If indeed the spiritual dimension takes over the bodily one at the end of life, it behooves the caregiver to accompany the patient in this journey. Meaningful attendance may be provided by listening to the patient instead of dismissing the communication with a sympathetic but rushed smile, by asking pertinent questions and by investigating the patient's feelings and beliefs if this can be engaged in a conversation. Attentive interaction may foster the patient's trust and disassemble the wall of loneliness and disregard so common in demented individuals. It may also widen the scope of the caregiver. Irrespective of whether the caregivers hold any religious beliefs, they may recognize the most effective promotion of the patient's quality of life in cultivating the spiritual dimension. To do that, the caregivers are compelled to get in touch with their own spiritual dimension. Appropriately, the spiritual dimension is becoming increasingly accepted by official medicine as an area of therapeutic interventions[26].

The philosophy of dementia involves several aspects of social and ethical philosophy, based on the assumption that a demented person is endowed with the full gamut of human rights. Two of the management-related ethical implications are discussed here.

It was previously illustrated how the mood of the demented mother of Alvarez Gardeazabal improved dramatically when she was returned to the country environment from the city that was foreign to her. The writer made the decision to allow her to stay in the country. Despite less supervision and availability of only rudimentary health care her life expectancy would have probably been longer and her quality of life would have definitely been better. These considerations are extremely important in managing cognitively impaired patients, and the legal system should have enough flexibility to allow to accommodate the preference of the demented beyond pure physical safety. One of the most tragic cases observed by the author included an 82 year old severely demented woman with breast cancer, that was not life-threatening. She clearly received the most loving care from her spouse who was able to see her in the timeless light of a life spent together. And this love was reciprocated by a succession of smiles that expressed a lifelong affection better than any word. Because they were of modest means and did not wish to importune the two married children living afar, the husband still had to work and she was left alone for eight hours a day. She was smelling of old urine at each visits and look disheveled, but certainly did not look unhappy. A well-meaning hospital employ reported the husband for neglect to the senior protective service. After learning that the lady was left alone 8 hours a day, the government representative ordered a coercive admission to an adult living facility and indicted the husband of neglect. In the nursing home the lady became confused, hostile, and aggressive, had to be heavily sedated, refused to eat, pulled the feeding tubes and the intravenous connections and eventually died of marasmus within three months from the forced admission. The husband fired the physicians who managed her cancer, had to be removed forcibly from the clinics as he insulted and threatened the personnel, quit his job and dissipated the next few months with alcohol before dying himself in a car accident. Clearly, the reasonable concern about the patient's safety shortened a lifelong love romance with a double tragedy.

Of course demented patients should be prevented from being a risk to others. But why should they not be allowed to represent a risk only for themselves in exchange of an enjoyable life? Aren't football players, motorbike riders, race car contestants, mountain climbers, boxers and many others risking their life more consistently than the old lady in order of enjoying the same life?

On the same line, demented individuals should be part of any medical decisions concerning them. At the very least they should be consulted even when they seem unable to communicate because nobody knows for sure how much they understand. The French movie "Le scaphandre et le papillon" (the diving bell and the butterfly)[27], narrates the true story of a man with the so called "locked in syndrome" whom a speech specialist train to communicate with the movement of an eyelid. It became clear that this person understood everything occurring around him. If the patient is able to communicate it is important to try to assess how much they understand the situation, and if they have adequate understanding the final medical decision should be theirs.

Conclusions

Dementia is a syndrome involving cognitive decline such that a persona cannot survive alone. In most cases it is related to a degenerative brain disorder. Medications may at most delay the progression of the cognitive decline, but cannot reverse it.

Through a number of case studies this chapter examines two common features of dementia: loss of the consciousness of time, and tendency to revisit the most meaningful events of a person's life and to dwell in them. Without doubt these symptoms originate from a dysfunction of certain areas of the brain. The author asks whether this dysfunction may not unleash a spiritual experience that may be considered a foretaste of eternity. An eternity conceived as a dynamic dimension, comparable to a virtual exposition or to a cyclorama, where experiences distant in time and space may be lived simultaneously. This vision of eternity contrasts with the Faustian pretense to stop the time or with the Scholastic construct of perpetual present. This first implies an endless repetition of the same event; the second may imply the suppression of individuality in a kind of nirvana.

In any case the experiences of the patient are real and remind the practitioner that the demented patient is endowed with a full humanity. These philosophical considerations have two important management implications. The patient should be humored and listened to, rather than disregarded with benign incredulity and with a rushed and benevolent smile. The concern for the patient's physical safety should be balanced by the attention to the patient unstable emotional status. The safety of close supervision in an adult living facility might hasten rather than prevent the patient's demise.

References

1. Pietro Aretino | Italian author | Britannica
2. Paolo D'Angelo: La nevrosi di Manzoni. Il Mulino saggi. Bologna, Italy
3. Alessandro Manzoni, biografia (biografieonline.it)
4. Alssandro Manzoni: i promessi sposi con il commento di Attilio Momigliano. Sansoni editore. Firenze 1960
5. Simon Weil: La pesanteur et al grâce. Agora, Paris, 1991

6. Lodovico Balducci : Chiaroscuro. I Diamanti Poesia. Aletti Editore, Villanova di Guidonia, Roma, 2021
7. Gianni Bonadonna: Appuntamento col Padreterno. *Collana Le Querce (diari) Montedit, Vardellino (BG), 2014*
8. Livingston G, Huntley J, Sommerlad A, et al. Dementia prevention, intervention, and care: 2020 report of the Lancet Commission. Lancet. 2020 Aug 8;396(10248):413-446. doi: 10.1016/S0140-6736(20)30367-6. Epub 2020 Jul 30. PMID: 32738937; PMCID: PMC7392084.
9. Mehta RI, Schneider JA. Neuropathology of the Common Forms of Dementia. Clin Geriatr Med. 2023 Feb;39(1):91-107. doi: 10.1016/j.cger.2022.07.005. Epub 2022 Oct 18. PMID: 36404035.
10. Baratono S, Press D. What Are the Key Diagnostic Cognitive Impairment and Dementia Subtypes and How to Integrate all of the Diagnostic Data to Establish a Diagnosis? Clin Geriatr Med. 2023 Feb;39(1):77-90. doi: 10.1016/j.cger.2022.08.002. PMID: 36404034.
11. Harris JM, Jones M, Gall C, et al Co-Occurrence of Language and Behavioural Change in Frontotemporal Lobar Degeneration. Dement Geriatr Cogn Dis Extra. 2016 Jun 1;6(2):205-13. doi: 10.1159/000444848. PMID: 27350781; PMCID: PMC4913762.
12. Jellinger KA. Dementia with Lewy bodies and Parkinson's disease-dementia: current concepts and controversies. J Neural Transm (Vienna). 2018 Apr;125(4):615-650. doi: 10.1007/s00702-017-1821-9. Epub 2017 Dec 8. PMID: 29222591.
13. Oliveira LM, Nitrini R, Román GC. Normal-pressure hydrocephalus: A critical review. Dement Neuropsychol. 2019 Apr-Jun;13(2):133-143. doi: 10.1590/1980-57642018dn13-020001. Erratum in: Dement Neuropsychol. 2019 Jul-Sep;13(3):361. PMID: 31285787; PMCID: PMC6601311.
14. Arendt JFH, Horváth-Puhó E, Sørensen HT, et al Plasma Vitamin B12 Levels, High-Dose Vitamin B12 Treatment, and Risk of Dementia. J Alzheimers Dis. 2021;79(4):1601-1612. doi: 10.3233/JAD-201096. PMID: 33459639; PMCID: PMC7990402.
15. Rotstein A, Kodesh A, Goldberg Y, et al Serum folate deficiency and the risks of dementia and all-cause mortality: a national study of old age. Evid Based Ment Health. 2022 May;25(2):63-68. doi: 10.1136/ebmental-2021-300309. Epub 2022 Mar 15. PMID: 35292483.
16. Chan HJ, Yanshree, Roy J, Tipoe GL, et al: Therapeutic Potential of Human Stem Cell Implantation in Alzheimer's Disease. Int J Mol Sci. 2021 Sep 21;22(18):10151. doi: 10.3390/ijms221810151. PMID: 34576314; PMCID: PMC8471075.

17. Jones RB. Impairment, disability and handicap--old fashioned concepts? J Med Ethics. 2001 Dec;27(6):377-9. doi: 10.1136/jme.27.6.377. PMID: 11731599; PMCID: PMC1733473.
18. Acts of the Apostles, chapter 9
19. Associazione Medici cattolici italiani: il medico di fronte al miracolo. San Paolo, Cinisello Balsamo, 2004
20. Angelo Stagnaro: Why was Emile Zola so frightened of Our Lady of Lourdes? National Catholic Register, November 29, 2022 Why Émile Zola Was So Frightened of Our Lady of Lourdes| National Catholic Register (ncregister.com)
21. Marcel Proust: A la recherche du temps perdu. Bibliothèque de la Pléiade, Gallimard éditeur, Paris, 1989
22. Johann Wolfgang von Goethe: Goethe's Faust Anchor Books, New York, 1962
23. William Hansen, *Classical Mythology: A Guide to the Mythical World of the Greeks and Romans* (Oxford University Press, 2005), pp. 32, 48–50, 69–73, 93, 96, 102–104, 140; as trickster figure, p. 310.
24. St. Thomas Aquinas's commentary on *De anima*, Bk. I, 402a1–403b2, §1. Archived
25. Allen Speight: The philosophy of Hegel. Routledge, New York, 2004
26. Puchalski CM. The FICA Spiritual History Tool #274. J Palliat Med. 2014 Jan;17(1):105-6. doi: 10.1089/jpm.2013.9458. Epub 2013 Dec 18. PMID: 24351125.
27. Le Scaphandre et le Papillon — Wikipédia (wikipedia.org)

ABOUT THE EDITORS

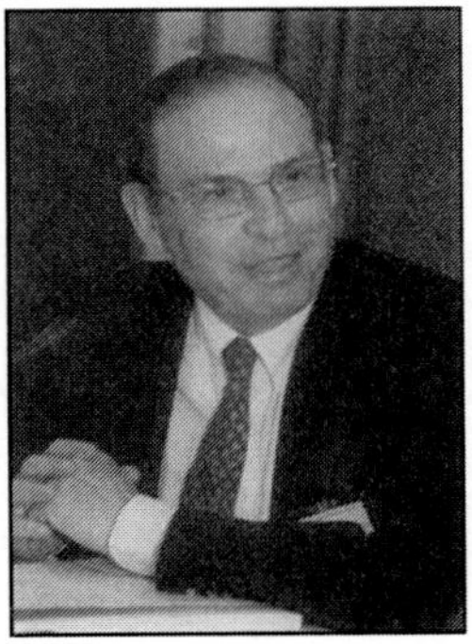

Michael Silbermann, DMD, Ph.D. - Editor

Michael Silbermann, D.M.D., Ph.D., received his DMD at the Hebrew University in Jerusalem, Israel, and his Ph.D. at Tufts University Medical School in Boston, MA, USA and completed his postdoctoral research at the University of Southern California in Los Angeles, CA and spend a year as a visiting scientist at the NIH in Bethesda, MD, USA.

Professor Silberman has held several senior national and international administrative academic roles, especially in the field of biomedical research. He was Chairman of the Department of Anatomy and Cell Biology, Faculty of Medicine, and Dean of the Faculty of Medicine at the Technion in Haifa, Israel. He served as Chief Scientist for the Ministry of Health in Israel, Chairman of the Board of Governors at the United States-Israel Binational Science Foundation, and Executive Director of the Middle East Cancer Consortium since its establishment in 1996. Professor Silberman was the first representative of the State of Israel at the European Commission in the Program Committee for Bio-Medical Research at the European Union in Brussels. In addition, he served as a mentor to 32 Master's and Doctoral students.

Professor Silberman has published over 380 articles in international peer reviewed journals, presented over 560 presentations in international meetings and organized over 70 international workshops. He was Editor-in-Chief of the Journal of Palliative Care and Medicine and the Journal of Palliative Medicine and Hospice Care, as well as serving on the Editorial Board of the Journal of Cancer & Clinical Research. Citations 6708, h-index 43; i10-index 163.

Ann Berger MD, MSN - Co-Editor

Dr. Ann Berger completed her undergraduate degree with a B.S. in nursing from New York University, which was then followed by receiving a MSN in Oncology Nursing from University of Pennsylvania. After working as an Oncology Clinical Nurse Specialist for several years, Dr. Berger completed her medical training at Medical College of Ohio in Toledo, Ohio. Following medical school, Dr. Berger completed an internship and residency at Hartford Hospital in Connecticut and a Fellowship in medical oncology and pain/palliative care at Yale University in Connecticut.

Dr. Berger has had over 30 years of experience in pain and palliative care. Currently she is chief of pain and palliative care at National Institutes of Health, clinical center where she has patient care, education, administrative, and research responsibilities. Dr. Berger is cochair of the National Institutes of Health clinical center wellness initiative for health care professionals and support staff. She is also intramural advisor for several scientific interest groups including the resilience sig, consciousness sig, psychedelic sig and religion and spirituality sig.

Dr. Berger has lectured nationally and internationally. Dr. Berger's research involves developing ways to measure psychosocial spiritual healing. Her other area of research is the use of integrative modalities for wellness for health care professionals and others such as teachers. She has also published extensively (articles, chapters and books) in the field of pain and palliative care and wellness for health care providers. *Dr. Ann Berger contributed to this book in her personal capacity.*